# Women's Health and Fitness Guide

Michele Kettles, MD
Colette L. Cole, MS
Brenda S. Wright, PhD

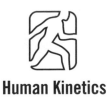

**Human Kinetics**

**Library of Congress Cataloging-in-Publication Data**

Kettles, Michele, 1964-
    Women's health and fitness guide / Michele Kettles, Colette L. Cole, Brenda S. Wright.
        p.  cm.
    Includes bibliographical references and index.
    ISBN-13: 978-0-7360-5769-1 (soft cover)
    ISBN-10: 0-7360-5769-2 (soft cover)
  1.   Women--Health and hygiene. 2.   Physical fitness for women. 3.   Exercise for women.
I. Cole, Colette L., 1966- II. Wright, Brenda S., 1946- III.  Title.
    RA778.K455 2006
    613.7'045--dc22

                                    2006006677

ISBN-10: 0-7360-5769-2
ISBN-13: 978-0-7360-5769-1

The Web addresses cited in this text were current as of April 2006, unless otherwise noted.

**Acquisitions Editor:** Michael S. Bahrke, PhD; **Developmental Editor:** Renee Thomas Pyrtel; **Assistant Editors:** Kevin Matz and Jillian Evans; **Copyeditor:** Joyce Sexton; **Proofreader:** Anne Rogers, **Indexer:** Robert Swanson; **Permission Manager:** Dalene Reeder; **Graphic Designer:** Robert Reuther; **Graphic Artists:** Denise Lowry; **Photo Manager:** Sarah Ritz; **Cover Designer:** Robert Reuther; **Photographer (cover):** Sarah Ritz; **Photographer (interior):** Sarah Ritz, except where otherwise noted. Photos on pages 1 (basketball), 11, 13, 17, 43, 53 (tennis), 58, 61, 99, 109, 112, 121, 126, 128, 152, 158, and 167 (volleyball) © Human Kinetics; **Art Manager:** Kelly Hendren; **Illustrator:** Jason McAlexander; **Printer:** Sheridan Books

We thank the Cooper Fitness Center in Dallas, Texas, for assistance in providing the location for the photo shoot for *Women's Health and Fitness Guide.*

Printed in the United States of America        10   9   8   7   6   5   4   3   2   1

**Human Kinetics**
Web site: www.HumanKinetics.com

*United States:* Human Kinetics, P.O. Box 5076, Champaign, IL 61825-5076
800-747-4457
e-mail: humank@hkusa.com

*Canada:* Human Kinetics, 475 Devonshire Road Unit 100, Windsor, ON N8Y 2L5
800-465-7301 (in Canada only)
e-mail: orders@hkcanada.com

*Europe:* Human Kinetics, 107 Bradford Road, Stanningley, Leeds LS28 6AT, United Kingdom
+44 (0) 113 255 5665
e-mail: hk@hkeurope.com

*Australia:* Human Kinetics, 57A Price Avenue, Lower Mitcham, South Australia 5062
08 8277 1555
e-mail: liaw@hkaustralia.com

*New Zealand:* Human Kinetics, Division of Sports Distributors NZ Ltd., P.O. Box 300 226 Albany, North Shore City, Auckland
0064 9 448 1207
e-mail: info@humankinetics.co.nz

To my first and best inspiration in life for all things health and fitness related, my mother, Marjory Wilson. Run, Margie, run!

Michele Kettles, MD, MSPH

For my spiritual role models, my dad and mom. Thank you for giving me a life of unconditional love, prayer and support, personal sacrifice, and the encouragement to achieve dreams and be successful in all I do. Also for my lifelong best friends: my brother, Chuck, and my sister, Tammy.

Colette L. Cole, MS

For Delphine and Karen.

Brenda Wright, PhD

# Contents

# Foreword

Historically, American women live longer than men due primarily to the fact that women have some protection from heart disease until they go through menopause. But once women enter the menopausal years, heart disease rises rapidly, and by the time they are 65 years of age, it is well documented that more women are likely to have heart attacks and die from them than men.

The advances in prevention are a boon for women of all ages. We now know that regular physical activity and proper diet can help prevent heart disease in women and that regular medical evaluations that include treadmill stress tests, electron beam tomogram scans, and blood lipid profiles can diagnose heart disease in its early stages. Unfortunately, however, most women do not get the tests they need on an annual basis.

Preventive medicine in women consists primarily of gynecological evaluations that include pelvic examinations and mammograms. There is no question about the value of early detection of cervical cancer or breast cancer, but each year many more women die of heart disease than cancer. Yet preventive efforts concentrating on lifestyle changes to prevent heart disease in women are just not emphasized as much as they are in men. As healthcare providers, we need to lead the charge to promote proper diet and exercise to prevent heart disease and other chronic illnesses in women; otherwise, we will be providing way too much care too late.

The authors of *Women's Health and Fitness Guide* and I agree that adolescence, pregnancy, and menopause are challenges women must rise to—as opposed to excuses for gaining excess weight and losing fitness. Health and fitness professionals play a crucial role in guiding women safely through these life events. This book describes how to motivate young girls to be active, ensuring a healthy transition through adolescence. A chapter on fitness details the significant risks women, and their babies, face if fitness is neglected during pregnancy. Finally, understanding the changes related to menopause and how exercise can promote healthy, independent senior living is an integral part of this book. As our population ages, we must continue to foster lifelong fitness goals for senior women.

Osteoporosis is another disease that can be prevented through lifestyle modifications. Many women die each year from the complications of osteoporotic fractures and many more lose their ability to live independently after hip fractures. Once again, this is a preventable disease, and in older women at times it is reversible. Not only are there medications available that can be used to prevent and/or treat osteoporosis, but we now know that weight-bearing exercise associated with adequate intake of calcium, vitamin D, and magnesium can produce almost the same effect as medications.

Exercise can even play a role in mental illness. Depression is associated with an increase in many chronic physical diseases, including heart problems. It has been estimated that one out of eight American women is depressed, and many are using medications to control the depression. Yet studies performed at the Cooper Institute in conjunction with the University of Texas at Southwestern Medical School clearly show that regular aerobic exercise can be just as effective as antidepressants in treating mild depression.

In *Women's Health and Fitness Guide,* the authors expand on these topics and many more, discussing not only the etiology of the medical problems, but also providing excellent guidelines and instructions as to how to prevent and even treat these conditions. If we all embraced these recommendations and passed them on to our female patients and clients, the cost of healthcare would be dramatically reduced. But if a major effort along these lines is not implemented, the future for optimal health and longevity in American men and women is very dismal. Remember, it is much cheaper and more effective to maintain good health than to regain it once it is lost.

–Kenneth H. Cooper, MD, MPH
Founder of Cooper Aerobics Center, author of 18 books, including *Aerobics* (M. Evans and Co., Inc. 1968). He is credited with starting more people exercising than any other person.

# Preface

> Common sense is the knack of seeing things as they are, and doing things as they ought to be done.
>
> Harriet Beecher Stowe

## About Women

This book is about women. In the fitness industry, women are often treated as if their bodies are the same as men's. Of course, women aren't the same as men. We have fundamental differences in our anatomy, physiology, and psychology as compared to men, and these differences affect how we should be treated as people, patients, and athletes. Women have unique health risks that translate into distinct approaches for the prevention and management of disease. Fitness has an important role to play in almost every chronic disease that a woman faces—cardiovascular disease, type 2 diabetes, cancer, obesity, arthritis, osteoporosis, or depression. The information in part I of this book consists of concise, relevant, current data on women's health and fitness research. It lays the foundation for the research-based recommendations that follow.

The chapters in part II look at the behavior of physical activity and exercise from the perspective of three significant life events—puberty, pregnancy, and menopause. Adolescent girls and young women have issues and needs different from those of their mothers and grandmothers. Recognizing the physical, mental, emotional, and social challenges women are likely to face during each transition period of their life encourages self-awareness for the woman and provides critical insights for her trainer or health advisor. A knowledgeable and observant health or fitness professional can use the broad short- and long-term goals that we identify for each transition period as the starting point for developing and promoting effective fitness programs. We also provide age-appropriate information and tips to help encourage the behavior of physical activity.

Part III addresses the specific components of a balanced fitness program—cardiovascular fitness, muscular strength and endurance, and flexibility—but with a new twist. In addition to reviewing the key principles of each exercise component, we provide a sound rationale and advice for rethinking traditional exercise in favor of functional and integrated exercises. We believe that exercise should prepare us to perform the tasks and activities of everyday living. Fortunately, today's woman has numerous options for getting and staying fit—new exercise machines, innovative classes, recreation and sport, and a renewed emphasis on lifestyle activities.

In part IV, the chapter on program design draws on the research and recommendations from previous chapters and puts everything together. But there is no generic, "one size fits all" program when it comes to balanced fitness. Each woman is unique. From initial assessments and consultation to exercise selection, sequence, and progression, we take you through the step-by-step process that leads to a safe, effective, and enjoyable program. Because women, especially younger women, are more susceptible to anterior cruciate ligament (ACL) tears and other injuries, this book concludes with a chapter about how to avoid and treat these potential problems.

## For Women

Ultimately, the information in this book is for women. But the book itself is directed to professionals, both women and men, who promote health and fitness among women. Your role is critical in helping bridge the gap between science and reality. Whether you are an educator, coach, personal trainer, dietitian, or health care provider, women will look to you for answers and advice. Your technical expertise is invaluable in helping them sort through the hearsay, testimonials, and observations they are bombarded with each day. But, respect the boundaries of your scope of practice and be alert to the signs and symptoms that warrant referral to another specialist.

## By Women

*Women's Health and Fitness Guide* was written by a team of three women. Each brings a unique perspective to the work. Michele Kettles, MD, MSPH, is a practicing physician at the world-renowned Cooper Clinic in Dallas, Texas. She sees patients daily, advising them about clinical and lifestyle issues, especially the benefits of fitness, in improving health and preventing disease. Brenda Wright, PhD, is a health promotion consultant with more than 25 years of experience in the field. Much of her professional work involves translating technical messages to ensure that they reach the lay audience. Colette Cole, an award-winning personal trainer at the Cooper Fitness Center, designs fitness programs and trains women with a variety of needs. Her clients include elite athletes, women recovering from serious injuries or surgeries, and those managing conditions such as breast cancer or osteoporosis, as well as women who see fitness as a means to improve daily function or appearance. Together, these three authors cover an array of fitness issues aimed at helping women achieve clinical, public health, and performance goals.

## How to Use This Book

We have attempted to organize *Women's Health and Fitness Guide* in a straightforward manner, always progressing from research to practice. Our total bibliography includes more than 250 references. Because the book is intended for a wide audience of professionals, we've included a glossary at the end. Terms that are defined in the glossary appear in bold when first used in the text. Especially in relation to exercise, a picture is "worth a thousand words." So, we've included lots of photographs and illustrations. Also, numerous sidebars have been positioned throughout the book to summarize key findings and recommendations that are discussed in detail in the text. Because readers may serve as both teachers and technicians, we have provided a variety of tools and handouts (in the appendixes) for you to use or pass along to your clients as appropriate.

In conclusion, we hope that *Women's Health and Fitness Guide* will be a resource that you will refer to again and again as you meet new challenges in your efforts to promote health and fitness among women.

# Acknowledgments

We thank our colleagues at the Cooper Aerobics Center for their collaboration and stimulation over the years and for their support in this endeavor. We recognize the pioneering work of Dr. Kenneth Cooper and scientists at the Cooper Institute who established the database that confirms the benefits of fitness related to health and longevity and that made "aerobics" a household word. Millie Cooper, Dr. Cooper's wife and co-author of *Aerobics for Women* (1972), deserves significant recognition for her role in motivating and encouraging women to be active. She was one of the first spokespersons for fitness among women worldwide.

As with every book, the contributions of numerous people make it a reality. Dr. Michael Bahrke, acquisitions director in the scientific, technical, and medical division of Human Kinetics, worked closely with us to develop our plan for a book on women's fitness. Kara Witzke of Norfolk State University had originally proposed such a book, but because of professional responsibilities decided not to pursue the project. Her outline was very helpful as we began to define the scope and sequence of the book. We hope we have achieved her original goal of creating a resource grounded in current research for health and fitness professionals who work with women. Dr. Steve Blair of the Cooper Institute suggested that Brenda and Michele might collaborate on the book. When the outline was completed and the project approved, Michele invited Colette to join the writing team to provide the unique expertise of a personal trainer.

Several well-qualified health and fitness professionals reviewed the proposal and manuscript during its development. We thank these individuals for their help in shaping the content and approach of the book: Kara Witzke and Marilyn Strawbridge.

One of the features of the book that we are most proud of is the photography. Hundreds of new photographs were taken at the Cooper Fitness Center in Dallas. We extend a special thanks to our photographer, Sarah Ritz, whose skill and patience are unequalled; our developmental editor, Renee Thomas Pyrtel, whose keen eye and organizational genius made the photo shoot a pleasure; our wonderful models, Mukidah Wiggins, Rosson Grover, Carla Sottovia, Kristen Wells, Donna Fisher (and baby-to-be Fisher), Christian Brunet-Maianu, Marius Maianu, Sara Heard, Julie Farrell, Elva Eichenwald, Gail Richardson, Nick Enthoven, Elysia Hernandez, and Dr. Riva and baby Evan Graeme. We appreciate everyone's willingness to be a part of this book.

The combined efforts of a talented team at Human Kinetics gave the book physical reality. Special thanks go to Renee Thomas Pyrtel, Sarah Ritz, Kevin Matz, and Dalene Reeder. Working together as a team, we feel we have created a book that can help health and fitness professionals help women of all ages improve their fitness and quality of life.

–Michele Kettles, Colette Cole, and Brenda Wright

The support of my husband and children was wonderful during this project; thank you so much, Mike, Jack, and Sophie; now you may have a turn on the computer! I thank my mother, Marjory Wilson, my sister Jennifer Anderson, and my aunt Meg Burkardt, who listened, advised, inspired, and motivated me throughout this project. I truly could not have done it without you.

To my coauthor, Colette, thank you from the bottom of my heart for saying yes to this project; nobody could have done it better—nobody. To my coauthor, Brenda, thank you for sharing your expertise and experience; your eloquence is truly a gift.

I thank Steve Blair, PhD, of the Cooper Institute who initially brought this project to my attention. I thank my assistant, Stephanie Phillips, who tirelessly retrieved articles and performed many administrative tasks with enthusiasm. Diane Proud, Cooper Fitness Center running coach, graciously and patiently answered my questions. To all of my patients at the Cooper Clinic, you make my work a joy, it is a privilege to be your doctor. Finally, I thank Dr. Kenneth Cooper, who has written more books than I can count, for his amazing foresight in establishing the Cooper Aerobics Center.

–Michele Kettles

Foremost, I thank my Lord and Savior, Jesus Christ, for His everlasting strength, sacrificial love, mercy, and grace in my life.

Thank you to my Aunt Syvio and Mammaw for being such a positive and strong influence as women of devotion, strength, and kindheartedness.

To the rest of my family and their own, thank you for a lifetime of deep friendship, devotion, and endless times of laughter.

I would like to thank my closest friends, Donna Fisher, Joanne Keeney, and Cecilia Keil, for your constant support, patience and understanding, love, and encouragement to accomplish a personal and professional ambition that at times was more than challenging and at others seemed never-ending. I am truly grateful for the immeasurable times of faithful friendship. My sincere hope is that your own ambitions and dreams have been and will be achieved by the same support and friendship.

I want also to thank Michele Kettles for the combined professional opportunity to educate and help others through this book. Additionally, I especially treasure the true friendship qualities you possess and shared with me before and throughout this project. I look forward to years of friendship and training together.

I need to thank all of my clients at the Cooper Fitness Center for their constant support and consistent dedication not only to their health, but also to me. May we have many more years together to progress and achieve goals. Now go stretch!

Thank you, Brenda Wright, for your expertise and help in content organization and author voice.

I thank my fellow fitness staff for the personal accountability and level of determination to excel that drives other fitness professionals to succeed at the Cooper Fitness Center. Special thanks to Donna Fisher, Carla Sottovia, Lisa Hanley, Laura Alton, Jill Turner, Steve Farrell, and Ruth Ann Carpenter for their valuable time and professional input.

To Renee (RTP), through career opportunities and mere chance emerges a unique, reverent friendship. May it continue to develop. Whenever possible, work should be fun—and this was! Thank you for giving more than I expected.

–Colette Cole

I thank Michele for taking the lead in managing this project as a whole. It's always a challenge coordinating a team of three authors, especially when one lives in Costa Rica. It has been an honor for me to work with both Michele and Colette.

–Brenda Wright

# How Women Are Unique

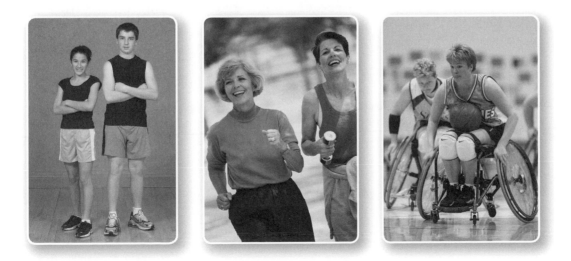

# CHAPTER 1

# Sex Differences in Anatomy, Physiology, Psychosociology, and Mortality

## Topics in This Chapter

- ◆ Male versus female pelvis
- ◆ Q angle
- ◆ Normal body fat ranges for women by age
- ◆ The female knee
- ◆ Male versus female dynamics of landing
- ◆ Cardiovascular and strength issues
- ◆ Menstrual cycle and performance
- ◆ Fat and carbohydrate utilization
- ◆ Competition versus connectedness
- ◆ Female mortality statistics

It's too bad that society isn't to the point yet where the country could just send up a woman astronaut and nobody would think twice about it.

Sally Ride

This chapter discusses the anatomic, physiologic, and psychosocial differences between men and women that affect function. Because of the increased risk of lower extremity injury for girls and women, we take a special look at sex differences of the knee. Next, sex differences in the cardiovascular system are explained in detail. We also review the latest data on how phases of the menstrual cycle affect exercise performance. Finally, we discuss interesting data on sex differences in fat and carbohydrate metabolism. Knowledge of these basic differences sets the stage for developing comprehensive fitness programs for females.

Fitness reduces risk for many of the leading causes of morbidity and mortality for women in the United States, including cardiovascular disease and stroke, hypertension, **dyslipidemia,** diabetes, cancer, dementia, osteoporosis, and obesity. Toward a better understanding of this relationship, we review the latest morbidity and mortality statistics for women.

## Female Anatomy

The differences between male and female anatomy start with the structure of the pelvis and follow through to the knee. The female pelvis is smaller on average than the male pelvis. To accommodate childbirth, the cavity of the female pelvis is shallower, wider, and more circular, with a shorter and wider sacrum, more movable coccyx, and larger superior and inferior openings (see figure 1.1). These are general statements. It is important to remember that pelvic shapes vary not just between men and women but also within each sex.

The differences in the pelvis result in hip joints that are smaller and more forward facing in women. In a lateral projection (see figure 1.2), you will note that the acetabula are more lateral and that the female pelvis projects downward (anterior pelvic tilt) as compared to the male pelvis.

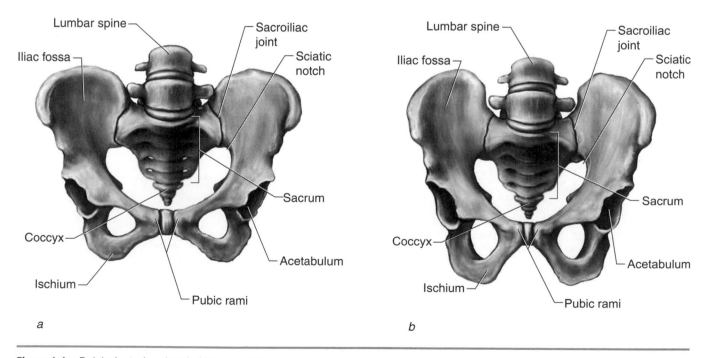

*a*           *b*

**Figure 1.1**   Pelvis (anterior views). Note the difference in the placement of the acetabulum for *(a)* the female pelvis, which is at a slightly more lateral, downward angle than *(b)* the male pelvis, which is more frontal and has a less downward pitch.

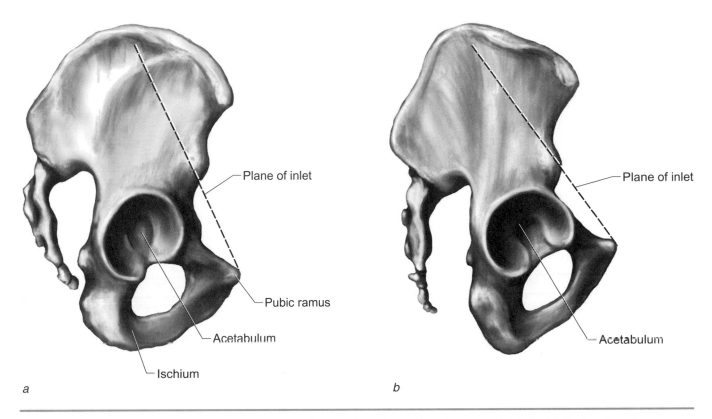

a

b

**Figure 1.2** Pelvis (right lateral views). Note the longer distance from the pubis to the sacral table in *(a)* the female pelvis compared to *(b)* the male (anterior pelvic tilt). Also note the relative placement of the coccyx in relation to the pubis in each figure.

Reprinted, by permission, from A. Cowlin, 2002, *Women's fitness program development* (Champaign, IL: Human Kinetics), 4.

The longer vertical distance between the sacral table and pubis symphysis of the female confers a slightly lower center of gravity. Anterior pelvic tilt results in compensations including excessive lumbar **lordosis** and hip adduction and internal rotation. These compensations follow through to the knee and foot, causing knee valgus ("knocked knees"), external tibial torsion, and forefoot pronation.

Another important anatomical difference is the larger "Q angle" (quadriceps angle) in women. The Q angle is an estimate of the effective angle at which the quadriceps averages its pull on the knee. To measure the Q angle, a line is drawn from the anterior superior iliac spine to the center of the kneecap. Another line is drawn from the center of the kneecap to the insertion of the patellar tendon on the tibial tuberosity (see figure 1.3). The angle should be measured in the standing position. Horton and Hall (1989) measured Q angles in 50 males and 50 females, average age 22.6 years. In men, the angle was 11.2 ± 3.0 degrees. In women, this angle was 15.8 ± 4.5 degrees. This variation in alignment

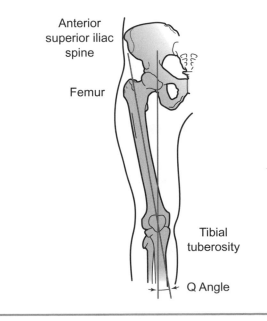

**Figure 1.3** The Q angle is measured at the intersection of two straight lines originating from the center of the patella and ending at the anterior superior iliac spine and the insertion of the patellar tendon on the tibial tuberosity.

Reprinted, by permission, from P. Houglum, *Therapeutic exercise for musculoskeletal injuries*, 2nd ed. (Champaign, IL: Human Kinetics), 826.

between men and women has a direct effect on injury risk to the knee. Further sex differences in the knee are discussed later in this chapter.

When muscle force, degree of tension, or a greater angle of pull affects the tracking pattern of the patella at the patellofemoral groove, abnormal patellofemoral function can occur. A greater Q angle increases the lateral pull on the patella during knee flexion and extension. It can cause discomfort and pain from contact pressures between the femur and patella. Muscle imbalances of the **vastus medialis** and **vastus lateralis** can also cause lateral pulling on the patella. Women tend to be weaker in their vastus medialis (VMO); this is likely due to both anatomic (wider Q angle) and conditioning differences from men. The VMO controls medial movement to the patella and is the only dynamic medial stabilizer to the patella. Lack of flexibility in the hamstrings, quadriceps, **iliotibial band,** and calf muscles may also contribute to patellofemoral stress syndrome, which is far more common in women than men.

Figure 1.4 provides an excellent visual summary of the anatomic differences between men and women in the lower body. Taken together, these differences result in significant alignment variance between the sexes. And, as discussed

## Important Skeletal Differences Between Men and Women

Compared to men, women have

- ◆ smaller, shallower, wider, and more circular pelvic cavity;
- ◆ anterior pelvic tilt;
- ◆ smaller, forward-facing hip joints (acetabula);
- ◆ greater degree of genu valgum;
- ◆ larger Q angle;
- ◆ shorter arms and legs relative to height; and
- ◆ smaller bones overall and lower bone density.

As a result of these anatomical differences, women have

- ◆ slightly lower center of gravity,
- ◆ more patellofemoral stress syndrome,
- ◆ more risk for anterior cruciate ligament injury, and
- ◆ different postures for stability and activity.

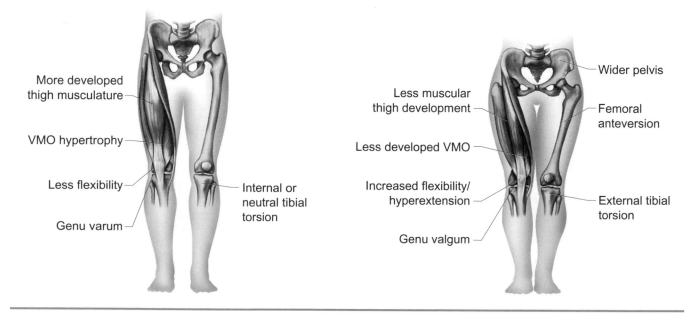

**Figure 1.4** The male alignment, shown on the left, is overall straighter, the pelvis narrower, and the thigh musculature more developed. The male has less flexibility, genu varum, and internal or neutral tibial torsion. The female alignment, shown on the right, has a relatively wider pelvis, and the thigh musculature is less developed. The female has increased flexibility, hyperextension of the knees, genu valgum, and external tibial torsion.

Reprinted, by permission, from F.H. Fu and D. Stone, 1994, "Special concerns of the female." In *Sports injuries: mechanisms, prevention, treatment* (Philadelphia, PA: Lippincott, Williams, and Wilkins), 159.

later in the chapter, this divergence is related to injury risk.

The acetabula position and the lower center of gravity differences between men and women translate into different postures for stability and activity. One stable preparatory stance for movement for a female is to have the ankles directly under the acetabula. This usually means that the feet are 6 to 8 inches (15 to 20 centimeters) apart (Cowlin 2002). In this position, when a woman squats, the knees are directly

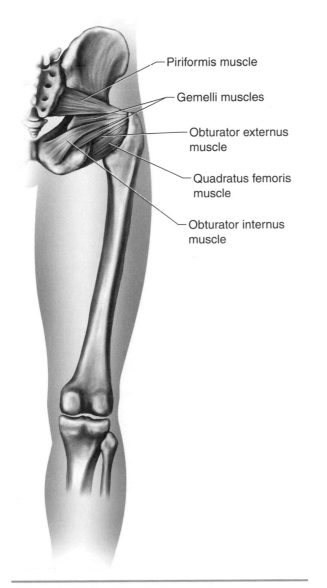

- Piriformis muscle
- Gemelli muscles
- Obturator externus muscle
- Quadratus femoris muscle
- Obturator internus muscle

**Figure 1.5** The six deep rotators, seen here from the posterior aspect of the right hip joint, rotate the femur in the acetabulum in an outward circle. In a wide stance, the deep rotators guide the knee safely over the feet in the typical female anatomy.

Reprinted, by permission, from A. Cowlin, 2002, *Women's fitness program development* (Champaign, IL: Human Kinetics), 7.

over the toes instead of rotated inward. When the knees are rotated inward, this creates an unstable position. A wider stance can be used to increase stability by engaging the outward rotators (see figure 1.5). Outward rotation is initiated from the hip and follows through to the knee and ankle.

# Female Physiology

Prior to puberty, the development of motor skills is similar for boys and girls. With the onset of puberty and the influence of sex hormones, boys and girls undergo fundamental changes that affect physical performance. These changes include effects on bone development, strength, body fat, aerobic power, and metabolism.

## Differences in Bone Development and Body Composition

Women are generally shorter than men because their higher levels of estrogen cause earlier fusing of the epiphyseal growth plates. So, compared to men, women have shorter arms and legs relative to height. Women have smaller bones overall and lower bone density. Women's center of gravity is lower, but not hugely so. In fact, center of gravity is more accurately predicted by height and body type than by sex (Ireland and Ott 2004).

During puberty, boys gain lean muscle mass and lose body fat under the influence of testosterone. Girls, on the other hand, gain muscle and fat during puberty under the influence of estrogen. The average adult woman has 10 percent more fat than the average man (Holschen 2004). Even the distribution of fat tissue varies, with women having more subcutaneous fat in the arms and legs. Men have generally been described as "android" or having a higher percentage of their body fat in the abdomen or "central" distribution. The "gynoid" fat distribution implies a gluteofemoral predominance of body fat and is more common in women. The android fat pattern is associated with higher cardiovascular risk, even in children and adolescents (Daniels et al. 1999).

Humans need some body fat for normal function, and women need more than men, especially for pregnancy and lactating. Fat is also important for cushioning to prevent osteoporotic fracture from falls later in life, a problem that affects far more women than men. Note the normal body fat ranges for women by age group in table 1.1.

## The Female Knee

The anatomy of the knee is complex (see figure 1.6). The cruciate ligaments are located inside the knee joint and stabilize the knee by controlling front-to-back motion of the tibia in relation to the femur. The anterior cruciate ligament (ACL) prevents the tibia from sliding forward beneath the femur. Since the ACL helps to stabilize the knee joint, any injury of the ligament can result in chronic instability of the joint (Woo et al. 2001).

Knee anatomy doesn't differ significantly between the sexes, but there are significant neuromuscular, biomechanical, postural, and hormonal differences between men and women that may affect this joint during exercise performance.

### ◆ TABLE 1.1 ◆
### Body Composition—Females

| | AGE | | | | | | |
|---|---|---|---|---|---|---|---|
| Percentile | 20-29 | 30-39 | 40-49 | 50-59 | 60-69 | 70-79 | |
| 99 | 9.8 | 11.0 | 12.6 | 14.6 | 13.9 | 14.6 | Very lean* |
| 95 | 13.6 | 14.0 | 15.6 | 17.2 | 17.7 | 16.6 | |
| 90 | 14.8 | 15.6 | 17.2 | 19.4 | 19.8 | 20.3 | Excellent |
| 85 | 15.8 | 16.6 | 18.6 | 20.9 | 21.4 | 23.0 | |
| 80 | 16.5 | 17.4 | 19.8 | 22.5 | 23.2 | 24.0 | |
| 75 | 17.3 | 18.2 | 20.8 | 23.8 | 24.8 | 25.0 | Good |
| 70 | 18.0 | 19.1 | 21.9 | 25.1 | 25.9 | 26.2 | |
| 65 | 18.7 | 20.0 | 22.8 | 26.0 | 27.0 | 27.7 | |
| 60 | 19.4 | 20.8 | 23.8 | 27.0 | 27.9 | 28.6 | |
| 55 | 20.1 | 21.7 | 24.8 | 27.9 | 28.7 | 29.7 | Fair |
| 50 | 21.0 | 22.6 | 25.6 | 28.8 | 29.8 | 30.4 | |
| 45 | 21.9 | 23.5 | 26.5 | 29.7 | 30.6 | 31.3 | |
| 40 | 22.7 | 24.6 | 27.6 | 30.4 | 31.3 | 31.8 | |
| 35 | 23.6 | 25.6 | 28.5 | 31.4 | 32.5 | 32.7 | Poor |
| 30 | 24.5 | 26.7 | 29.6 | 32.5 | 33.3 | 33.9 | |
| 25 | 25.9 | 27.7 | 30.7 | 33.4 | 34.3 | 35.3 | |
| 20 | 27.1 | 29.1 | 31.9 | 34.5 | 35.4 | 36.0 | |
| 15 | 28.9 | 30.9 | 33.5 | 35.6 | 36.2 | 37.4 | Very poor |
| 10 | 31.4 | 33.0 | 35.4 | 36.7 | 37.3 | 38.2 | |
| 5 | 35.2 | 35.8 | 37.4 | 38.3 | 39.0 | 39.3 | |
| 1 | 38.9 | 39.4 | 39.8 | 40.4 | 40.8 | 40.5 | |
| n = | 1,360 | 3,597 | 3,808 | 2,366 | 849 | 136 | |

Total n = 12,116

*Very lean: No less than 10-13% body fat is recommended for females.

Reprinted, by permission, from The Cooper Institute, 2005, *Physical fitness specialist course and certification* (Dallas, TX: The Cooper Institute), 7.

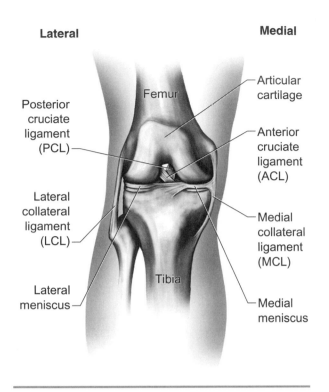

**Lateral**

Femur

Posterior
cruciate
ligament
(PCL)

Lateral
collateral
ligament
(LCL)

Lateral
meniscus

**Medial**

Articular
cartilage

Anterior
cruciate
ligament
(ACL)

Medial
collateral
ligament
(MCL)

Tibia

Medial
meniscus

**Figure 1.6** Anatomy of the knee, anterior view with patella and patellar tendon omitted.

## Neuromuscular, Biomechanical, and Postural Factors

The authors of one study compared young male and female soccer and basketball players by assessing medial knee motion and lower extremity valgus angle during landing from a jump. The values were compared between sexes according to maturational stage. The female athletes landed with a greater medial motion and valgus angle than did the male athletes following the onset of maturation. This indicates that as a result of puberty, young girls experience bone and muscle changes that decrease neuromuscular control of the knee joint (Hewett et al. 2004).

Research has shown that females land in a more upright position than males do (Ireland and Ott 2004), exposing the ACL to higher forces and stress. Bending at the knee and hip during directional change and jumping movements reduces the force placed on the

tibia by engaging the hamstring muscle. Note in figure 1.7a that the man has more flexion of the knee and hip of the landing leg. The woman's more erect posture (figure 1.7b) favors use of the quadriceps over the hamstring, increasing torque on the ACL.

Figure 1.7 also illustrates the increased valgus angulation (the knees are closer together) that females experience during landing. When a woman flexes her hip, as into the lunge position, the hip also rotates inward. For males, there is no iliofemoral rotation during a lunge or landing. The movement involves purely flexion and extension.

The main reason for increased risk of ACL injury in females seems to be increased torque on the ACL, which results from the factors just described. Being smaller than men on average, women also have smaller ligaments that, given the same activity as in men, may be more susceptible to tears. Additional factors that may influence ACL injury risk, including notch width and shape (figure 1.8), are not necessarily sex specific.

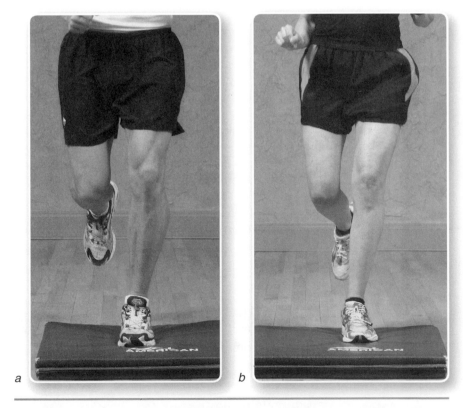

*a*      *b*

**Figure 1.7** Dynamics of landing. The male *(a)* has less valgus angulation at the knee and more flexion at the hip and knees. The female *(b)* has more valgus angulation at the knee and less hip and knee flexion; note how this shifts her body weight more forward. Also, note the significant difference in thigh and calf musculature between these two highly conditioned athletes.

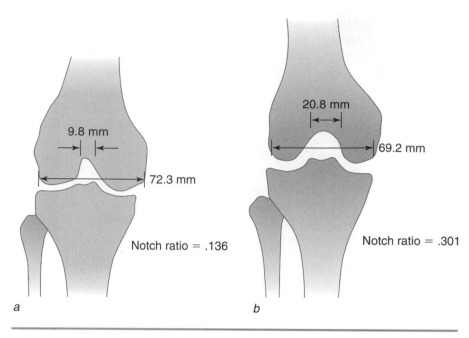

9.8 mm

72.3 mm

Notch ratio = .136

a

20.8 mm

69.2 mm

Notch ratio = .301

b

**Figure 1.8** *(a)* and *(b)* Intercondylar notch width and shape may vary by sex and be associated with a relative increased risk of anterior cruciate ligament (ACL) injury. To measure the notch width index (NWI) at the level of the popliteal groove, one divides the notch width by the width of the condyles. An NWI less than 0.21 signifies stenosis and a relatively increased risk of ACL injury.

Reprinted from *The female athlete*, M.L. Ireland and A. Nattiv, pg. 394, Copyright ©2003, with permission from Elsevier.

### Hormonal Issues

It is generally accepted that women have more ligamentous laxity than men, but whether this increased laxity increases injury risk is controversial. An American College of Sports Medicine study measured changes in knee laxity as a function of changing sex hormone levels over one complete menstrual cycle (Shultz et al. 2004). Twenty-five nonathletic females ranging from 18 to 30 years of age who reported normal cycles over the past six months were tested. Estradiol, progesterone, and testosterone levels were

## The Female Knee

As compared to men, women have

- ◆ neuromuscular changes resulting from puberty,
- ◆ more upright landing posture,
- ◆ valgus angulation with landing, and
- ◆ smaller ligaments with variable laxity.

measured. The results revealed that changes in all three sex hormones mediate changes in knee laxity across the menstrual cycle. From the data, it is impossible to predict when any individual woman would be at increased risk for knee laxity. Timing of peak hormone levels in the cycle was variable between women. Laxity resulting from hormone peak levels generally occurred three to four days after the peak.

## Cardiovascular and Strength Differences

Due to lesser muscle mass gains, women have less powerful upper and lower bodies than men, with upper body strength being 30 to 50 percent lower in women. The strength difference is not as pronounced in the lower body. The distribution of muscle fiber *types* doesn't vary much between sexes, but women have fewer and smaller muscle fibers (Pollock et al. 1998). The strength difference appears to be more a function of muscle mass than a fundamental difference between male and female muscle fibers.

Women's hearts are smaller than men's hearts. This means that women pump less blood with each heartbeat (lower stroke volume) and that their resting and exercise heart rates are higher than men's. Women also have about 10 percent less hemoglobin on average than men, again due to the influence of testosterone. Hemoglobin transports oxygen. More hemoglobin means that oxygen is transported to the muscles faster. The maximum amount of oxygen that the muscles use per minute, the $\dot{V}O_2$max, is a strong predictor of performance and is determined largely by heart size and fat-free weight (Hutchinson et al. 1991). With training, the sexes have similar increases in their aerobic capacity; but generally, men and boys have higher $\dot{V}O_2$max than women and girls (Pollock et al. 1998). Interestingly, the effects of training on aerobic capacity are not influenced by pre-, peri-, or postmenopausal status, according to a position stand from the American College of Sports Medicine (Pollock et al. 1998).

## Performance Difference Related to Menses

Women experience many hormonal influences that affect physical performance. They have higher levels of the hormones relaxin and elastin, allowing for more laxity in the joints. This is especially important for childbirth, but may increase injury risk during pregnancy and postpartum. The role of relaxin in injury risk is discussed in more depth in chapter 5.

During the menstrual cycle, hormone levels fluctuate. Estrogen is most influential early in the cycle. Later, when progesterone peaks, many women note such symptoms as irritability, bloating, cramping, and headache accompanying their menstrual flow. More information on the menstrual cycle is provided in chapter 4.

One small study compared women during three phases of the menstrual cycle (menstruation, midfollicular, midluteal) and showed no difference in measures of maximal anaerobic performance during cycling and jumping between various parts of the cycle or between oral contraceptive (OC) users and nonusers (Giacomoni et al. 2000). However, the authors note that the presence of symptoms of premenstrual or menstrual syndrome (fatigue, fluid retention, weight gain, mood changes, and **dysmenorrhea**), with or without OC use, was associated with decreased multijump performance.

Another small study, done in 2003, showed no decrement in performance for trained athletes during menses when tested to fatigue on a cycle ergometer (Bergen et al. 2003). In this study, untrained women exercised significantly longer during the midluteal phase as compared to during menses. And it was noted that all women gained weight during menses.

One study of five female rowers showed that when they were taking a low-dose OC, anaerobic power, output, and capacity were highest during pill days 26 to 28, when estrogen and progesterone doses were lowest (Redman et al. 2004). Finally, a study of young sedentary women showed improved aerobic capacity and endurance performance with OC as compared to a control group. The authors suggest that improved performance in this group may have been a function of improvement in stroke volume and relative increases in fat versus carbohydrate metabolism (Redman and Weatherby 2004).

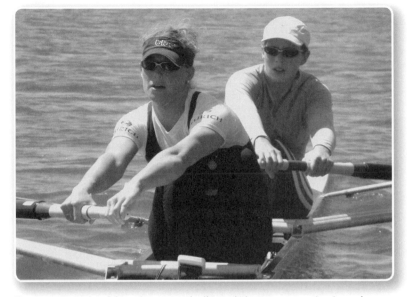

One small study of female rowers indicated that power, output, and capacity are highest when estrogen and progesterone doses of oral contraceptive are the lowest.

These studies suggest that exercise performance is not affected by menses unless menstrual symptoms are present or women are untrained. It is unclear whether OCs improve the performance of trained and untrained athletes, although there is speculation about mechanisms for such an effect. It may be fair to say that if OC use reduces premenstrual and menstrual symptoms, then performance could be enhanced. It is important to note that these studies are small, use different outcome measures, have widely different participants, and have varying outcomes. More research is needed before we can draw clear conclusions about the influence of OCs on athletic performance.

## Differences in Metabolism

During aerobic exercise women burn more fat (as a percentage of total energy expenditure) than men (Tarnopolsky et al. 1990, 1995, 1997) at all levels of exercise intensity (Venables et al. 2005). By default, this means that men use a higher percentage of carbohydrates for total energy during exercise than women. A 1995 study (Tarnopolsky et al.) suggested that when men and women load carbohydrates prior to an event, men are able to store more carbohydrates as glycogen than women are. A follow-up study by the same lead author strongly suggested that the difference in carbohydrate-loading capacity between men and women was actually more a function of absolute and relative carbohydrate intake (Tarnopolsky et al. 2001). As a final point of interest, one study addressed the effect of hormone therapy on postmenopausal women in relation to fat and carbohydrate metabolism during exercise at 80 percent of $\dot{V}O_2max$ (Johnson et al. 2002). As compared to postmenopausal women not taking hormone therapy, those women taking estrogen showed no difference in the percentages of fat and carbohydrate utilized during 30 minutes of treadmill exercise. It is also important to note that other factors contribute to the relative use of carbohydrates and fat for fuel, including diet, muscle glycogen content, exercise duration, and training status.

Although these differences in metabolism are interesting, they don't necessarily confer an advantage to one sex over the other. Some have argued that the difference in fat burning renders women better endurance athletes. If that were true, women would be beating men at endurance events such as marathons, which is not the case. The gender gap in running performance *has* narrowed for the marathon; the fastest woman marathoner is only 8.4 percent slower than the fastest male. But overall, running performance at the elite level for various distances still shows a gender gap on average around 11 percent, and this hasn't changed much in recent decades (Holden 2004).

Of course, not all exercise is aerobic. During sprints or when the body needs energy right away, anaerobic metabolism is the primary system at work. Stored carbohydrate in the muscles, or glycogen, can be burned for energy by enzymes in the muscles without oxygen. Men have an advantage in this area as well, likely due to their larger muscle fibers (Batterham and Birch 1996; Naughton et al. 1997). Fortunately, anaerobic capacity can be improved with speed work. Doing workouts that require anaerobic metabolism improves the ability to burn energy without oxygen.

# Female Psychosociology

Another area of interest regarding women's fitness is the psychosocial realm. Many have argued that women approach exercise and competition differently than men. As Kathleen DeBoer states, "Males and females have different worldviews. The paradigms that shape values, the situations that cause fear, and the circumstances that define success are distinct" (Ireland and Nattiv 2002 page 40). In short, many women value belonging to a group more than independence and fear isolation more than failure, while many men value success over connectedness and fear failure more than loneliness.

Of course, these are generalizations; but for coaches, trainers, or any fitness professional, it is important to acknowledge that men and women are different psychosocially and may perform better if their coaching and training incorporate these general worldviews. On a practical level, in some cases, this means encouraging women in team sports to play their best in order to support the team, not necessarily to stand out.

It is also absolutely critical to understand that women transition through life stages. Their health and fitness goals during these stages may vary considerably from those of men and from those of other women depending on their ages. Part II of this book explores how health and fitness goals can be targeted during the adolescent, childbearing, menopausal, and senior years.

## Important Physiological Differences Between Men and Women

As compared to men, women have

- 10 percent higher body fat,
- about 30 to 50 percent less upper body strength,
- smaller hearts,
- lower stroke volume,
- about 10 percent lower hemoglobin,
- lower $\dot{V}O_2max$,
- menstrual symptoms that can affect performance, and
- smaller muscle fibers.

# Female Morbidity and Mortality

To better understand how fitness can impact morbidity and mortality of women in the United States, it is important to understand which diseases they are at risk for. Table 1.2 shows the

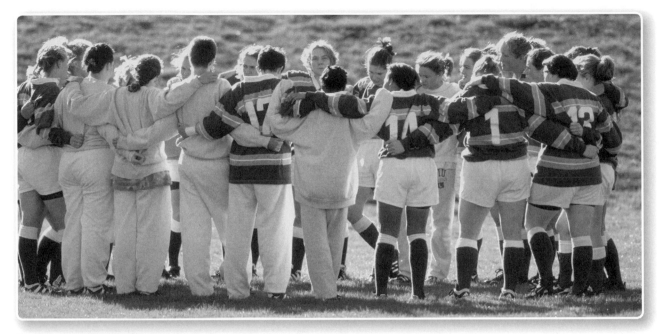

Feeling connected with a group may be a prime motivator for women to pursue physical activity and excel in competition.

leading causes of death for women based on data from 2000. Death rates vary by age and race, so the table shows a breakdown of death rates by race. For adult women, diseases of the heart and cancers are the top killers. In all groups of women, except American Indians, stroke is the third leading cause of death. Of course, some of the leading causes of death are not influenced by fitness, such as lung diseases (emphysema, chronic obstructive pulmonary disease), which are usually consequences of smoking.

Of course, when we discuss the health of women, cause of death does not represent the only data of importance. Our public health goal

◆ TABLE 1.2 ◆

## Leading Causes of Death by Race, Females, All Ages, United States, 2000*

|    | White | Black | American Indian | Asian/Pacific Islander |
|----|-------|-------|-----------------|------------------------|
| 1  | Heart disease | Heart disease | Heart disease | Cancer |
| 2  | Cancer | Cancer | Cancer | Heart disease |
| 3  | Stroke | Stroke | Accidents | Stroke |
| 4  | Lung disease | Diabetes | Diabetes | Accidents |
| 5  | Alzheimer's | Kidney disease | Stroke | Diabetes |
| 6  | Flu/pneumonia | Accidents | Liver disease | Flu/pneumonia |
| 7  | Diabetes | Lung disease | Lung disease | Lung disease |
| 8  | Accidents | Infection | Flu/pneumonia | Kidney disease |
| 9  | Kidney disease | Flu/pneumonia | Kidney disease | Hypertension |
| 10 | Infection | HIV | Infection | Infection |

*Data for races other than white and black should be interpreted with caution because of inconsistencies between reporting race on death certificates and on censuses and surveys.

Adapted from *National Vital Statistics Report*, Vol. 50, No. 15, September 16, 2002.

is not only to prevent women from dying prematurely, but also to help them enjoy optimal high quality of life for all the years they live. That's why it's important to address the risk factors that cause these diseases and to address diseases that affect quality of life, such as osteoporosis and arthritis, but don't necessarily cause premature death.

## ◆ Conclusion ◆

The most striking differences between men and women that affect exercise are related to lower extremity alignment. Girls and women are at particular risk for lower extremity injury, and it is essential that health and fitness professionals understand why. A strong foundation of knowledge on sex differences in anatomy and physiology will allow the professional to use information from the rest of this book to create an efficient and appropriate exercise program. Cardiovascular, strength, and metabolic differences, as well as psychosocial variables, also play important roles in female athletic performance. Women can be educated regarding all of these differences so that they can pursue any level of fitness they desire.

Achieving fitness should be strongly encouraged, as it is one of the many variables that prevent the development of risk factors for disease. Just as for men, cardiovascular disease is the number-one cause of death for women in the United States. In chapter 2, we review studies that have shown how physical activity reduces the occurrence of this disease, and many others, to improve quality of life for women.

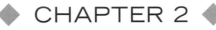 

# Exercise and Disease Prevention

## Topics in This Chapter

- ◆ Findings from the Nurses' Health Studies (NHS and NHSII)
- ◆ Exercise and coronary events in women
- ◆ Mechanisms by which aerobic exercise lowers risk of cardiovascular disease and stroke
- ◆ Exercise and blood pressure
- ◆ Resistance training and lipids
- ◆ Exercise and inflammation
- ◆ Exercise and insulin sensitivity

- ◆ Theories about exercise and cancer prevention—hormone levels, immune system function, insulin sensitivity, body composition
- ◆ What studies show about exercise and the prevention of cancer, dementia, osteoporosis, and obesity

I'm more aware than ever that I'm at risk for this disease (osteoporosis). And I'm also aware that I can take steps now to keep my bones strong for a lifetime. That's why no matter how busy I get, I work hard to maintain my active lifestyle and healthy diet.

Miriam E. Nelson, PhD,
author of *Strong Women, Strong Bones*

One problem with early research on ways to prevent disease was that it focused on men only. As we've reviewed in the previous chapter, women are different from men in many important ways. Assuming that what reduces risk of disease for men will also work for women is problematic. Risk factors vary in importance between men and women and are affected differently by lifestyle change. For example, elevated highly sensitive C-reactive protein (a marker of blood vessel wall inflammation) is a stronger predictor of cardiovascular disease risk for women than men (Ridker 2001). Also, regular physical activity appears to have a more powerful protective effect against type 2 diabetes for women than for men (Haapanen et al. 1997).

Fortunately, in the past few years, many studies have been done to examine women's health separately from men's. Landmark studies such as the Nurses' Health Study allow us to draw conclusions about female health behaviors and make specific recommendations for women. In this chapter, we review the findings of some high-profile studies that examine women's fitness and how it relates to health. Specifically, we address how physical activity reduces risk for developing cardiovascular disease and stroke, diabetes, cancer, dementia, osteoporosis, and obesity.

## Nurses' Health Studies

The Nurses' Health Study (NHS) was established in 1976 by Dr. Frank Speizer with funding from the National Institutes of Health. Originally this study was designed to examine the long-term effects of oral contraceptives on women's health.

Nurses, aged 30 to 55, were chosen for the study because it was thought that their level of medical knowledge would assist in obtaining the most accurate results possible. The nurses were surveyed (by mail) over the years about various health behaviors and health outcomes. Dietary information was collected as well, starting in 1980. Over the years, blood samples were also obtained from the study participants.

In 1989 the Nurses' Health Study II (NHSII) was established by Dr. Walt Willett. In this study, a younger group of nurses, aged 25 to 42, was enrolled to further explore the relationship between oral contraceptive use and health, as well as to examine diet and lifestyle risk factors (such as physical activity) and their impact on health.

Combined, the studies follow almost 250,000 women. The nurses in both studies continue to be surveyed every two years, and the data collected have resulted in hundreds of publications on women's health. The survey response rate for both groups of nurses is 90 percent. (This is an incredibly high rate of return of surveys as compared to rates in other studies that use this methodology.) The data collection has expanded to include food frequency questionnaires and quality of life information, as well as blood and urine samples. The Nurses' Health Studies have been and will continue to be one of the most valuable sources of information on women's health ever devised.

## Exercise and Cardiovascular Disease and Stroke

Cardiovascular disease, stroke, and **peripheral vascular disease** are largely preventable. Key among the interventions that lower risk is physical activity. Observational studies have shown that regular physical activity in women lowers risk of coronary heart disease and stroke (Blair et al. 1996; Iiu et al. 2000; Lee et al. 2001; Manson et al. 1999; Manson et al. 2002).

The largest **prospective study** to examine this issue was part of the Nurses' Health Study. In this analysis, 72,488 women were followed for eight years. At the beginning of the study, these women were free of heart disease and cancer. Periodically throughout the study, the

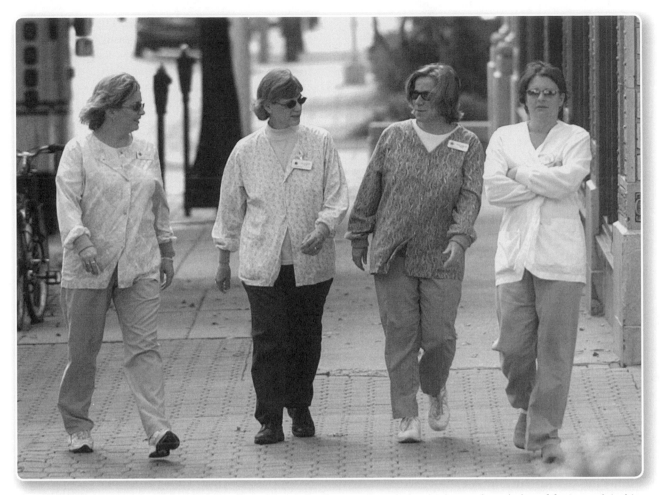

By participating in the Nurses' Health Studies, thousands of nurses have helped advance knowledge of factors related to women's health.

nurses answered detailed questionnaires regarding health habits, including exercise. The study showed that increasing levels of aerobic exercise led to decreasing numbers of cardiovascular events. Specifically, there was a 30 to 40 percent reduction in coronary events in women who were regular walkers. The more exercise, the better. The lowest event rate was in women who walked 3 or more hours per week. Women who initially were sedentary but became active over the course of the study had a lower risk of coronary events than women who remained sedentary (Manson et al. 1999).

Similar findings were noted in 70,000 postmenopausal women in the Women's Health Initiative Observational Study. In this investigation, women who sat for prolonged periods had a higher risk of cardiovascular events. The benefit of aerobic exercise in decreasing risk of events

was noted, and the degree of benefit related to the duration of exercise (Manson et al. 2002). Total stroke and **ischemic stroke** were reduced in the Nurses' Health Study in a dose-dependent fashion based on intensity of regular exercise (walking); in other words, the more intense the exercise, the lower the risk for stroke (Hu et al. 2000). Intensity of exercise can be defined generally (using the Borg scale, for example) or on an individual basis, and this topic is addressed specifically in chapter 7.

The mechanisms by which aerobic exercise lowers risk of cardiovascular disease and stroke include reduction in blood pressure, improvement in lipid profile, reduction of inflammation in the blood vessel walls, treatment and prevention of type 2 diabetes mellitus, and reduction in body weight. We'll explore each of these risk factors individually.

## Exercise and Coronary Events—Summary of Important Findings

◆ Women who walked regularly had a lower risk of coronary events.

◆ Women who sat for prolonged periods had higher risk of cardiovascular events.

◆ Sedentary women who became active had a lower risk of coronary events than women who remained inactive.

◆ The benefit of aerobic exercise in reducing the risk of coronary events was related to the duration of the exercise.

◆ The benefit of aerobic exercise in reducing the risk of stroke was related to the intensity of regular exercise.

## Exercise and Blood Pressure

Regular exercise prevents the development of high blood pressure in women (Blair et al. 1984). But women who already have high blood pressure may be fearful of exercise, thinking that it may aggravate their condition. Many studies show the opposite. After a few weeks, participation in a regular exercise program clearly lowers blood pressure in women with or without hypertension (Cox et al. 2001; Fagard 1995; Tanaka et al. 1997; Whelton et al. 2002). The amount of blood pressure change

### ◆ TABLE 2.1 ◆
### Blood Pressure and Lifestyle Modification

| Modification | Approximate SBP reduction |
| --- | --- |
| Weight reduction | 5-20 mmHg/10 kg weight loss |
| DASH eating plan | 8-14 mmHg |
| Dietary sodium reduction | 2-8 mmHg |
| Physical activity | 4-9 mmHg |
| Moderation of alcohol consumption | 2-4 mmHg |

DASH, Dietary Approaches to Stop Hypertension; SBP, systolic blood pressure.

Data from the *Seventh Report of the National Joint Committee on Prevention, Detection, Evaluation, and Treatment of High Blood Pressure.*

varies, from about 4 to 9 mmHg (millimeters of mercury, or "points" in common parlance) lower for the systolic and 3 to 5 mmHg lower for the diastolic.

Of interest, the type, frequency, and intensity of aerobic exercise don't seem to matter. All aerobic exercise lowers blood pressure. The blood pressure–lowering effect is more pronounced in women with hypertension than in those who are normotensive. Regular aerobic exercise often leads to weight loss, and this in turn further improves blood pressure. Of course, as noted in table 2.1, other lifestyle changes can improve blood pressure, too.

## Exercise and Lipids

Many studies of men and women have shown that lowering low-density lipoprotein cholesterol with medication prevents cardiovascular events. Of course, many women would prefer to make lifestyle changes to reduce their cholesterol levels instead of taking medicine. Is this feasible? It is.

A 2002 study by researchers at Duke University showed that aerobic exercise improves many measures in the cholesterol panel (Kraus et al. 2002). A total of 111 sedentary, overweight men and women with abnormal cholesterol were assigned to one of three exercise groups. One group performed high-amount, high-intensity exercise; another performed low-amount, high-intensity exercise; and the final group performed low-amount, moderate-intensity exercise. High-amount, high-intensity exercise was defined as the caloric equivalent of jogging about 20 miles (32 kilometers) per week at 65 to 80 percent of peak oxygen consumption. Low-amount, high-intensity exercise was the equivalent of jogging about 12 miles (19 kilometers) per week at 65 to 80 percent of peak oxygen consumption. And low-amount, moderate-intensity exercise referred to walking about 12 miles per week at 40 to 55 percent of peak oxygen consumption. There was an initial conditioning period of two to three months during which exercise was slowly increased in frequency and intensity. The study groups' cholesterol results were compared to each other as well as to those of a control group of non-exercisers. After six months at the respective exercise programs, cholesterol parameters were

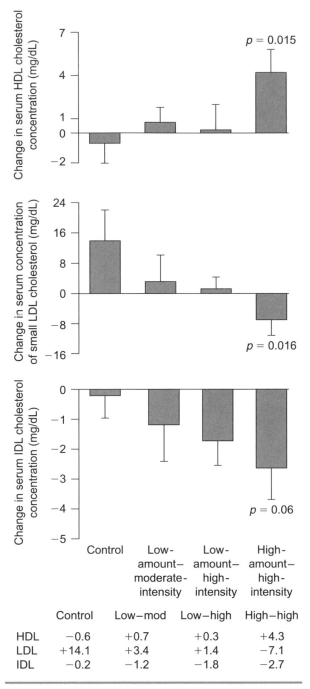

| | Control | Low–mod | Low–high | High–high |
|---|---|---|---|---|
| HDL | −0.6 | +0.7 | +0.3 | +4.3 |
| LDL | +14.1 | +3.4 | +1.4 | −7.1 |
| IDL | −0.2 | −1.2 | −1.8 | −2.7 |

**Figure 2.1** Effects of exercise on plasma lipoproteins. Changes in serum concentration of high-density lipoprotein (HDL), low-density lipoprotein (LDL), and intermediate-density lipoprotein (IDL) cholesterol among 111 sedentary, overweight, nondiabetic men and women with mild to moderate dyslipidemia after six months of exercising to differing degrees. Compared with controls, all exercising groups had potentially beneficial changes in plasma lipoproteins, but only the high-amount, high-intensity group had a significant increase in HDL and a decrease in LDL cholesterol. To convert serum cholesterol values to mmol/L (millimoles per liter), multiply by 0.026.

reassessed. As shown in figure 2.1, each exercise group showed significant improvements in multiple cholesterol panel measures, with the most benefit seen for patients who exercised more often and more intensely.

In two ways this was a landmark study. First, it compared different levels of aerobic exercise and showed that more exercise confers more benefit. Second, it measured cholesterol parameters beyond the traditional lipid profile. Measurements of high-density lipoprotein (HDL) and low-density lipoprotein (LDL) cholesterol particle concentrations alone don't provide a complete picture of risk. Assessing cholesterol particle size and percentage of small particles is essential because lower risk of cardiovascular disease is associated with larger cholesterol particles. This study also clearly showed that frequent, intense aerobic exercise favorably affects these newly recognized cholesterol abnormalities.

While many studies evaluate the effect of aerobic exercise on cholesterol, one examined the relationship between resistance training and lipids (Prabhakaran et al. 1999). This study included 24 sedentary premenopausal women with abnormal cholesterol who were otherwise healthy. They were randomly assigned to either a supervised intensive 14-week resistance training program or a nonexercise group. The program included a variety of resistance exercises performed three days a week for 45 minutes. The results showed a significant decrease in total cholesterol, LDL cholesterol, and total cholesterol/HDL cholesterol ratio in the resistance-trained group. Body fat also decreased in the exercise group, and strength increased.

Of course, there are dietary changes, such as substituting monounsaturated fats for saturated fats and eating more fiber, that can positively affect the lipid panel as well. It is also critical to avoid trans fats or "hydrogenated oils" completely; they are found in many processed foods and are listed separately on nutrition labeling. But in at least one study, it was shown that dietary changes weren't effective without concomitant exercise (Stefanick et al. 1998).

## Exercise and Inflammation

Inflammation in the blood vessel walls is a newly identified risk factor for cardiovascular disease. Although data on this risk factor are limited, it

## Blood Pressure, Lipids, and Exercise—Summary of Important Findings

- Exercise lowers blood pressure in women with and without hypertension. The effect is more pronounced in women with hypertension than those who are normotensive.
- The type, frequency, and intensity of aerobic exercise don't seem to matter. All aerobic exercise lowers blood pressure in women.
- Exercise improves multiple cholesterol panel measures in women. Those who exercised more often and more intensely received the most benefit, including reduction in the percentage of small cholesterol particles.
- Resistance training decreases total cholesterol, LDL cholesterol, and total cholesterol/HDL cholesterol ratio in women.

appears to be a significant factor in promoting atherosclerosis, especially in women.

One marker of inflammation that is now widely used is the highly sensitive C-reactive protein (hs-CRP) level. As shown in figure 2.2, if hs-CRP level is chronically elevated in otherwise healthy women, there is a higher long-term risk of heart attack, ischemic stroke, and peripheral vascular disease. And, as shown in figure 2.3, elevated hs-CRP is a stronger predictor of risk than other conventional risk factors, such as total cholesterol, LDL cholesterol, or HDL cholesterol. Fortunately, lifestyle changes, such as improved diet, can lower hs-CRP levels. A diet low in saturated fat and higher in fiber, nuts, soy, and **plant sterols** proved beneficial (Jenkins et al. 2003).

Another study evaluated the role of exercise on hs-CRP in women who already had cardiovascular disease. Women who participated in a formal cardiac rehabilitation program lowered their hs-CRP (Milani et al. 2004).

There are no studies yet showing that regular exercise lowers hs-CRP in healthy women, but one study demonstrated that women with low fitness and type 2 diabetes had elevated hs-CRP levels (McGavock et al. 2004).

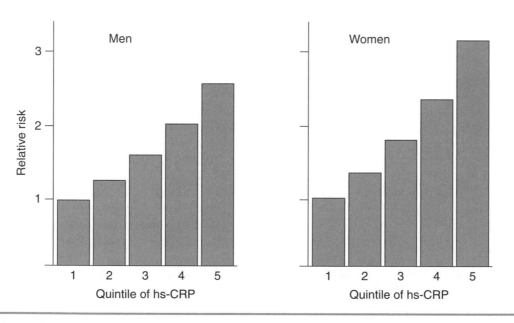

**Figure 2.2** Increasing concentrations of C-reactive protein predict the risk of myocardial infarction. In apparently healthy men (left panel) and women (right panel), the adjusted relative risk of future myocardial infarction is associated with increasing quintiles of high-sensitivity C-reactive protein (hs-CRP). Risk estimates are adjusted for age, smoking status, body mass index (kg/m$^2$), diabetes, history of hyperlipidemia, history of hypertension, exercise level, and family history of coronary disease.

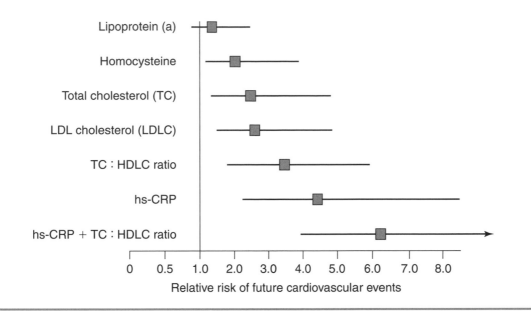

**Figure 2.3** High-sensitivity C-reactive protein improves risk prediction in healthy subjects. Shown is a direct comparison of the magnitude of relative risk of future cardiovascular events associated with high-sensitivity C-reactive protein (hs-CRP); levels of total cholesterol (TC), LDL cholesterol (LDLC), and HDL cholesterol (HDLC); lipoprotein (a); and homocysteine among apparently healthy subjects. Risk prediction is improved by the addition of hs-CRP to standard measurement of lipid levels. For consistency, relative risks and 95 percent confident intervals are shown for individuals in the top versus bottom quartile for each factor.

Reprinted, by permission, from P.M. Ridker, 2001, "High-sensitivity C-reactive protein: Potential adjunct for global risk assessment in the primary prevention of cardiovascular disease," *Circulation* 103: 1813-1818.

Inflammation clearly has a role in cardiovascular disease. Further research will better define this role. The best advice for women at this time is to control inflammation as well as other conventional risk factors for heart disease by maintaining an active lifestyle with consistent exercise and eating a diet low in saturated fat and higher in soy products, nuts, fiber, and plant sterols.

## Exercise and Type 2 Diabetes

There are two major types of diabetes: type 1 and type 2. Type 1 diabetes occurs when the pancreas stops producing insulin or does not produce enough insulin. (Insulin is a hormone that helps the cells use glucose for energy.) People with type 1 diabetes must take insulin injections for the rest of their lives. The exact cause of type 1 diabetes is not known, but exercise does not play a role in the prevention of type 1 diabetes. The role of exercise in the management of type 1 diabetes is discussed in chapter 3.

People with type 2 diabetes produce insulin, but the cells of the body are not able to use the insulin; they develop "insulin resistance." Type 2 diabetes is one of the top 10 leading causes of death in the United States for women of all races. Type 2 diabetes disproportionately affects most minority groups, especially American Indians and Alaska Natives (U.S. Department of Health and Human Services 2003). There are clear data showing that regular physical activity reduces the risk of type 2 diabetes. This important message must be communicated to help women prevent type 2 diabetes and its many complications such as cardiovascular disease, damage to eyes and loss of vision (retinopathy), damage to kidneys and kidney failure (nephropathy), nerve dysfunction (neuropathy), and infections (especially in the feet, leading to amputation).

As shown in figures 2.4 and 2.5, weight gain and increased body mass index (BMI) are associated with increased risk of developing type 2 diabetes. Note the especially sharp increase in risk of diabetes in women, as compared to men, with increasing BMI. Type 2 diabetes doesn't develop overnight. It is typically the result of years of low fitness, poor eating habits, and weight gain.

## Acute and Chronic Complications of Diabetes

- ◆ Cardiovascular disease
- ◆ Retinopathy
- ◆ Nephropathy
- ◆ Neuropathy (peripheral and autonomic)
- ◆ Infections

Women at risk of developing type 2 diabetes usually show a steady increase in their fasting blood glucose over years. The American Diabetes Association (ADA) recently lowered the level at which fasting blood glucose is considered abnormal. Normal fasting blood glucose is <100 milligrams per deciliter. If fasting blood glucose is in the range of 100 to 125 milligrams per deciliter, it is considered "impaired fasting glucose." People with impaired fasting glucose have a higher risk of developing diabetes in the future as compared to those with normal blood glucose (ADA 2004). Once fasting blood glucose reaches 126 milligrams per deciliter (on two separate readings), a person is diagnosed with diabetes. Based on current ADA guidelines, persons with

diabetes are presumed to have heart disease. It is essential to prevent diabetes to minimize cardiovascular risk. Clearly, it is in every woman's best interest to follow a lifestyle conducive to preventing diabetes.

How much exercise is necessary to prevent type 2 diabetes? Once again, interesting data come from the Nurses' Health Study. Typically, studies that examine the relationship between fitness and type 2 diabetes evaluate levels or amounts of aerobic exercise. One investigation from the Nurses' Health Study (Hu et al. 2003) looked at this question from a different viewpoint. In that investigation, 68,497 nurses were surveyed about their sedentary behaviors, such as watching television, in addition to exercise activities, such as walking.

At the start of the study, none of the women had diabetes. The women were followed from 1992 to 1998. A clear association between sedentary behaviors and development of diabetes was found. By the end of the study, 2.2 percent of the women (1,515 cases) were newly diagnosed with type 2 diabetes. Each increment of 2 hours per day of TV watching was associated with a 14 percent increase in risk of diabetes. Each increment of 2 hours per day of sitting at work was associated with a 7 percent increase in risk of diabetes. In contrast, standing or walking around the home for 2 hours per day was

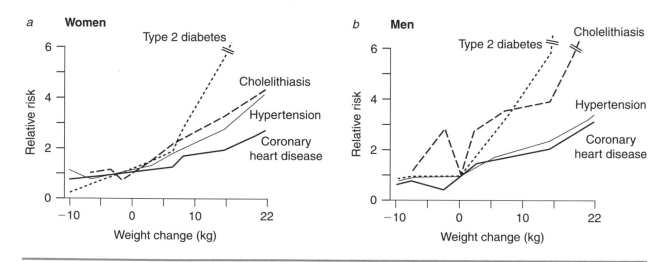

**Figure 2.4** Adult weight change and the risk of disease. Even a modest increase in weight as an adult is associated with an increased risk of type 2 diabetes, hypertension, coronary heart disease, and cholelithiasis. *(a)* Data for women in the Nurses' Health Study, initially 30 to 55 years of age, who were followed for up to 18 years. *(b)* Data for men in the Health Professionals Follow-up Study, initially 40 to 65 years of age, who were followed for up to 10 years.

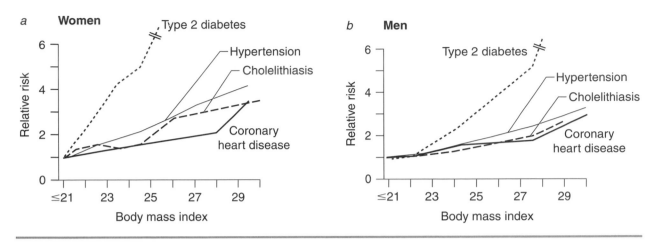

**Figure 2.5** Body mass index and the risk of disease. Increasing body mass index (BMI kg/m²), even within the normal range of BMI (21 to 24.9), is associated with an increased risk of type 2 diabetes, hypertension, coronary heart disease, and cholelithiasis. (a) Data for women in the Nurses' Health Study, initially 30 to 55 years of age, who were followed for up to 18 years. (b) Data for men in the Health Professionals Follow-up Study, initially 40 to 65 years of age, who were followed for up to 10 years.

associated with a 12 percent reduction in risk for diabetes. Walking briskly for 1 hour per day was associated with a 34 percent reduction in risk for type 2 diabetes.

For this group of women, it was estimated that 43 percent of new cases of diabetes could have been prevented by reducing television viewing to less than 10 hours per week and adding 30 minutes per day of brisk walking. It is important to note that sedentary behaviors predicted risk for diabetes independent of exercise level. That is, sedentary behaviors must be reduced and exercise activity increased to reduce risk for type 2 diabetes.

Authors of another investigation from the Nurses' Health Study (Hu et al. 1999b) followed 70,102 nurses from 1986 to 1992. In this study, walking and other forms of exercise were measured to determine the influence on future risk for developing type 2 diabetes. This study showed that the more frequent and more vigorous the exercise, the lower the risk of developing diabetes. These aren't the only studies published on this topic. In fact, there is another study of women in this database that confirms these findings (Manson et al. 1991), as well as studies from other databases, examined next.

The Diabetes Prevention Program Research Group published a study in 2002 showing that an intensive program of lifestyle change, including instruction in weight reduction through healthy diet and regular physical activity, reduced the risk of developing type 2 diabetes in male and female patients who were at risk. The at-risk patients entered the study with known abnormalities of blood glucose, but did not meet criteria for diabetes. At least 150 minutes per week of physical activity was recommended for the group receiving intensive lifestyle coaching. The other two groups received standard lifestyle recommendations, and one of these groups also received medication to improve blood glucose. As shown in figure 2.6, clearly the most benefit in reducing risk of type 2 diabetes was seen in the group receiving intensive lifestyle change. It is important to note that the benefit for this group even exceeded the benefit seen in the group treated with medication.

An interesting study out of Finland followed both men and women to determine if physical activity prevented type 2 diabetes. Not only did the researchers find that regular physical activity was associated with decreased risk of type 2 diabetes; they also noted that regular physical activity had a more powerful protective effect for women than for men (Haapanen et al. 1997). The level of physical activity in this study was less important than the overall amount of activity performed. Again, it appears that minimizing sedentary behaviors and increasing

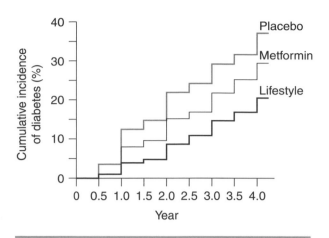

**Figure 2.6** Cumulative incidence of diabetes according to study group. The diagnosis of diabetes was based on the criteria of the American Diabetic Association. The incidence of diabetes differed significantly among the three groups ($p < 0.001$) for each comparison.

Adapted, by permission, from Diabetes Prevention Program Research Group, 2002, "Reduction in the incidence of type 2 diabetes with lifestyle intervention or metformin," *New England Journal of Medicine* 346: 393-403. Copyright ©2002 Massachusetts Medical Society. All rights reserved.

## Risk Factors for Type 2 Diabetes in Women

- ◆ Family history (genetics)
- ◆ Older age (over 55)
- ◆ Obesity
- ◆ Sedentary lifestyle
- ◆ High-calorie diet

insulin can more readily transfer glucose from the blood into the cell.

A clear relationship exists between regular exercise and type 2 diabetes risk. All women should be encouraged to participate in regular exercise to minimize risk of impaired fasting glucose and type 2 diabetes. Walking for 30 to 60 minutes on most days of the week and minimizing sedentary behaviors both favor good blood glucose control.

## Exercise and Type 2 Diabetes—Summary of Important Findings

- ◆ The more frequent and vigorous the exercise, the lower the risk of developing type 2 diabetes.
- ◆ Sedentary behaviors (sitting, watching TV) predicted risk for diabetes independent of exercise level. Sedentary behaviors must be reduced and exercise activity increased to reduce risk for type 2 diabetes.
- ◆ Regular physical activity has a more powerful protective effect against type 2 diabetes for women than for men.
- ◆ In women at risk for type 2 diabetes, regular physical activity as part of intensive lifestyle change had a greater benefit than treatment with glucose-lowering medication.

leisure-time physical activity or moderate activity are beneficial in reducing risk of developing type 2 diabetes.

The physiology behind exercise and type 2 diabetes prevention is as follows: With low fitness and weight gain, the muscles in the body become less sensitive (more resistant) to insulin. Insulin is used to transport glucose into the cells. If the cells become less sensitive to insulin, less glucose enters the muscles and more glucose stays in the blood. Exercise increases insulin sensitivity, probably through several mechanisms. One known mechanism is by increasing the number of insulin-responsive glucose transporters from inside cells to cell surfaces (Devlin 1992). With more transporters available on the cell surfaces,

## Exercise and Cancer Prevention: Theory

Several mechanisms have been proposed to address how physical activity may decrease cancer risk. However, it is important to keep in mind that physical activity is just one lifestyle behavior that may influence cancer risk. Often, women who exercise adopt other healthy habits that may reduce cancer risk, such as avoiding tobacco, minimizing alcohol, following a healthy diet, and seeking regular preventive care. How exercise influences cancer risk may also vary by age, menopausal status, race, and family history. For example, exercise may be less likely to reduce cancer risk in a woman with a strong family history of the disease. In order to understand how physical activity may reduce cancer risk, it is important to explore possible biologic mechanisms. The key mechanisms we will review here include the effects of exercise on hormone levels, immune system function, insulin sensitivity, and body composition.

## Exercise, Hormone Levels, and Cancer Risk

Exercise has an effect on hormone levels in the body, including estrogen, progesterone, and testosterone. Exercise can delay the onset of menses, contribute to delaying the regularity of menses, or both. When the onset of menses is delayed, risk of breast and endometrial (uterine) cancer may be reduced, because early age of **menarche** is associated with increased risk of breast cancer. The number of menstrual cycles a woman experiences is also related to risk—the more menstrual cycles a woman has in her lifetime, the higher the risk of breast cancer (Vihko and Apter 1986).

In premenopausal adult women who exercise, there are multiple hormonal differences from nonexercisers. Exercising women have lower levels of estrogen and progesterone, as well as shorter luteal phases and more missed periods, amenorrhea, or both. Again, these changes could theoretically lead to lower risk of breast and endometrial cancer. But with prolonged amenorrhea (greater than three months) there is increased risk for bone loss and osteoporosis.

Exercise may also influence how estrogen is metabolized. Estrogen is metabolized by two pathways in the body. One pathway forms far more potent estrogen metabolites than the other. Preliminary data suggest that exercise favors production of the less potent estrogen metabolites, therefore decreasing risk of both breast and endometrial cancer.

Estrogen and androgen levels are lower in postmenopausal women who exercise, too. One study in particular focused on the change in hormone levels that occur with exercise in postmenopausal women. The Physical Activity for Total Health Study led by Anne McTiernan, MD, PhD, recruited healthy, postmenopausal women who were overweight and sedentary, then randomized them to an exercise or control group. The women were not on hormone therapy, were nonsmokers, and drank alcohol only in modera-

tion. During the year of follow-up, it was found that hormone levels (testosterone, free testosterone, estrone, estradiol, and free estradiol) in the exercising women were lower than in the control group. The effect was limited to women who lost body fat (McTiernan et al. 2004).

## Exercise, the Immune System, and Cancer Risk

Another mechanism by which exercise may influence cancer risk is through affecting the immune system. Most cancers don't appear to be immunogenic, meaning that they aren't caused by the immune system. But they may be influenced by the immune system. If this is true, then anything that affects the immune system could influence cancer risk. If exercise enhances the immune system, then it may decrease cancer risk. Therefore, people who don't get enough exercise may be at higher cancer risk. On the other hand, if excessive exercise suppresses the immune system, then cancer risk may rise with increased physical activity.

Regular, moderate exercise appears to enhance the immune system not only by increasing the number of immune cells at work, but also by making the cells more active (Shephard et al. 1995). This is especially important with aging, because immune function declines with age. This immune senescence may account for increasing cancer risk with age. One study examined this issue and showed that elderly women (and men) who were regular exercisers had improved immune cell function as compared to elderly nonexercisers (Mazzeo 1994).

## Exercise, Insulin Resistance, and Cancer Risk

The presence of type 2 diabetes is a predictor of risk for colon, liver, pancreas, endometrium, and breast cancer (Bugianesi 2005; Hu et al. 1999a; Moore et al. 1998a). Insulin resistance, which may be present for years before the development of diabetes, is strongly influenced by physical activity (Moore et al. 1998b). Exercise training reduces insulin resistance, thereby decreasing risk of diabetes. It is theorized that via reducing insulin resistance, exercise may lower risk of colon, liver, pancreas, endometrial, and breast cancer. Actual studies testing this hypothesis are reviewed later in the chapter.

### Exercise, Energy Balance, Body Composition, and Cancer Risk

Final factors to consider in the relationship between exercise and cancer risk have to do with energy balance and body composition. It is proven that calorie restriction increases longevity and lowers cancer risk in animals (Dirks and Leeuwenburgh 2005). Calorie restriction in humans, however, is controversial; and side effects may occur such as hypotension, loss of **libido,** menstrual irregularities, infertility, osteoporosis, cold sensitivity, loss of strength and stamina, slower wound healing, depression, and irritability. It is thought that increased calorie expenditure through exercise may be equivalent to calorie restriction for cancer risk reduction. However, this theory hasn't been proven.

Obesity and central body fat are risk factors for many cancers, including breast, endometrial, colon, and non-Hodgkin's lymphoma (Frezza et al. 2005; Rapp et al. 2005). Obviously, exercise helps reduce obesity and may specifically reduce central body fat. Decreasing central adiposity likely has multiple positive metabolic effects, including improved blood sugar control, that reduce cancer risk. Keep in mind that weight loss from caloric restriction (without concomitant exercise) may favor diffuse, as opposed to central, body fat loss.

## Ways Exercise May Reduce Cancer Risk

- ◆ Reduction of hormone levels
- ◆ Immune system augmentation
- ◆ Decreased insulin resistance
- ◆ Reduction in central adiposity

# Exercise and Cancer Prevention: Studies

The second leading cause of death in women is cancer, all types combined. Of course it's important to discuss cancer by type, as the risk factors for one type of cancer may be very different from those for another. Figure 2.7 shows that lung cancer has become the leading cancer concern for women. Unfortunately, it is the burden of smoking from prior decades that has led to the surge in lung cancer deaths since 1970. As fewer women smoke cigarettes over time, the number of lung cancer deaths will slowly decrease. This is a cancer that does not appear to be directly affected by exercise. In figure 2.8, note that the number of women diagnosed with breast cancer is greater than the number diagnosed with lung cancer, but more women die of lung cancer because it is far less curable than breast cancer. This is just another reason to discourage smoking.

There aren't data on the relationship between every type of cancer and exercise, but let's review what has been done. Does being physically active have any effect on developing colorectal, breast, ovarian, endometrial, or pancreatic cancer?

### Exercise and Colorectal Cancer

Colorectal cancer risk is clearly decreased in women who are regularly physically active. Numerous studies of both occupational and leisure-time physical activity have shown decreased colon cancer risk, with higher levels of activity reducing risk by about 50 percent (Colditz et al. 1997). In one specific investigation from the Nurses' Health Study, both low BMI and high physical activity were associated with decreased colon cancer risk. Specifically, for women who exercised regularly, as in walking at a normal or brisk pace for 1 hour per day, colon cancer risk was reduced 46 percent (Martinez et al. 1997). A meta-analysis by Samad and colleagues (2005) also confirms reduction of colon cancer risk with physical activity. Specifically, recreational physical activity reduced colon cancer risk by 29 percent in women. In this meta-analysis, physical activity did not reduce risk of *rectal* cancer in either sex.

### Exercise and Breast Cancer

For breast cancer, the study results are mixed. Three studies were published from the Nurses' Health Study database. The first, in 1998 (NHS II), showed no link between physical activity in late adolescence or in the recent past and breast cancer risk among young adult women (Rockhill et al. 1998). One significant limitation of this study was the relatively short follow-up period of six years. Another limitation was reliance on

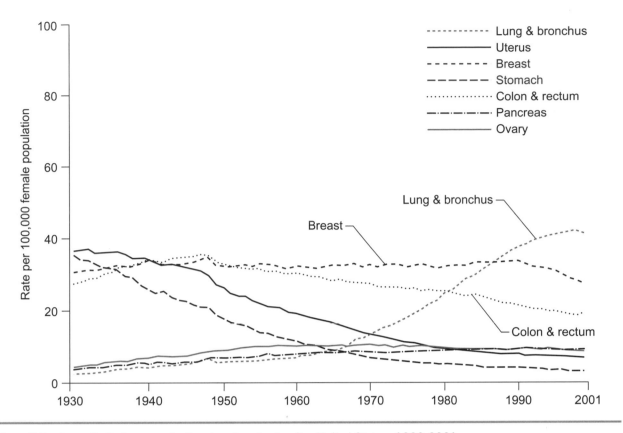

**Figure 2.7** Age-adjusted cancer death rates, females by site, United States, 1930-2001.
Per 100,000, age-adjusted to the 2000 U.S. standard population. Uterus cancer death rates are for uterine cervix and uterine corpus combined. Note: Due to changes in ICD coding, numerator information has changed over time. Rates for cancers of the lung and bronchus, colon and rectum, and ovary are affected by these coding changes. Note in particular the rise in lung cancer deaths. This is directly attributable to the burden of prior smoking.

exercise history from just a few discrete points in time, as opposed to a lifetime exercise history.

The second study, published in 1999, used several different measures of adult physical activity and included pre- and postmenopausal women (Rockhill et al. 1999). The results showed that women who engaged in moderate or vigorous physical activity for 7 or more hours per week, as opposed to those who were active less than 1 hour per week, had a statistically significantly lower risk of breast cancer. The relative risk was 0.82, meaning that breast cancer was reduced 18 percent in vigorous exercisers. In this study, women were followed for 16 years, and physical activity was assessed on multiple questionnaires throughout the years of follow-up.

Finally, a third study from this database (NHS II) was published in 2003 by Colditz and colleagues. A surprising result from this investigation was that premenopausal women with a higher BMI (greater than or equal to 30) had an increased risk of breast cancer from regular physical activity. The theory behind this finding is as follows: Overweight and obesity are associated with anovulation. Anovulation reduces risk of breast cancer. Regular exercise in obese women may actually increase their frequency of ovulation and therefore increase breast cancer risk. A limitation of this study was the low number of women who engaged in regular vigorous exercise.

A recent investigation outside the Nurses' Health Study database examined the relationship between breast cancer and physical activity. A case control study suggested that any exercise activity reduced risk of breast carcinoma in situ, but only in women without a family history of breast cancer (Patel et al. 2003). The study included white, Hispanic, and black women aged 35 to 64. Lifetime exercise history was determined by personal interview.

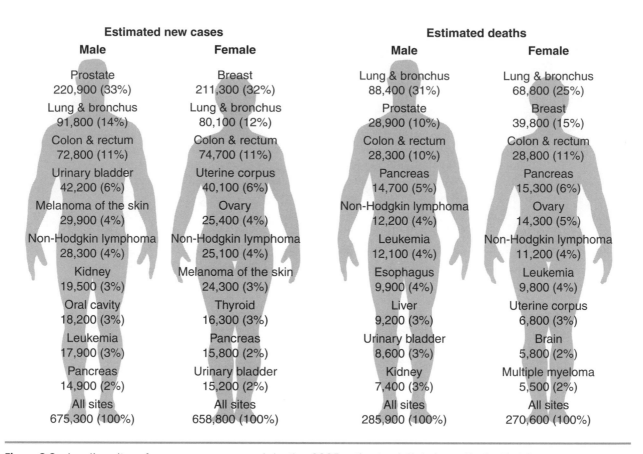

**Figure 2.8** Leading sites of new cancer cases and death—2005 estimates.* Note in particular that far more women are diagnosed with breast cancer than lung cancer, but almost twice as many die from lung cancer. The reason is that lung cancer is often diagnosed at later stages and less effective treatments are available. Note: Percentages may not total 100 due to rounding.
*Excludes basal and squamous cell skin cancers and in situ carcinoma except urinary bladder.

The reduction in risk for breast cancer in physically active women without a family history of breast cancer was 35 percent. Higher levels of physical activity did not confer any additional benefit. This confirmed results from an earlier similar study done at the same university, published in 1994 (Bernstein et al.), that showed reduced risk of breast cancer of 58 percent in women who exercised 3.8 or more hours per week over their lifetime. The population in the earlier study differed in that the women were all under age 40.

The results from research regarding the relationship between breast cancer and physical activity are mixed. We haven't cited every study done in this area, but the ones mentioned mirror what has been published from studies of other groups of women. Although we would like to say that regular physical activity lowers breast cancer risk, and in some studies it does, it has not been consistently shown to be beneficial. One main reason for the apparent contradictory findings may be inaccurate or inadequate exercise history.

## Exercise and Ovarian Cancer

Ovarian cancer risk was also examined in the Nurses' Health Study cohort. One study in 2001, by Bertone and colleagues, did not show any association between recreational physical activity and ovarian cancer risk. However, there was a suggestion that women who engaged in frequent vigorous activity had a modest increase in ovarian cancer risk. Dr. Bertone was lead author of another study in 2002, with a different patient population, that showed no association between any level of physical activity and ovarian cancer risk. In other databases, including studies done in other countries, results are mixed. Some studies show no effect, some show a protective effect, and others show increased risk of ovarian cancer with regular exercise. A recent study published on this issue was done in 2004. It showed no overall significant association between physical activity and risk of ovarian cancer, although the results were suggestive of a protective effect (Hannan et al. 2004). It is unclear whether exercise has any significant impact on risk of ovarian cancer.

## Exercise and Endometrial (Uterine) Cancer

Data on whether regular exercise reduces endometrial cancer are unclear. A prospective cohort study done in the United States showed a nonsignificant reduction in endometrial cancer risk in women who were physically active as compared to those with the lowest levels of activity (Colbert et al. 2003). This work was limited by its focus on recent physical activity as opposed to lifelong exercise patterns. A case control study done in Washington State showed that more women in the control group (women without cancer) were regular exercisers than cases (women with cancer) (Littman et al. 2001). In this study, there was little evidence of a trend of decreasing risk with increasing activity. According to a statement in a review article from Australia, obesity and diabetes increase the risk of endometrial cancer, while low-fat diets and exercise appear to decrease risk (Purdie and Green 2001).

## Exercise and Pancreatic Cancer

The Nurses' Health Study also addressed the relationship between physical activity and pancreatic cancer. Finding anything that reduces risk of pancreatic cancer is helpful because this is a rapidly fatal cancer. Often diagnosed in later stages because it is asymptomatic early on, pancreatic cancer kills about 15,000 women on average every year in the United States.

Two prospective studies examined the relationship between pancreatic cancer and exercise. A 2001 publication by Michaud and colleagues showed that in the Nurses' Health Study, obesity significantly increased the risk of pancreatic cancer and physical activity appeared to decrease the risk of pancreatic cancer, especially among women who were overweight. By contrast, a

## Exercise and Cancer— Summary of Important Findings

- ◆ Colorectal cancer risk is clearly decreased in women who are regularly physically active. Higher levels of activity reduce risk by about 50 percent!
- ◆ The results regarding the relationship between breast cancer and physical activity are mixed.
- ◆ Results are mixed regarding ovarian cancer. Some studies show no effect, some show a protective effect, and others show increased risk of ovarian cancer with regular exercise.
- ◆ Physical activity may decrease the risk of endometrial cancer.
- ◆ Physical activity may decrease the risk of pancreatic cancer, especially among women who are overweight.

2003 study by Lee and colleagues showed no association between physical activity or overweight/obesity and pancreatic cancer in men and women. However, there weren't enough women in the study to be analyzed separately from the men. The jury is still out as to whether physical activity reduces pancreatic cancer risk in women; but the Michaud study is compelling. It involved women only and showed a significant 30 to 40 percent reduction in risk.

# Exercise and Dementia

The number of adults over age 65 is growing rapidly in the United States. Age is one of the risk factors for dementia, and women generally live longer than men. Also, dementia may be most successfully treated in its earliest stages. For all these reasons, women need to follow lifestyles conducive to long-term cognitive health. Fortunately, this is a disease that may be modified by physical activity.

Several groups have examined the relationship between physical activity and cognitive function.

It appears that physical activity may lower risk for dementia. Several prospective studies support this finding (Barnes et al. 2003; Lytle et al. 2004; Weuve et al. 2004), and one did not (Verghese et al. 2003). Exercise may protect the brain by reducing risk for stroke, as mentioned in the section on cardiovascular disease, via a favorable effect on blood pressure, blood cholesterol, and blood glucose. Through control of these risk factors, blood flow to the brain is protected or even enhanced, thereby theoretically preserving function.

The Weuve publication used data from the Nurses' Health Study, including data on 18,766 women between the ages of 70 and 81 years who began the study in 1986. One of the most exciting findings from this study was that the level of physical activity needed to preserve cognitive function was not vigorous or extensive. Even simply walking, for at least 1.5 hours per week at a 21 to 30 minute per mile pace, was associated with better cognitive performance than lower levels of activity. Higher levels of activity conferred even more benefit. The authors note that the differences in cognition between women with higher and lower activity were equivalent to the differences seen between women two to three years apart in age. In other words, women who exercised more had cognitive skills that were better than their lower-activity peers and more similar to those of women two to three years younger.

These data on preventing cognitive decline come from observational studies. While the data suggest a possible benefit from physical activity, we cannot draw definitive conclusions without confirmatory data from randomized clinical trials.

## Exercise and Osteoporosis

Osteoporosis is defined as decreased density of the bone with loss of the normal bony microarchitecture. Figure 2.9 shows a section of bone with osteoporosis. Individuals with osteoporosis have less dense bone that is unstable and therefore more prone to fracture, even with minimal or no trauma. Osteoporosis is a preventable disease, and performing regular exercise is one of the critical behaviors needed to maintain healthy bone.

Preventing osteoporosis is important because for many women a fracture has significant consequences beyond the initial injury. There is an increased risk of mortality following osteoporotic fracture; however, it is unclear if the fracture itself is the cause of premature death as opposed to other causes or underlying chronic conditions. After hip fracture, some women are unable to return to their prior levels of independence

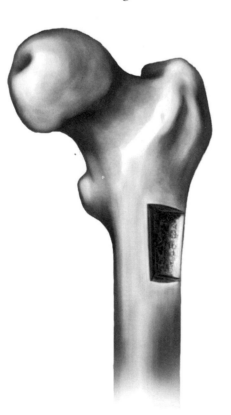
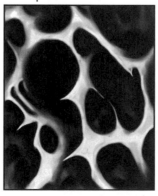
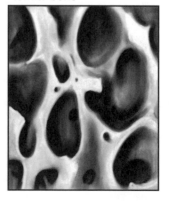

Osteoporotic bone     Normal bone

**Figure 2.9** Normal bone is shown on the right. Note the differences from osteoporotic bone on the left. Not only is the bone less dense, but there is also loss of the normal bony microarchitecture.

and activity. Spine fractures cause significant pain, and one fracture leads to another due to changes in spine alignment from the initial fracture. Women with osteoporosis are at risk for fracturing ribs, wrist, and other sites, too. The most common osteoporotic fracture sites are the spine, hip, and distal wrist because of their high concentration of trabecular (spongy) bone. The key to preventing death and disability due to osteoporosis is to prevent the first fracture.

Regular exercise is a cornerstone of building and maintaining healthy bone. Both weight-bearing activities and strength training are important for best results. Weight-bearing exercises such as walking, running, and aerobics provide compression forces on bone, while strength training provides bending forces. Both types are important for bone strength and integrity. Observational studies show that women who perform regular exercise have lower risk of osteoporotic fracture than those who do not. Bone health benefits from walking were noted in a Nurses' Health Study investigation (Feskanich et al. 2002). Risk of hip fracture decreased with increasing levels of physical activity. For postmenopausal women (not on hormone therapy) who walked at least 4 hours per week and did no other exercise, hip fracture risk was 41 percent lower than in those walking less than 1 hour per week. Similarly large reductions in risk for hip fracture were found in a study, by Gregg and colleagues in 1998. In this study, a variety of activities, including household chores, were associated with decreased fracture risk at the spine and hip.

## Exercise and Obesity

As shown in figure 2.10, overweight and obesity have reached alarming levels in the United States. Overweight and obesity are associated with increased risk of cardiovascular disease, metabolic syndrome, hypertension, abnormal cholesterol, sleep apnea, arthritis, diabetes, cancer, and premature death (Blair et al. 1996; Farrell et al. 2004; Grundy et al. 1999; Rockhill et al. 2001). Increasing the level of physical activity in children and adults is essential to prevent weight problems and to reverse this trend.

There are differences in the percentages of men and women affected by obesity based on race. Mexican Americans have an equal distribution of obesity between men and women. African American women have a higher rate of obesity as compared to African American men. For Caucasians, the opposite is true; more white men are affected by obesity than white women. We don't know exactly why these differences exist.

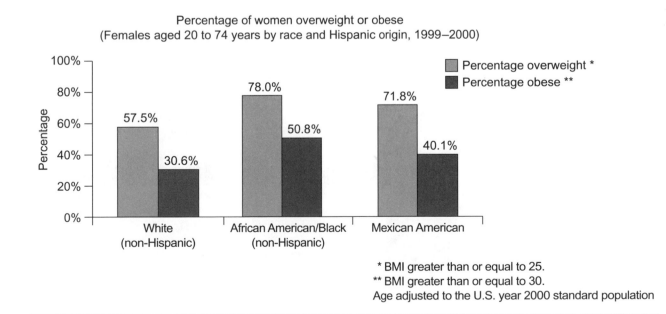

**Figure 2.10** Overweight and obesity rates vary by race. African Americans and Mexican Americans are disproportionately affected.

Centers for Disease Control and Prevention, National Center for Health Statistics, National Health and Nutrition Examination Survey, Health, United States, 2002.

From figure 2.11, we see that physical inactivity increases with age, contributing to weight gain with age. After age 65, more than half of adults become physically inactive.

In the past, pregnancy and oral contraceptive use were thought to play causal roles in weight gain for women. But, as outlined next, these don't appear to be significant factors. Changes associated with menopause, on the other hand, may play a significant role.

Weight gain is expected during pregnancy. After a first pregnancy, according to a study by Smith and colleagues (1994), women do end up heavier than their **nulliparous** peers, even 12 months postpartum, but only by 4 to 7 pounds (1.8 to 3.2 kilograms). In that study, African American women retained more weight post-pregnancies than Caucasian women. Of interest, this study indicated that it was first pregnancies and not later pregnancies that were primarily associated with weight gain. It is also important to note that weight gain after a first pregnancy resulted in a more central pattern of adiposity, as measured by waist-to-hip ratio. In one prospective study of childbearing with 10 years of follow-up, the overall risk of weight gain was quite small for American women; this study included Caucasians only (Williamson et al. 1994).

In the past, when oral contraceptives were taken in higher doses, weight gain with use was a side effect. With the current low-dose preparations, weight changes (gain or loss) do not differ between users and nonusers of oral contraceptives (Reubinoff et al. 1995).

The metabolic changes that occur during menopause appear to promote redistribution of body fat. The use of estrogen for control of menopausal symptoms does not appear to cause weight gain. Hormonal changes of menopause result in central or abdominal fat increases in postmenopausal women not on hormone therapy. We know from many clinical studies that an increase in central or abdominal fat is associated with increased risk of cardiovascular events. This explains why women, although at similar risk for heart disease later in life compared to men, don't start to experience this increased risk until five years or so after menopause.

Of course, overweight and obesity are often a problem for women long before menopause. If pregnancy and oral contraceptives don't cause significant weight gain, what is causing so many women to gain weight? Well, it is no more complicated than the old standby formula: "Calories in" are greater than "calories out." That is, women are consuming more calories than they are burning.

Let's discuss the "calories out" portion of this formula. Americans' lifestyles have become more and more sedentary. Multiple studies have shown that decreased energy expenditure is strongly associated with weight gain (Prentice and Jebb 1995; U.S. Department of Health and Human Services 1996; Williamson et al. 1993). Once again, the Nurses' Health Study is relevant. A 2003 publication from Hu and colleagues showed that of all sedentary behaviors,

## Healthy Eating Resources

All this talk about exercise shouldn't lead one to assume that dietary factors don't matter. Of course they do. The "calories in" portion of the formula is probably just as important as the "calories out" portion. Here are several resources on healthy eating:

Carpenter RA, Finley CE. 2004. *Healthy eating every day.* Champaign, IL: Human Kinetics.

Clark N. 2003. *Nancy Clark's sports nutrition guidebook, third edition.* Champaign, IL: Human Kinetics.

Kostas GG. 1996. *The guilt-free comfort food cookbook.* Nashville: Thomas Nelson.

Willet WC. 2001. *Eat, drink and be healthy: The Harvard Medical School guide to healthy eating.* New York: Free Press.

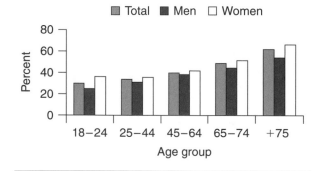

**Figure 2.11** Percentage of men and women who are physically inactive, by age group.

From 1997-98 National Health Interview Survey.

prolonged television watching was the most predictive of obesity and type 2 diabetes risk. For every 2-hour increment spent watching TV, there was a 23 percent increase in obesity and a 14 percent increase in risk of type 2 diabetes (Hu et al. 2003). These risks held true even after adjustment for age, smoking, exercise, and diet. In that same study, each hour per day of brisk walking was associated with a 24 percent reduction in obesity and a 34 percent reduction in type 2 diabetes. From their cohort study, the authors estimated that 30 percent of new cases of obesity and 43 percent of new cases of type 2 diabetes could be prevented if people viewed less than 10 hours per week of television and walked briskly for at least 30 minutes per day.

What about genetics? Aren't some women genetically predisposed to be overweight or obese? In a study of 970 healthy female twins, total body fat and central abdominal fat were lower in the women who reported vigorous weight-bearing activity (Samaras et al. 1999). Even in women who had an overweight twin, higher levels of physical activity resulted in lower total body fat and lower abdominal fat. These findings suggest that physical activity protects against weight gain even if an individual is genetically predisposed to it.

## ◆ Conclusion ◆

It is best to prevent disease in the first place rather than to treat it after the fact. This chapter outlined numerous ways in which physical activity can help prevent chronic diseases in women—diseases that affect both longevity and quality of life. Specifically, regular physical activity reduces risk of cardiovascular disease and stroke, type 2 diabetes, hypertension, colon cancer, dementia, and obesity. Risk for these diseases is reduced via improvements in blood pressure, cholesterol measures, and insulin sensitivity and via reductions in inflammation and central adiposity. Risk of osteoporotic fracture is reduced in women who regularly exercise, too.

Even with the best efforts toward prevention, some women will develop chronic diseases because of risk factors they cannot control or because of poor lifestyle habits earlier in life. As we emphasize many times in this book, a woman is never too old, or too sick, to benefit from physical activity. In fact, physical activity is often just what the doctor orders to help manage chronic conditions when they occur. The next chapter addresses the role of physical activity in the treatment and management of chronic diseases in women.

# CHAPTER 3

# Exercise and Disease Management

## Topics in This Chapter

- ◆ Fitness benefits for women with heart disease
- ◆ Exercise and blood pressure medications
- ◆ Blood pressure response to exercise and recovery
- ◆ Blood sugar response to exercise in diabetes
- ◆ Exercise tips for women taking insulin
- ◆ Exercising with complications of diabetes
- ◆ Metabolic syndrome

- ◆ Exercise during cancer treatment
- ◆ Managing arthritis with exercise
- ◆ Exercise and joint replacement
- ◆ Exercise and bone health
- ◆ Managing fibromyalgia and depression with exercise
- ◆ Exercise and obesity
- ◆ Fitness for physically challenged women
- ◆ Risks of aerobic exercise

If you think you can, you can. And if you think you can't, you're right.

Mary Kay Ash, Chairman, Mary Kay Cosmetics Inc.

Chapter 2 reviewed current scientific data showing how exercise can prevent chronic diseases. Many of your clients may already have some of these diseases, so their needs are different from those of low-risk women. After reading this chapter, you can confidently explain to women how exercise is not only necessary for disease prevention, but also critical in disease management. Whether a woman has cardiovascular disease, hypertension, diabetes, cancer, arthritis, osteoporosis, frailty, depression, or obesity, research shows she can benefit by being regularly physically active.

## Cardiovascular Disease

Quite a lot of data on men show that higher levels of fitness reduce risk of recurrent cardiovascular events. In women with heart disease, far fewer prospective studies have been done. In chapter 2, we discussed how fitness protects against the development of cardiovascular disease in women, but what if a woman already has cardiovascular disease? Does she benefit by having a higher fitness level? The answer is yes. Although there are fewer data on this issue for women, it is clear that higher fitness (as measured by $\dot{V}O_2$**peak**) reduces risk for cardiac mortality in women with heart disease (Kavanagh et al. 2003).

In Kavanagh's study, 2,380 women with known coronary artery disease, referred for cardiac rehabilitation, completed bicycle exercise testing. The women were followed for an average of six years. There were 209 deaths from all causes (8.8 percent of total) and 95 deaths from cardiac causes (4 percent of total, 45 percent of all deaths). $\dot{V}O_2$peak from the baseline bicycle testing was a strong independent predictor of cardiac mortality. As illustrated in figure 3.1, the specific $\dot{V}O_2$peak cutoff point above which there is significant survival benefit is 13 milliliters per kilogram per minute. For every 1 milliliter per kilogram per minute increase in $\dot{V}O_2$peak, there

was a 10 percent reduction in cardiac mortality. A similar study done in 2002 (Arruda-Olson et al.) showed that achieving a workload of $\leq 6$ METs (metabolic equivalents) on standard treadmill testing was associated with increased risk of cardiac events for women (and men) who were known or suspected to have coronary artery disease. In women, an increase of 1 MET in workload was associated with a 14 percent reduction in risk of cardiac events. Clearly, a higher level of fitness has a protective effect for women, even if they have coronary artery disease.

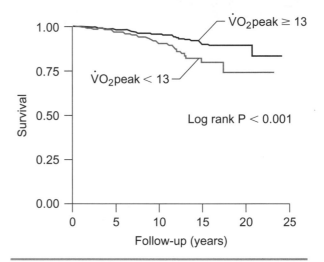

**Figure 3.1** Kaplan-Meier survival curves for cardiac deaths by peak oxygen intake.

Reprinted from *Journal of the American College of Cardiology*, Vol. 42, T. Kavanaugh et al., 2003, "Peak oxygen intake and cardiac mortality in women referred for cardiac rehabilitation," pgs. 2139-2143, Copyright 2003, with permission from the American College of Cardiology Foundation.

Certainly, any woman who is newly diagnosed with cardiovascular disease should participate in an appropriate cardiac rehabilitation program. Participation in a cardiac rehabilitation program after a myocardial infarction confers a marked survival advantage for women as compared to nonparticipants (Witt et al. 2004). Unfortunately, Witt's study showed that women are less likely to participate in cardiac rehabilitation than men. The best-case scenario for a woman at risk for heart disease is to maintain physical fitness to improve her chance of survival should heart disease develop; *and*, if despite her best efforts at prevention she develops heart disease, then participation in cardiac rehabilitation is critical. For more information on cardiac rehabilitation, refer to the American College of Sports Medicine's (ACSM's) guidelines for exercise testing and prescription (Whaley et al. 2006)

# Hypertension

In chapter 2 we reviewed data showing that regular exercise prevents the development of high blood pressure in women and improves blood pressure control in those with and without hypertension. Remember, the type, frequency, and intensity of aerobic exercise don't seem to matter. All aerobic exercise lowers blood pressure. The blood pressure–lowering effect of exercise can last for up to 22 hours after endurance exercise and is greatest in those with the highest baseline blood pressure (Pescatello et al. 2004).

## Blood Pressure Medications and Exercise

Treatment with certain medications for high blood pressure may interfere with exercise. Use of **beta-blockers** makes it difficult to elevate the heart rate during exercise. But with regular exercise, men on beta-blockers can compensate for this effect and improve exercise performance. There are no studies to show if this is true of women.

Another class of medication used for treatment of hypertension, **diuretics,** may also pose problems. Probably because these medications decrease the amount of fluid in the blood vessels, patients often notice decreased exercise tolerance. Using lower doses of both beta-blockers and diuretics (in combination with other medications, if needed) may help to prevent these problems.

Other medications used for control of high blood pressure, such as **angiotensin converting enzyme (ACE) inhibitors, angiotensin receptor blockers (ARB),** and **calcium channel blockers,** do not appear to interfere with exercise, but a gradual cool-down period following exercise is prudent to prevent hypotension in any woman on medication for high blood pressure.

## Short-Term Versus Long-Term Effects of Exercise

The short-term effects of exercise on blood pressure are different from the long-term effects. During exercise there is a rise in systolic pressure. For women, a rise in systolic pressure up to 190 mmHg (millimeters of mercury) is normal. This peak increases with age. (For men, a rise in systolic pressure up to 210 mmHg is considered normal.) In some women, the systolic blood pressure rises above this acceptable level. Several studies have reviewed the long-term consequences of having an exaggerated blood pressure response to exercise, but they are not conclusive. Studies of men with exaggerated systolic blood pressure response to exercise have shown increased risk of left ventricular hypertrophy (enlargement of the pumping chamber of the heart) and cardiovascular death, but similar studies have not been done in women (Gottdiener et al. 1990; Mundal et al. 1994). In fact, after six years of follow-up, the largest study that looked at this issue showed no increase in mortality in women (with known or suspected coronary artery disease) who had exaggerated systolic blood pressure response to exercise (Campbell et al. 1999). These women, as compared to women with heart disease who had a normal blood pressure response to exercise, were less likely to have blocked heart arteries when tested by nuclear scan.

Changes in diastolic pressure are usually minimal during exercise. For most women, the

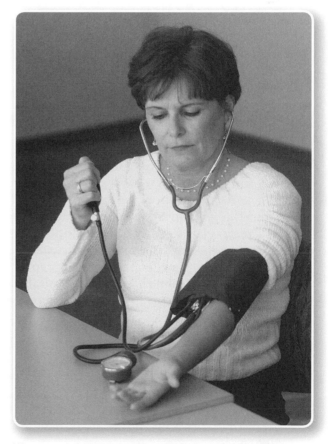

Women can learn to monitor their own blood pressure at home manually or with an automatic blood pressure device.

diastolic blood pressure remains stable, or even decreases slightly with physical activity. Of interest, in women who have an exaggerated diastolic blood pressure response to exercise, there is one study showing increased risk for future development of hypertension (Singh et al. 1999).

Because the prognostic importance of blood pressure response during exercise is still not clearly understood in women, it is prudent to recommend more frequent resting blood pressure checks for any woman with exaggerated systolic or diastolic response to exercise.

What may be even more important than how blood pressure responds during exercise is how blood pressure responds in recovery. One study has shown that women with heart disease who have a delayed decline in systolic blood pressure after exercise have a worse prognosis than those with a more rapid decline (McHam et al. 1999). A delayed decline was defined in terms of the ratio of systolic blood pressure at 3 minutes to systolic blood pressure at 1 minute of recovery—with a ratio greater than 1 indicating delayed decline. There are no data regarding the prognostic significance of delayed systolic blood pressure decline in women without heart disease.

### Exercise Recommendations for Hypertensive Women

Women with hypertension can exercise safely and should be reassured that regular exercise will improve control of their blood pressure. For some women, the goal of decreasing or eliminating blood pressure medication is motivational, and it is realistic to encourage some women in this regard. The primary form of exercise for hypertensive women should be aerobic. Resistance exercises are appropriate, too, but should involve lower weights with higher repetitions. Valsalva maneuvers should be avoided. Exercise should be postponed if blood pressure is significantly elevated (systolic >200 or diastolic >110).

Given the current state of literature on exercise and hypertension, the ACSM recommends the following exercise prescription (Pescatello et al. 2004):

> *Frequency:* on most, preferably all, days of the week
>
> *Intensity:* moderate intensity (40 to <60 percent of $\dot{V}O_2R*$)

---

## Blood Pressure Response to Exercise—Important Findings

◆ Women who show an exaggerated diastolic blood pressure response to exercise may be at risk for the future development of high blood pressure and thus should have more frequent resting blood pressure checks.

◆ In women with heart disease, an exaggerated systolic blood pressure response to exercise was associated with better prognosis.

◆ Delayed systolic blood pressure recovery after exercise is predictive of severe disease in women with known coronary artery disease.

> *Time:* ≥30 minutes of continuous or accumulated physical activity per day
>
> *Type:* primarily endurance physical activity supplemented by resistance exercises

# Diabetes

Aerobic exercise should definitely be included as part of the therapeutic program for patients with type 1 and type 2 diabetes. The benefits of regular exercise for people with diabetes include improved glycemic control and decreased risk of cardiovascular disease. As discussed in chapter 2, regular exercise improves body composition, blood pressure, and cholesterol. Controlling these risk factors is especially critical for women with diabetes to prevent disease complications.

### Glucose Metabolism

When people who do not have diabetes exercise, they first use glucose from muscles for energy. As exercise continues, glucose is taken from other sources, such as conversion of glycogen in muscles and uptake of blood glucose. As blood glucose falls, insulin secretion decreases while glucagon secretion increases. Glucagon facilitates production of glucose in the liver. If exercise continues further, other hormones, such as epinephrine, norepinephrine, growth hormone,

---

*A detailed explanation of exercise intensity, including target heart rate ranges and use of VO₂R, is provided in chapter 7.

and cortisol, begin to play a role. Lipolysis (breakdown of fats) is stimulated by these hormones. Muscles use the resulting free fatty acids for energy. The longer exercise goes on, the more lipolysis occurs and the lower insulin secretion drops. Figure 3.2 illustrates the relative contribution of these different fuels for energy consumption during exercise.

When people with type 1 diabetes exercise, the physiologic responses differ. Glucose levels can be driven too low by injected insulin that can't be turned off. Also, exercise can speed absorption of insulin from injections due to increased temperature and blood flow. This is especially true if the injection was given into the arm or leg being exercised or if the injection was inadvertently given intramuscularly (Frid et al. 1990; Koivisto and Felig 1978). In poorly controlled type 1 diabetes, exercise can cause paradoxical elevations of blood glucose. In these patients, lack of insulin impairs glucose uptake; and unchecked counterregulatory hormones including epinephrine, growth hormone, and cortisol stimulate hepatic glucose production. Lipolysis is enhanced as well, leading to **ketosis** as shown in figure 3.3.

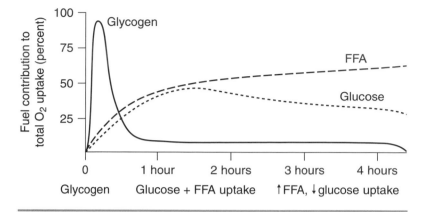

**Figure 3.2** Substrate utilization during prolonged exercise in normal subjects. Muscle glycogen breakdown is important initially, but stores are rapidly depleted. Glucose (derived from circulating glucose and hepatic glycogenolysis and gluconeogenesis) and free fatty acids (FFA) then become increasingly important. However, the fall in plasma glucose concentration reduces the secretion of insulin and raises that of counterregulatory hormones (such as epinephrine and norepinephrine). As a result, prolonged exercise is associated with a gradual fall in utilization of glucose and increase in that of FFA.

Adapted with permission from: D.K. McCulloch. Effects of exercise in diabetes mellitus in adults. In: UpToDate Rose, BD (Ed.), UpToDate, Wellesley, MA, 2005. Copyright 2005 UpToDate, Inc. For more information visit www.uptodate.com.

Because of the possibility of significant fluctuations in blood glucose, it is imperative that people with insulin-dependent diabetes (type 1 or type 2) perform frequent checks of blood glucose before, during, and after exercise.

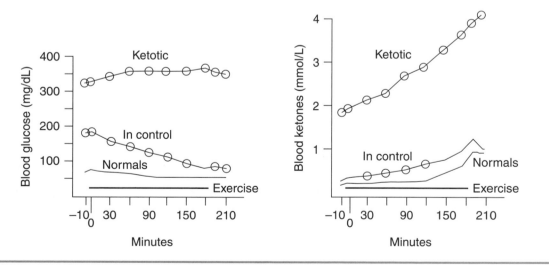

**Figure 3.3** Comparison of the effects of exercise in normal subjects and patients with type 1 diabetes that is in control or poorly controlled (ketotic). Exercise modestly lowered blood glucose concentrations and raised blood ketone concentrations in the normal subjects and in well-controlled diabetic patients. In the latter group, the fall in blood glucose is somewhat more prominent since exogenous insulin prevents plasma insulin concentrations from falling, thereby maintaining both muscle glucose utilization and inhibition of hepatic glucose output. In comparison, the lack of availability of insulin in poorly controlled diabetic patients prevents the fall in blood glucose and augments the increase in ketogenesis. To convert blood glucose values to mmol/L (millimoles per liter), multiply by 0.056.

*Diabetologia*, Vol 13, 1977, pg. 355, Metabolic and hormonal effects of muscular exercise in juvenile type diabetics, M. Berger et al., ©1997. With kind permission of Springer Science and Business Media.

For the most part, people with type 2 diabetes do not experience large fluctuations in blood glucose, especially when treatment is with diet and exercise alone. But, on the basis of one study of people with type 2 diabetes who were treated with oral hypoglycemic drugs, exercise may lower blood glucose acutely. A study by Poirier and colleagues (2000) showed this effect, but only if exercise occurred after eating.

The reactions discussed so far are short-term effects of exercise and are important to understand to avoid complications from diabetes during exercise. See "Exercise Tips for Women Taking Insulin" for more specific guidance on safe exercise.

## Long-Term Effects of Exercise

Now let's explore the data on the long-term effects of exercise in people with diabetes. The results of regular exercise differ for people with type 1 and type 2 diabetes. People with type 2 diabetes are insulin resistant. Regular exercise improves insulin sensitivity. This appears to be modulated via an increased number of glucose transporters on the muscle cell surface (Devlin 1992; McAuley et al. 2002). Because exercise improves insulin sensitivity, there is a clear long-term benefit of improved glycemic control in people with type 2 diabetes who exercise (Boule et al. 2001). However, this beneficial effect requires ongoing exercise. People with type 2 diabetes also decrease their risk of cardiovascular events and death by doing regular exercise, even with as little as walking for 2 hours a week (Gregg et al. 2003). Walking for more hours per week lowers risk further. In the Nurses' Health Study, women with type 2 diabetes lowered their risk of developing cardiovascular disease by 40 percent by doing 4 hours a week of moderate to vigorous activity, including walking (Hu et al. 2001).

People with type 1 diabetes do not experience an improvement of glycemic control with regular exercise. Presumably the reason is the lesser role of insulin resistance in type 1 diabetes. There are, however, still benefits of regular exercise for people with type 1 diabetes. They can achieve similar glycemic control with perhaps less insulin. They may show improvement in other risk factors for cardiovascular disease, such as high blood pressure and high cholesterol, as well as experience improved well-being.

## Exercise Tips for Women Taking Insulin

◆ Blood glucose should be measured before, during, and after exercise so that the changes in blood glucose can be documented and then predicted for subsequent exercise sessions.

◆ If blood glucose is over 250 mg/dL (milligrams per deciliter), exercise should be delayed until better control is achieved. Another insulin injection may be necessary.

◆ If blood glucose is less than 100 mg/dL, the woman should have a snack of at least 15 grams of carbohydrate (such as a piece of fruit) and retest 15 to 30 minutes later. She should not exercise until blood glucose is greater than 100 mg/dL.

◆ On days when exercise is scheduled, it may be possible or necessary to decrease the usual scheduled dose of insulin for that time of day.

◆ The insulin should be injected in a site other than the muscles to be exercised in order to prevent increased insulin absorption. The insulin should be administered 60 to 90 minutes before exercise to minimize the problem of increased absorption. For cycling, the arm should be injected; for exercise that involves arms and legs, such as tennis, the abdomen should be the injection site. Absorption of insulin from the abdomen is faster than from the arm or leg at rest, but this difference is reversed with exercise.

◆ The woman should eat food with 15 to 30 grams of carbohydrate (such as glucose tablets, hard candies, juice) 15 to 30 minutes before exercise and approximately every 30 minutes during exercise.

◆ To avoid late hypoglycemia, she should eat slowly absorbed carbohydrates (dried fruit, granola bars, trail mix) immediately after exercise.

◆ The woman should exercise with a buddy or carry a cell phone and should always wear proper, visible diabetes identification.

## Complications of Diabetes

In some people with diabetes, the type of exercise may be limited by complications of diabetes. As mentioned in chapter 2, complications of diabetes include peripheral and autonomic neuropathy, peripheral arterial disease and **claudication,** retinopathy, and nephropathy. The following are recommendations for exercise modifications for women with chronic complications of diabetes.

### For Patients With Peripheral Neuropathy

- Because neuropathy impairs feeling in the feet, people with this complication should examine their feet every day for sores or injuries. Any foot problem should be discussed with a physician immediately.
- Traumatic weight-bearing exercise (such as running) should be minimized for those with significant neuropathy.
- Wearing well-fitted footwear is a must. Poor shoe fit may lead to foot ulcers and infections that can result in amputation.
- Women with this complication also need to dress appropriately to prevent cold stress to the feet.

Autonomic neuropathy impairs the normal temperature and blood pressure regulation of the body. As for any exerciser, people with diabetes should be careful to stay well hydrated and appropriately dressed during exercise. This is especially important for people with autonomic neuropathy.

### For Patients With Autonomic Neuropathy

- Perceived exertion should be used to guide intensity of exercise.
- It is important to exercise with a buddy to help monitor for signs and symptoms of abnormal blood sugar, abnormal blood pressure, and ischemia.

### For Patients With Peripheral Arterial Disease

- With peripheral arterial disease, the arteries to the feet and legs become obstructed. Women with this complication may experience claudication (pain or burning in the calves/legs) with exercise.
- The mainstays of treatment for peripheral arterial disease are smoking cessation and supervised exercise.

- Non-weight-bearing exercise or lower-intensity exercise (or both) may help prevent symptoms.

### For Patients With Retinopathy

- Patients with retinopathy should avoid weightlifting because the increase in blood pressure that occurs during straining could increase risk for bleeding in the retina (eye).
- Jarring or Valsalva maneuvers should also be avoided.

For patients with nephropathy (kidney damage), high-intensity or strenuous exercises should probably be discouraged. In these patients there is risk for increasing amounts of protein in the urine.

## Benefits and Potential Risks of Exercise for Women With Diabetes

Benefits of regular exercise for women with diabetes:

- Improves insulin sensitivity (in type 2 diabetes)
- Improves cardiovascular fitness
- Reduces risk for developing cardiovascular disease
- Lowers blood pressure
- Improves cholesterol panel
- Improves sense of well-being

Potential risks of exercise for some women with diabetes:

- Hypoglycemia (for those taking insulin or certain oral diabetes medications)
- Hyperglycemia
- **Ketoacidosis** (for those with type 1 diabetes)
- Cardiac complications
- Retinal bleeding in the eye
- Protein in the urine
- Excessive rise or fall of systolic blood pressure
- Steeper rise in body temperature
- Greater risk of foot injuries and problems

## Exercise Recommendations for Diabetic Women

Before starting an exercise program, a woman with diabetes should undergo a detailed medical evaluation with appropriate diagnostic studies. A careful medical history and physical examination should focus on the symptoms and signs of disease affecting the heart and blood vessels, eyes, kidneys, and nervous system. According to the American Diabetes Association, an exercise stress test may be important for a woman planning to begin a vigorous exercise program who has any of the following conditions:

Known heart or vascular disease

Symptoms of heart disease, such as chest discomfort with physical activity

Age over 35

Type 2 diabetes of more than 10 years' duration

Type 1 diabetes of more than 15 years' duration

Any additional risk factor for coronary heart disease

Retinopathy

Nephropathy

Peripheral vascular disease

Autonomic neuropathy

Sedentary lifestyle

Seniors with diabetes should also be screened for any musculoskeletal problems before beginning an exercise program.

For your patients or clients with diabetes, recommend regular exercise. To benefit, exercise doesn't need to be vigorous or extensive. A program of regular walking, 2 to 4 hours a week, has a significant impact. Of course, any aerobic activity is acceptable; but review precautions as outlined next. Emphasize the importance of warming up and cooling down. Meeting with a diabetes educator or dietitian for guidance prior to starting a new exercise program can also be of tremendous benefit. For the patient who needs a more supervised setting, referral to a university or hospital wellness or rehabilitation program is appropriate.

It is also important to understand the general exercise precautions and modifications for women with diabetes. Be sure that clients know and heed warning symptoms for potential emergencies:

- *Warning symptoms of heart problems.* These include, but are not limited to, chest discomfort (pressure, pain, burning), sudden or unusual shortness of breath, nausea, lightheadedness, arm or neck pain, sudden anxiety, unusual sweating, rapid heart rate.

- *Warning symptoms of overheating.* Overheating can lead to heatstroke, which can be fatal. Symptoms of overheating include dizziness, cramps, nausea, headache.

- *Warning symptoms of hypoglycemia.* Be sure that clients who take insulin or oral diabetes medications know the symptoms of hypoglycemia and the steps to take immediately in the event of a hypoglycemic attack. Symptoms of hypoglycemia include shakiness, nervousness, sweating, chills and clamminess, rapid heartbeat, trouble concentrating, headache, dizziness, light-headedness, moodiness, clumsiness, tingling in the face or lips, extreme hunger, or irritability.

You should also know the precautions and modifications necessary for strength training:

- Strength training exercises with very heavy weight (for women with cardiac, vascular, eye, or neurological complications) are to be avoided. Women should substitute lighter weights and do more repetitions. They should start with one set and progress to 15 to 20 repetitions.

- Prolonged isometric contractions are to be avoided.

- Women should breathe normally and not grunt or exhale forcefully; they should avoid holding their breath.

- Exercises that hold weights above the head for more than a few seconds, or that involve straining or jarring movements, are to be avoided.

When developing the exercise plan, include moderate-intensity exercise of longer duration rather than higher-intensity exercise of shorter duration. Plan a consistent exercise session and advise against spontaneous or abrupt changes in physical activity. Clients should exercise every day, at about the same time of day, at similar intensity and for the same duration (this is especially important for those with type 1 diabetes because they may need to modify insulin dosage according to the volume of exercise they perform). Encourage clients to keep a record of their exercise sessions and review records frequently. Remind clients to always wear a diabetes identification bracelet or shoe tag and keep it visible during exercise.

## Metabolic Syndrome

There is no consensus on the definition of metabolic syndrome. However, most authorities agree that the following components are part of the syndrome: elevated blood pressure, elevated blood glucose, central obesity (excessive fat in and around the abdomen), low high-density lipoprotein (HDL) cholesterol, elevated triglycerides, and a proinflammatory state (elevated highly sensitive C-reactive protein) (National Heart, Lung, and Blood Institute 2001). Obviously, women with metabolic syndrome are at increased risk of heart disease, stroke, and peripheral vascular disease due to this accumulation of risk factors. It is imperative to note that *all* of the risk factors listed are exquisitely sensitive to exercise! In fact, researchers at the Cooper Institute in Dallas, Texas, have coined their own name for this problem: physical inactivity syndrome. Encouraging increased physical activity in women with this syndrome is critical to reduce risk of complications.

There aren't any specialized recommendations for exercise prescription for this group. Due to their generally low levels of cardiorespiratory fitness, an exercise program should progress slowly in intensity, frequency, and duration. Goals include exercising five to seven days per week (primarily aerobic) for 45 to 60 minutes and gradually increasing intensity to 50 to 75 percent $\dot{V}O_2R$.

# Cancer

Women with cancer may think they should avoid exercise, especially if they are fatigued or are having other symptoms from chemotherapy or radiation. But evidence is emerging to suggest that staying physically active during treatment for cancer actually decreases fatigue and other symptoms (Schmitz et al. 2005). Breast cancer presents some unique challenges for women during and after treatment.

A study by Mock and colleagues (2001) addressed the effect of regular exercise on fatigue and quality of life for women undergoing chemotherapy or radiation. Fifty-two women with a new diagnosis of breast cancer were randomly assigned to a control group or a walking program. The exercise group experienced improved quality of life and less fatigue as compared to the control group. The amount of exercise needed was minimal. A total of 90 minutes per week was sufficient to reduce fatigue and emotional distress, as well as improve functional ability and quality of life.

Women with breast cancer who undergo surgery including lymph node dissection may experience lymphedema causing swelling of the arm. Lymphedema is very unpredictable. It can occur immediately postoperatively or anytime thereafter. Gentle exercise can help to reduce lymphedema, but vigorous exercise including heavy lifting, pulling, or high repetitions should be avoided. Each woman will respond differently to the amount or intensity of exercise. Determining beneficial exercise levels will depend on each

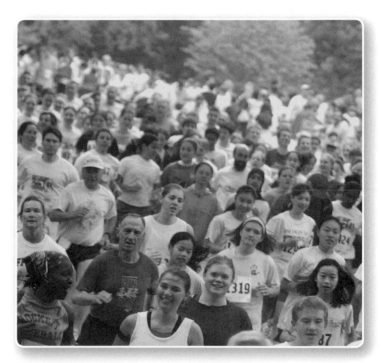

Several popular walking events are held each year to raise support for cancer research. This is particularly appropriate since walking is excellent exercise for women with cancer.

woman's reaction to the exercise. Some physical therapists are trained in Complex Decongestive Therapy (CDT), a specialized technique to treat lymphedema that includes skin care, massage, bandaging, exercise, and fitting for a compression sleeve. See the following suggestions when recommending an exercise program for a woman at risk for lymphedema.

Certainly other cancers affect women and therefore their exercise programs. For more information on exercise after a cancer diagnosis, see Anna Schwartz's book, *Cancer Fitness: Exercise Programs for Patients and Survivors* (2004).

## Exercise Recommendations for Women at Risk for Lymphedema

- Any slight increase in swelling, aching, or heaviness should not be ignored.
- Blood pressure should be checked in the unaffected arm.
- The woman should exercise with light weights.
- Weights should be lifted slowly and under control.
- Vigorous movements should be avoided.
- Highly repetitive motions should be avoided.
- Exercises should be alternated between upper and lower body.
- Progressions should be slower.
- A variety of cardiovascular modalities should be used when possible (swimming, biking, walking).
- Water exercises are very beneficial due to compressive forces on the limb and buoyancy. Consider water exercises if a woman experiences swelling with land exercise.

# Arthritis

There are many different kinds of arthritis. The most common type, osteoarthritis, is a disease that causes the breakdown of cartilage in joints, leading to joint pain and stiffness. It commonly occurs in the hips, knees, spine, fingers, and feet. It rarely affects the wrists, elbows, shoulders, ankles, or jaw. Osteoarthritis is one of the most common chronic conditions among seniors and is a major reason women give for not being physically active.

The specific cause of osteoarthritis is unknown, but scientists think there are several factors that increase the risk for developing arthritis, including the following:

- Defective genes that lead to defective cartilage and more rapid breakdown of the joints
- Joints that do not fit together correctly or that move incorrectly and thus wear badly (bowed legs are an example)
- Being overweight, especially for people who gained weight during their mid or later years (arthritis of the knees is a problem for people who are overweight)
- Accidents or sport-related injuries to the hips or knees
- Overuse of joints by repeating motions from certain jobs or tasks

## Osteoarthritis Versus Rheumatoid Arthritis

Osteoarthritis is sometimes confused with rheumatoid arthritis. It is possible to have both osteoarthritis and rheumatoid arthritis at the same time. For key differences, see table 3.1.

Osteoarthritis symptoms usually begin slowly. Most people feel mild aching and soreness, especially when they move. A few people develop constant nagging pain, even when they're resting. The pain of osteoarthritis usually occurs only in the joint or in the area around the joint. In some cases, people feel pain far from the affected joint. This feeling is called referred pain.

Unfortunately, most osteoarthritis is chronic, which means it may last a lifetime. People usually have ups and downs. There are times when they feel no symptoms at all. These periods are called remissions. The times when the osteoarthritis gets worse are called flares. All of this is true of rheumatoid arthritis as well.

## Symptoms of Osteoarthritis

Though you are not expected to diagnose arthritis in your clients, you should be aware of the symptoms so that you can direct them to see a health

◆ **TABLE 3.1** ◆

## Osteoarthritis Versus Rheumatoid Arthritis

| Osteoarthritis | Rheumatoid arthritis |
|---|---|
| Is not an autoimmune disease | Is an autoimmune disease |
| Usually begins after age 40 | Usually begins between ages 25 and 50 |
| Usually develops slowly, over many years | May develop suddenly, within weeks or months |
| Affects a few joints and may occur on both sides of the body | Usually affects many joints, primarily the small joints, on both sides of body |
| Usually causes only minimal redness, warmth, and swelling of joints; morning stiffness is common and may be severe but brief | Causes redness, warmth, swelling, and prolonged morning stiffness of the joints |
| Affects only certain joints; rarely affects wrists, elbows, or ankles | Affects many joints, including wrists, elbows, and shoulders |
| Doesn't cause a general feeling of sickness and fatigue | Often causes a general feeling of sickness, fatigue, weight loss, and fever |

care provider if needed. Note that osteoarthritis affects each joint somewhat differently, but general symptoms include the following:

- ◆ Pain following overuse
- ◆ Pain following periods of inactivity
- ◆ Difficulty in moving the joint easily
- ◆ Weaker muscles surrounding the affected joint
- ◆ Poor coordination and posture

Clients may display symptoms of osteoarthritis at specific joints such as the hips, knees, fingers, feet, and spine. In the hips, clients may feel pain around the groin or inner thigh, or referred pain in the buttocks, knee, or along the side of the thigh; and they may limp when walking. In the knees, they may experience "grating" or "catching" sensations with knee movement, pain when walking up or down stairs, or pain when getting up from a chair. In the fingers, they may have bony growths (spurs) in the joints or may notice redness, swelling, tenderness, or aching in the affected joints. Fingertips may be numb or may tingle. In the feet, women may feel pain and tenderness in the large joint at the base of the big toe and pain made worse when wearing tight shoes and high heels. In the spine, symptoms of osteoarthritis comprise pain at the base of the head; in the neck, legs, or lower back or down the arms; stiffness in the

neck or lower back; and weakness or numbness in the arms or legs.

## Managing Arthritis

Finding the right treatment for osteoarthritis often involves time and trial and error. What works for one woman might not work for another. People with arthritis are often tempted by promises of quick cures and treatments. Unfortunately, there is no cure for osteoarthritis at this time. Encourage clients not to be taken in by hoaxes. Some alternative remedies may not be dangerous, but others can be very harmful. No special diet, food, vitamin, or mineral is recommended for people with arthritis. Exercise, however, is strongly recommended. Specific guidelines are outlined in the next section.

One supplement, glucosamine and chondroitin, is widely used by women with arthritis. There is some limited evidence to support the use of glucosamine and chondroitin for reducing pain, improving function, and stopping progression of osteoarthritis of the knees in postmenopausal women (Bruyere et al. 2004). Prescription or over-the-counter anti-inflammatory medicines are often recommended for pain relief.

Joint replacement (mostly knee or hip) may be performed in older women, especially those with severe osteoarthritis. Rheumatoid arthritis or previous injury can also lead to joint replacement. Women with joint replacement may have limitations in joint mobility or contraindications to certain activities. Previously active women who have undergone joint replacement will need help and support to establish realistic goals for returning to activity. For most, biking, walking, swimming, and other low-impact exercises are permissible. High-impact exercises such as running, as well as heavy lifting, should be avoided.

## Exercise Recommendations for Women With Arthritis

It is often challenging for women with osteoarthritis to maintain long-term compliance with exercise programs. Nonetheless, regular exercise is recommended for this population since a review of randomized trials showed modest benefits from supervised exercise programs for patients with hip and knee osteoarthritis (van Baar et al. 1999).

A regular exercise program should include flexibility, resistance, and aerobic activities, preferably in that order to minimize discomfort. Exercises can be performed in shorter bouts more frequently through the day to minimize discomfort. Resistance training can be tailored to the individual and may include machines, bands, or isometrics. Aerobic activities may be weight bearing or not; swimming or water exercise classes are excellent options. Women with arthritis may experience muscular pain after beginning a new exercise program; advising them of this will help them to learn the difference between joint pain from disease and normal postexercise muscle fatigue. Give women a copy of the handout in appendix B, "Living with Osteoarthritis" on page 228.

Women with hip and knee arthritis may have deficiencies in gait or strength. These deficiencies as well as limitations in flexibility, power, and endurance are important to address to preserve and improve function. Addressing gait problems may help prevent falls and fractures, fostering independence. By improving range of motion and strength, women can increase mobility and

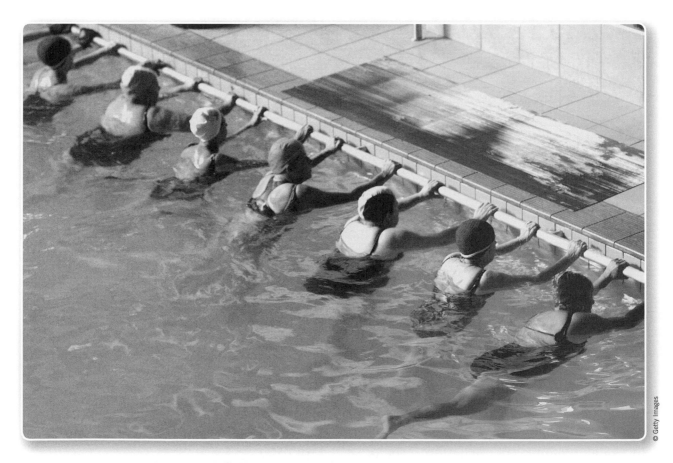

Water aerobics is an excellent option for women with arthritis.

reduce pain (Baker et al. 2001; Thomas et al. 2002). Improving power and endurance not only allows women to regain skills they may have lost from progressive disease, but also reduces morbidity and mortality from cardiovascular and other diseases (Blair et al. 1989).

To achieve these benefits while protecting joints, various low-impact exercises, such as cycling, swimming, tai chi, walking, and resistance training, are options. These are generally better choices than running or stair climbing, especially for women with arthritis of the knees. Keep in mind that regular physical activity also improves quality of life and self-efficacy for those with osteoarthritis (Baker et al. 2001). For more information on exercise for women with osteoarthritis, review the consensus practice recommendations from the American Geriatrics Society (2001). Refer your patients to www.arthritis.org, the Web site for the Arthritis Foundation.

# Osteoporosis

In chapter 2 we noted observational studies showing that women can reduce fracture risk by participating in a regular exercise program. Observational studies are subject to certain biases, so it is important to note that there haven't been any **randomized controlled clinical trials** showing that exercise reduces fracture risk. Such studies would be quite difficult to perform as they would require a large number of participants followed over a long period of time.

Further, it is unclear if women can significantly improve bone density with exercise. Exercise intervention studies generally target specific anatomic sites for measuring bone density and employ high-intensity exercises. Transient elevations of bone density at specific sites from such efforts have unclear clinical significance. Yet there is consensus that regular exercise forestalls *age-related* bone loss (Kelley et al. 2001; Todd and Robinson 2003). Importantly, it is uncertain whether exercise has any impact on *menopause-related* bone loss.

If exercise hasn't been proven to reduce fracture risk and only forestalls age-related bone loss, then why is it consistently recommended for bone health? The reason is that *in*activity

## Exercise and Bone Health—Important Findings

- ◆ Low bone density increases fracture risk.
- ◆ There have been no randomized controlled clinical trials showing that exercise reduces fracture risk.
- ◆ It is unclear if women can significantly improve bone density with exercise.
- ◆ There is consensus that regular exercise forestalls age-related bone loss.
- ◆ It is uncertain if exercise has any impact on menopause-related bone loss.
- ◆ Inactivity has clearly been shown to increase fracture risk, especially in people who are elderly.

has clearly been shown to *increase* fracture risk, especially in the elderly (Marks et al. 2003). Low bone density also increases fracture risk, so it is especially important for postmenopausal women with low bone density to consistently participate in an exercise program to prevent further loss. Women with low bone density may hesitate to exercise, fearful they may fall and fracture. But a review and meta-analysis (Chang et al. 2004) showed that a variety of exercises can reduce risk of falls in postmenopausal women. Reducing falls is one of the critical ways physical activity may reduce fracture risk. Give women a copy of the handout in appendix B, "Reduce Risks for Falls and Fractures" on page 232.

For these reasons we recommend the following exercise prescription from the American College of Sports Medicine to *preserve* bone health in healthy women without osteoporosis (Kohrt et al. 2004):

- ◆ *Frequency:* weight-bearing endurance activities three to five times per week; resistance exercise two to three times per week
- ◆ *Intensity:* moderate to high, in terms of bone-loading forces
- ◆ *Time:* 30 to 60 minutes a day of a combination of weight-bearing endurance activities and resistance exercise that targets all major muscle groups

◆ *Type:* weight-bearing endurance activities (tennis; stair climbing; jogging, at least intermittently during walking), activities that involve jumping (volleyball, basketball), and resistance exercise (weightlifting)

Women with significantly low bone density or osteoporosis should participate in aerobic activity three to five days per week and resistance training two to three days per week (unless pain precludes activity). When doing resistance exercises, certain maneuvers, such as spinal flexion, bending at the waist, or twisting, should be avoided. Resistance exercises should start with low weights and low repetitions to minimize fracture risk.

# Fibromyalgia

Fibromyalgia is a disorder characterized by multiple symptoms; the most common are musculoskeletal pain and extreme fatigue. Women may also experience generalized stiffness, multiple tender points, and sleep difficulty, among other symptoms. The cause of fibromyalgia is unknown. It is, however, reported to affect as many as 10 million people in the United States (White and Harth 2001). More women are affected than men, and typical onset occurs between the ages of 20 and 40. There is currently no cure for this condition.

Treatment plans focus on reducing and managing symptoms with regular exercise, medication, massage, cognitive behavioral therapy, and relaxation. Women with fibromyalgia may avoid physical activity, fearing it may exacerbate their symptoms. But preliminary studies suggested that tai chi, aerobic, and resistance exercises reduced symptoms and improved quality of life in fibromyalgia sufferers (Karper et al. 2001; Taggart et al. 2003). A review article on exercise and fibromyalgia concluded that consistent low- to moderate-intensity exercise can help reduce fatigue and pain and improve overall fitness and quality of life in patients with fibromyalgia (Clark 2001). High-impact activities, such as running or stair climbing, as well as heavy resistance training, may aggravate symptoms and should be avoided in most women with fibromyalgia.

# Depression

Exercise has been studied as a treatment for depression. However, good-quality research has been limited. A literature review in 2001 (Lawlor and Hopker) concluded that the lack of quality research precluded any judgment as to whether exercise is effective in reducing symptoms of depression. But two randomized controlled clinical trials merit further mention.

One study of women and men aged 50 and older with major depression showed that treatment with an antidepressant or group exercise (or both) resulted in significant and equivalent improvement in mood (Blumenthal et al. 1999). The exercise consisted of three sessions per week with 30 minutes of walking/jogging at 70 percent maximum heart rate reserve. Treatment with an antidepressant resulted in quicker relief of symptoms than exercise alone, but at 4-month and 10-month follow-ups, all groups did equally well (Babyak et al. 2000). One limitation of this study was the possible influence of social interaction. Perhaps the patients improved due to interaction within the group, not specifically because of the exercise. Another limitation was the lack of a no-treatment control group.

A more recent study (Dunn et al. 2005) used two different "doses" of exercise to determine not only if exercise reduces depressive symptoms, but also how much exercise is needed. This study was small (80 participants), but did include a control group. The exercise groups performed either "low-dose" or "public health dose" exercise, defined as 7.0 calories (kcal) per kilogram per week or 17.5 kcal per kilogram per week, respectively. The frequency of exercise was three or five times a week. The placebo group performed flexibility activities. The group performing the "public health dose" of exercise experienced a depression remission rate of 42 percent, which was statistically significant as compared to rates in the "low-dose" exercise group and placebo group. The frequency of exercise did not affect results; there was no difference in effectiveness whether exercise was done three or five times a week. The total energy expenditure appeared to be the most significant variable, and the "public health dose" of exercise is equivalent to at least 30 minutes of moderate-intensity exercise. This study is encouraging, even though it had some minor limitations.

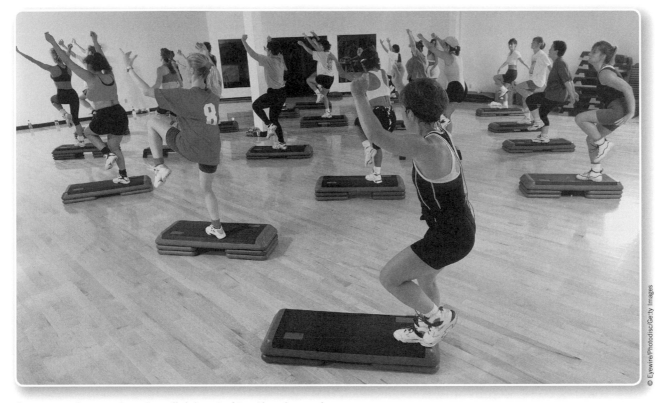

Group exercise may be a beneficial part of treating depression.

Aerobic exercise should be encouraged for women with depression even though the data aren't conclusive. And, of course, women stand to gain many other proven significant benefits from regular aerobic activity. Group classes may be more appealing to women with depression than exercising on their own and may help them to be more "accountable" for exercise.

## Obesity

One of Dr. Kenneth Cooper's favorite sayings is "It is easier to maintain good health than it is to regain it once it is lost." Preventing obesity is easier than treating it. Although a complex set of genetic and behavioral factors influences the development of obesity, a simple formula governs weight loss. To lose weight, women must burn more calories than they consume. The formula is simple, but the application of the formula requires self-education, discipline, and consistency.

Any woman with a significant amount of weight to lose (more than 15 pounds or 6.8 kilo-grams) should meet with a dietitian to design an appropriate individualized dietary plan. Obese women should also see a physician for a full physical exam for clearance for exercise. Meeting with a personal trainer is helpful for proper exercise program design and accountability. Because obese women are at higher risk for orthopedic injury, their exercise programs should generally start at lower intensity and gradually increase in duration of activity. Employing non-weight-bearing activities or varying activities (or both) helps to prevent overuse injury. For women who have been exercising but aren't losing weight, a consultation with a trainer is appropriate. Often, more variety (cross training) or intensity is needed in the program to continue progress toward a weight loss goal.

It is important to be sure that women with a weight loss goal follow appropriate dietary guidelines. If they don't consult with a dietician for individualized advice, they may be following faddish, highly inadvisable programs. Health and fitness professionals should be aware of some basic dietary rules for weight loss even though they aren't the ones designing dietary programs.

A weight loss program should follow these guidelines from the ACSM (Franklin et al. 2000):

◆ Provide intake of not lower than 1,200 kcal per day for normal adults and allow for a proper distribution of foods to meet nutritional requirements. (Note: This requirement may not be appropriate for children, older individuals, and athletes.)

◆ Include foods acceptable to the dieter in terms of sociocultural background, usual habits, taste, costs, and ease in acquisition and preparation. However, these foods should be low in total fat, saturated fat, trans fat, cholesterol, and sodium.

◆ Provide a negative caloric balance (not to exceed 500 to 1,000 kcal per day), resulting in gradual weight loss without metabolic derangements such as ketosis.

◆ Aim for a maximal weight loss of 2.2 pounds (1 kilogram) per week.

◆ Include the use of behavior modification techniques to identify and eliminate diet habits that contribute to malnutrition.

◆ Include an exercise program that promotes a daily caloric expenditure of more than 300 kcal. For many participants, this may be accomplished best with moderate-intensity, long-duration exercise, such as walking.

◆ Provide that new eating and physical activity habits can be continued for life to maintain the achieved lower body weight.

# Women With Physical Challenges

There is an increasing amount of research on the benefits of regular physical activity for women with physical challenges. Physical challenge or disability can be broadly defined, but for our purposes in this text, it refers to limitations that don't relate to medical diseases or aging. Just as physical activity reduces risk of obesity and other diseases for able-bodied women, regular exercise benefits those with physical challenges.

A preparticipation physical should be completed for any woman with a physical challenge to guide design of an exercise program. For example, a vision-impaired woman who wants to jog needs a different plan than a spinal cord–injured

## Strategies to Share With Overweight or Obese Women

◆ Reduce overall calorie intake by minimizing "empty calorie" foods (high-fat and high-sugar foods and alcoholic beverages).

◆ Don't go hungry. Eat three meals and healthy snacks every day.

◆ Attend a behavior modification program or support group.

◆ Engage in moderate-intensity physical activity for a minimum of 45 minutes per day most days of the week.

◆ Include strength training to build and maintain muscle.

◆ Monitor weight only once a week. Weight fluctuates daily.

◆ For more strategies, refer to the handout in appendix B, "Healthy Eating Practices for Weight Management" on page 219.

female who wants to play wheelchair tennis. In addition to understanding the limitation from any particular challenge, it is important to take into account each woman's particular goals and preferences. Improved quality of life and independent living are primary goals. There may be concurrent illnesses, such as hypertension, that affect the exercise plan. Women who've exercised prior to developing a physical challenge will have different concerns than those who are starting to exercise for the first time.

Women with spinal cord injuries have some specific medical issues to address. Temperature regulation (hypo- and hyperthermia) is an issue due to inability to maintain core temperature and impaired sweating below the level of the injury. More complicated issues, such as **autonomic dysreflexia** and venous blood pooling, may also affect the injured woman, especially if she chooses to perform competitive sports. Spasticity and osteoporosis are additional challenges that may arise.

Despite the obstacles to an exercise program for physically challenged athletes, regular activity is a must, since this population (particularly spinal cord–injured women) is at increased risk of cardiovascular disease and obesity as compared to the general population (Kocina 1997). Through regular exercise, physically challenged women can improve physical functioning, improve muscle strength and endurance, reduce body fat, improve ventilatory efficiency, raise HDL cholesterol, and normalize insulin (Chen et al. 2005; LeFoll-de Moro et al. 2005; Mahoney et al. 2005; Noreau and Shephard 1995). The psychological benefits of exercise, including improved body image and self-esteem, apply to this population of women as well.

## Risks of Aerobic Exercise

Regular physical activity has a long list of benefits. However, exercise acutely and transiently increases the risk of cardiac events and sudden death. Keep in mind that male sex is a characteristic associated with exercise-related cardiovascular events; in other words, being male is an independent risk factor for sudden death and cardiovascular events during exercise.

One review of the literature concluded that 0.75 and 0.13 per 100,000 young male and female athletes and 6 per 100,000 middle-aged men per year die during vigorous exercise (Thompson 1996). In young persons, congenital abnormalities are the usual cause of death. In adults, coronary artery disease is the main culprit. It is important to note that *regular* exercise has a protective effect against sudden death during exercise (Mittleman et al. 1993). According to the ACSM, "Regardless of the presence or absence of heart disease, the overall absolute risk of cardiovascular complications during exercise is low, especially when weighed against the associated health benefits" (Franklin et al. 2000 page 13).

Of course, some individuals should undergo evaluation and testing prior to participating in an exercise program. We recommend using the AHA/ACSM Health/Fitness Facility Preparticipation Screening Questionnaire or PAR-Q (see appendix A) to determine which women need to consult with a physician before beginning an exercise program.

### ◆ Conclusion ◆

This chapter reviewed an extensive body of literature showing conclusively that fitness reduces risk of complications from many diseases. Many women with health challenges, from diabetes to cancer to physical disability, are fearful of exercise. It is the responsibility of the health and fitness professional to encourage exercise across a broad spectrum of diseases. Exercise programs can and should be modified to be disease appropriate. Information in this chapter gave specific guidance for program modification for women with cardiovascular disease, diabetes, hypertension, cancer, arthritis, osteoporosis, fibromyalgia, depression, and obesity.

There are some risks associated with exercise; fortunately, the rate of serious events is quite low. The benefit of exercise is so significant that all women should be strongly encouraged to participate consistently to gain tremendous health improvements.

In addition to being disease appropriate, exercise programs should be age appropriate. The next three chapters explore the changing exercise needs of girls and women as they transition through adolescence, childbearing years, menopause, and the senior years.

# PART II

# A Life-Stage Approach to Physical Activity and Fitness

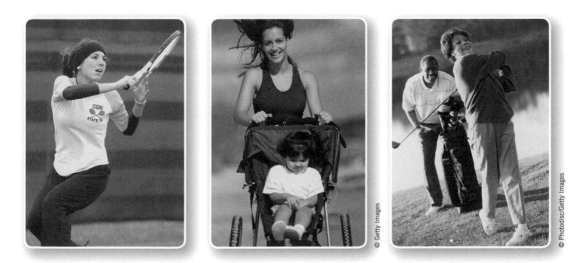

© Getty Images

© Photodisc/Getty Images

# CHAPTER 4

# Exercise During Adolescence

## Topics in This Chapter

Once you get into it, you're hooked.

Millie Cooper (on exercise)

Adolescence is a time of transition and exploration. We recommend fitness programs that appeal to the "whole" girl—her physical, mental, emotional, and social self. By including elements that girls value, we can help them develop lifelong habits of physical activity rather than slip into sedentary lifestyles that carry into adulthood. Issues such as how to develop a positive body image, build confidence and self-worth, and avoid weight problems and eating disorders are also critical at this time of life.

## Goals of Fitness Programs During Adolescence

The long-term, public health goal of fitness programming for adolescent girls and young women is for them to grow into fit, healthy, happy, well-adjusted women who enjoy life to its fullest for as many years as possible. As discussed in chapter 2, evidence is clear that physical activity and fitness can prevent cardiovascular disease, stroke, hypertension, abnormal cholesterol, obesity, type 2 diabetes, colon cancer, and osteoporosis in adult women.

The immediate goal of fitness programming for adolescent girls is to promote physical activity as part of a healthy lifestyle. Physical activity has the potential to help adolescent girls avoid risky behaviors, such as smoking, and their associated serious consequences. One study examined the relationship between changes in physical activity and changes in smoking among adolescents (Audrain-McGovern et al. 2003). Higher levels of physical activity reduced the odds of starting smoking or progressing to a higher level of smoking.

However, as helpful as regular physical activity could be at this critical time, we know that puberty marks the start of a decline in willingness among girls to participate in physical activity. As part of the National Heart, Lung, and Blood Institute Growth and Health Study, 1,213 African American girls and 1,166 Caucasian girls were followed from the ages of 9 or 10 to 18 or 19 years (Kimm et al. 2002). A validated questionnaire was used to measure leisure-time physical activity on the basis of metabolic equivalents (METs). Over the 10-year study, the median activity scores declined 100 percent for the African American girls and 64 percent for Caucasian girls. By the age of 16 or 17 years, 56 percent of the African American girls and 31 percent of the Caucasian girls reported no habitual leisure-time activity. Declines in physical activity during adolescence were associated with higher body mass index (both races), pregnancy (African Americans only), and cigarette smoking (Caucasians only). A follow-up study of the same girls again confirmed increased body mass index and increased adiposity with decreasing physical activity (Kimm et al. 2005). Clearly, it is essential to prevent the steep decline in activity during adolescence to reduce overweight and obesity.

In the short term, increasing participation in regular physical activity among adolescent girls is the tool—the means to the end. If physical activity habits are begun in childhood, continued in adolescence, and practiced over a lifetime, the long-term goal of disease prevention, optimal health, and quality of life could be attained by many more women.

## The Major Life Transition of Adolescence

Adolescence is the time between childhood and adulthood. For girls, complex changes occur in every aspect of their lives—physical, mental, emotional, and social. Each girl responds to the associated changes of adolescence in unique ways.

Usually between the ages of 8 and 16, girls start menstruating. Although they may be menstruating, they may not be ovulating (releasing a mature egg). The production of estrogen changes the skeleton, causing the growth spurt that occurs in girls during puberty. Estrogen is also responsible for changes in the uterus, sex organs, and breasts. The shape and size of a girl's body change as it prepares for the important role of reproduction.

### A Healthy Menstrual Cycle

Each young woman has her own experience of her menstrual cycle. What is true for one may not be true for her friend or her sister. It is important for young women to know that menstruation is not an illness. They need to learn to recognize the difference between the sensations of menses and being sick. If a girl hasn't started menstruating by age 16, she should see her doctor. Regular menstrual periods are important for producing the estrogen needed for normal development.

The menstrual cycle is one of the processes regulated by the hypothalamus, the master gland of the body. The hypothalamus sends signals to keep the body's energy in balance. If there is not enough energy to sustain the reproductive cycle and a possible pregnancy, the hypothalamus will take action to conserve energy, and menses may cease. The four phases of a normal menstrual cycle are outlined in the sidebar "A Normal Cycle in Four Phases."

### Achieving Peak Bone Mass

About 25 percent of peak bone mass (the genetically determined amount of bone mineral in the skeleton) is developed during puberty (ages 12 to 17). After puberty (at adult height), about 70 percent of peak bone mass has been developed. Bones grow denser and stronger rather than longer until age 25 to 35. Peak bone mass, which is achieved by age 30 to 35, reflects all of the good or bad influences on bone during puberty and early adulthood.

While osteoporosis is most common in women after menopause (about age 50 and older), it can occur in young women. In young women, osteoporosis is usually linked to delayed menarche, amenorrhea, eating disorders, or poor nutrition (especially lack of calcium). Other causes include taking certain medications, smoking, and abusing alcohol. Amenorrhea and eating disorders are discussed in detail later in this chapter. Clearly the best insurance against osteoporosis is to develop maximum bone mass at a young age. A handout with recommendations for developing maximum bone mass for girls and women, ages 14 to 35, is provided in appendix B (page 221).

### *Role of Hormones in Bone Development*

In addition to playing a key role in the changes in the reproductive system, estrogen works in these ways to help build and maintain bones:

- Helps the body absorb calcium
- Reduces calcium loss through the kidneys

## A Normal Cycle (23 to 35 Days) in Four Phases

- *Follicular phase*—FSH (follicle stimulating hormone) from the pituitary causes the ovary to develop eggs and make the hormone estrogen. Estrogen acts on the uterus to start a lining.

- *Ovulation*—As the eggs in the ovary develop and levels of estrogen rise, the pituitary gland sends a second hormone (LH or luteinizing hormone) to the ovary to release the egg. This is ovulation. Pelvic pain may be felt on one side for a few days. Body temperature will go up a few tenths of a degree.

- *Luteal phase*—This phase lasts an average of 14 days, until menstrual bleeding begins. This phase prepares the body for pregnancy. The egg travels from the ovary through the fallopian tube toward the uterus. The ovary produces a second hormone, progesterone. Progesterone and estrogen together prepare the uterine lining to receive a fertilized egg. If the egg is not fertilized, the ovary stops making estrogen and progesterone 14 days after ovulation. Symptoms during the luteal phase include breast tenderness, bloating, increase in acne, mood swings, and mild weight gain because of the production of progesterone; these symptoms disappear as soon as menstrual flow begins.

- *Menstrual bleeding* (usually four to six days)—The decline in levels of estrogen and progesterone causes the uterine lining to break down. The result is menstrual bleeding. Those who bleed heavily lose more iron and are at risk for anemia. Because of the menstrual blood loss, women need almost twice as much iron as men (15 to 18 milligrams a day). If women do not get enough iron from the foods they eat, they do not have the necessary iron to make new red blood cells and they become anemic. Fatigue and sluggishness are symptoms of anemia.

◆ Works directly on the cells that remodel the bone (the osteoclasts) and prevents bone resorption

◆ Improves the bone's response to exercise (young women who exercise and have normal levels of estrogen gain more bone than those with low estrogen levels who exercise)

Other hormones also seem to play a role in bone development in women, including young women. Cortisol (steroid hormone), made by the adrenal gland, causes breakdown of bone. Having a condition that produces high levels of cortisol, such as Cushing's syndrome, can cause bone loss. In addition, taking corticosteroids for more than three months of treatment for certain diseases such as rheumatoid arthritis, systemic lupus, inflammatory bowel disease (ulcerative colitis or Crohn's disease), severe asthma, or severe allergies makes bones thinner. Excess thyroid hormone, either produced by the thyroid gland or taken as hormone replacement, can also cause bone loss. Taking the right amount of thyroid hormone will not harm the bones.

### Role of Nutrition in Bone Development

Girls and young women need calcium to develop strong bones. Growing girls need 1,200 to 1,500 milligrams of calcium every day. Food is the best source of calcium. Three servings of high-calcium foods (as part of an otherwise healthy diet) would meet the daily requirement for calcium. See table 4.1 for a listing of the calcium content of various foods. Low-fat dairy foods (including milk, cheese, and yogurt), calcium-fortified foods (orange juice and ready-to-eat cereals), and soy products (such as soy milk and tofu, if labeled as fortified) are excellent sources of calcium. One cup of milk or yogurt contains about 300 milligrams of calcium. Girls and young women who have difficulty digesting lactose or milk sugar (a condition called lactose intolerance) can buy dairy products that have had the lactose removed. There is also a tablet to help digest dairy foods. Dark green vegetables (broccoli, spinach, collard greens) and canned fish with bones are also good sources of calcium. For girls who are strict vegetarians or vegans (who eat no foods from animal sources), there are numerous calcium-fortified foods to eat. Tofu and other soy products, fortified juices, and ready-to-eat cereals are available.

Young women who are concerned that they are not getting enough calcium from food should be encouraged to take a daily calcium supplement. A handout on calcium supplementation is provided in appendix B (page 222). The handout describes different types of calcium supplements and gives recommendations for how to get maximum absorption of calcium.

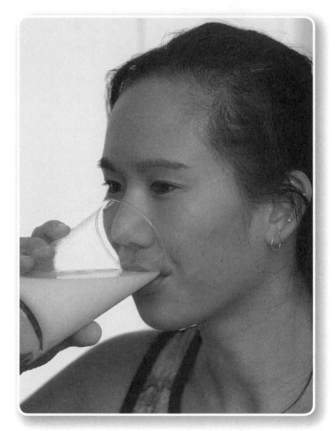

Three glasses of milk a day, in addition to a healthy diet, would meet the daily requirement for calcium.

Getting enough calcium from food doesn't mean that a girl's body will absorb all of the calcium. Certain diets can promote loss of calcium via the urine. High-protein diets can cause bone loss by increasing urinary calcium excretion. Diets high in caffeine cause diuresis, or increased urination, which means increased calcium loss. Girls and young women should limit themselves to no more than 200 milligrams of caffeine per day. See table 4.2 for the caffeine content of common foods and drugs.

Excess sodium also causes increased urinary excretion of calcium. Girls and women should

## Sources of Calcium-Rich Foods

| | Amount | Calcium (mg) | Calories |
|---|---|---|---|
| General Mills Total whole grain and raisin bran | 1/2 cup | 500 | 55-85 |
| Lactaid or Schepps calcium-fortified fat-free milk | 1 cup | 500 | 80 |
| GeniSoy Ultra soy protein powder | 1 scoop | 500 | 100-140 |
| Quaker Instant Oatmeal Nutrition for Women | 1 packet | 500 | 160 |
| Nestle Carnation Instant Breakfast, ready to drink | 1 carton | 500 | 240 |
| Blue Bell ice cream, no added sugar, low fat or fat free | 1/2 cup | 450 | 80-110 |
| Lucerne fat-free plain yogurt | 1 cup | 450 | 130 |
| Kraft 2% milk shredded cheese with added calcium (1 oz) | 1/4 cup | 400 | 80 |
| Tropicana grapefruit juice with calcium | 8 oz | 400 | 90 |
| Borden Plus Kid Builder 1% low-fat milk | 1 cup | 400 | 130 |
| Borden Plus fat-free skim milk | 1 cup | 350 | 90 |
| Minute Maid or Tropicana orange juice with calcium and vitamin D | 8 oz | 350 | 110 |
| Lucerne light fat-free flavored yogurt | 8 oz | 300-350 | 110-120 |
| Clif Luna Bar, most flavors | 1 bar | 350 | 180 |
| Nestle or Swiss Miss hot chocolate fat free and/or sugar free with calcium | 1 packet | 300 | 25-60 |
| Borden fat-free or 2% cheese slices | 1 slice | 300 | 30-50 |
| V-8 juice, calcium enriched | 8 oz | 300 | 50 |
| Tofu, Azumaya Lite | 2.8 oz | 300 | 60 |
| Milk, all types | 1 cup | 300 | 80-150 |
| Lucerne 2% cottage cheese, calcium fortified | 1/2 cup | 300 | 90 |
| Dannon fat-free, plain yogurt | 6 oz | 300 | 90 |
| Silk soy milk, calcium enriched (plain and vanilla) | 8 oz | 300 | 100 |
| Yoplait Nouriche light smoothie | 11 oz | 300 | 170 |
| West Soy (Plus) soy milk, regular or nonfat | 1 cup | 250-300 | 80-130 |
| Precious ricotta cheese, part skim | 1/4 cup | 250 | 100 |
| Kraft 2% milk cheese, singles | 1 slice | 200-250 | 50 |
| Part-skim mozzarella cheese sticks | 1 stick | 200 | 80 |
| Dannon Light'n Fit yogurt, creamy or regular | 6 oz | 200-250 | 80-100 |
| Yoplait light fat-free yogurt | 6 oz | 200 | 100 |
| Kraft or Smart Beat singles, fat free | 1 slice | 150 | 30 |
| Galaxy Veggie Soy, slices | 1 slice | 150 | 35 |
| Laughing Cow Mini Babybel cheese, individual | 1 piece | 150 | 70 |
| Philadelphia cream cheese, fat free or light | 2 tbsp | 100-150 | 30-60 |
| 1% fat cottage cheese | 1/2 cup | 100 | 80 |
| Yoplait GoGurt yogurt | 1 tube | 100 | 80 |
| Quaker instant oatmeal, plain or flavored | 1 packet | 100 | 100-170 |

Reprinted with permission from the Cooper Clinic Nutrition Department.

◆ **TABLE 4.2** ◆

## Caffeine Content in Common Foods and Drugs

| Food/Drug | Serving size | Caffeine (mg) |
|---|---|---|
| **Over-the-counter drugs** | | |
| Anacin | 1 tablet | 32 |
| Excedrin | 1 tablet | 65 |
| Dexatrim | 1 tablet | 80 |
| No Doz, maximum strength | 1 tablet | 200 |
| **Coffee** | 12 oz | |
| Brewed, drip method | | 200 |
| Instant | | 115 |
| Decaffeinated | | 6 |
| **Tea** | | |
| Brewed, leaf or bag | 12 oz | 25-110 |
| Iced | 12 oz | 40-75 |
| Instant | 8 oz | 15 |
| Green | 8 oz | 30 |
| **Soft drinks** | 12 oz | |
| Coca-Cola, regular or diet | | 45 |
| Pepsi | | 40 |
| Diet Pepsi | | 35 |
| Sunkist orange soda | | 40 |
| Barq's root beer | | 20 |
| Mello Yello, regular or diet | | 50 |
| Mountain Dew, regular or diet | | 55 |
| Snapple, decaffeinated lemon tea | | 5 |
| Snapple, lemon tea | | 30 |
| **Energy drinks** | 8 oz | |
| Adrenalin Rush | | 120 |
| KMX | | 38 |
| Red Bull | | 120 |
| **Caffeinated waters** | 1/2 liter | |
| Java water | | 125 |
| Water Joe | | 50-60 |
| Krank 20 | | 100 |
| **Chocolate foods and beverages** | | |
| Hershey bar (milk chocolate) | 1.5 oz | 10 |
| Cocoa or hot chocolate | 8 oz | 5 |

Adapted, by permission, from N. Clark, 2003, *Nancy Clark's sports nutrition guidebook*, 3rd ed. (Champaign, IL: Human Kinetics), 103.

consume no more than 2,400 milligrams of salt a day. Simple tips for avoiding excess salt include removing the salt shaker from the table, not adding salt when cooking, and avoiding highly processed foods (canned soups, frozen dinners) and salty snacks.

## Role of Exercise in Bone Development

Bones exposed to enough calcium, vitamin D, and estrogen become thicker and denser according to the loads placed on them. Physical activity loads the bones by causing the muscles to pull on bones and by applying the force of gravity during weight-bearing activity. The heavier the load, the denser the bone will become.

Exercise during puberty has a much greater bone-building benefit than exercise later in life. Gains made in puberty are maintained throughout life. After puberty, exercise affects only the bones used and must be in excess of normal activity to benefit the bones. Exercises that place stress on the bones—walking, running, gymnastics and dance, basketball, and jumping rope—are best. Strength-building exercises, such as lifting weights or body weight exercises, provide effective bone stimulation (Heinonen et al. 1993).

The authors of one study examined the relative importance of calcium intake, exercise, and oral contraceptive use in determining bone mass and bone strength in girls (Lloyd et al. 2004). The girls were followed from ages 12 to 22. They kept food records and completed questionnaires about their exercise activity and oral contraceptive use. Exercise during adolescence was significantly associated with increased bone density and bone strength. Calcium intake and oral contraceptive use were not. Of course, calcium and estrogen are necessary for normal bone development, but it appears that exercise plays a critical role in maximizing bone mass and strength among adolescent girls.

Another study conducted with adolescent girls tested the effects of **plyometric training** on bone mineral content, lower extremity strength, and balance (Witzke and Snow 2000). The test subjects exercised three times per week for 30 to 45 minutes per session over a period of nine months. They participated in hopping, jumping, bounding, box jumps, and various exercises using a weighted vest. The control group maintained their usual activities. Girls in both groups increased bone mass at the hip and lumbar spine, with the plyometric exercise group showing higher increases (especially at the greater trochanter of the hip). The researchers suggested that the significant increase in bone mass at the greater trochanter was due to the lateral movement involved in the exercises.

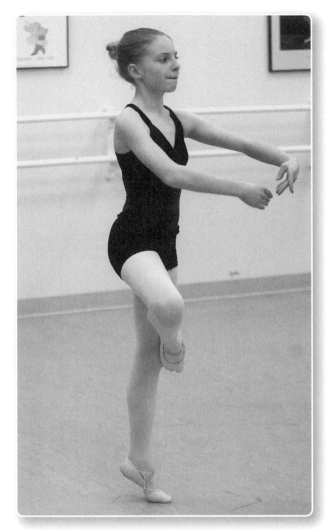

Weight-bearing exercise, such as ballet, promotes bone development.

## Factors Contributing to Weight Training Injuries in Young Females

◆ Skeletal immaturity
◆ Lack of supervision
◆ Improper training and overuse
◆ Poor technique and biomechanics

From Cowlin 2002.

of injury during physical activity. See "Factors Contributing to Weight Training Injuries in Young Females" in the sidebar. Proper instruction and supervision are critical in preventing weight training injuries in young females.

# Benefits and Barriers to Physical Activity During Adolescence

Before planning programs, it is important to talk with adolescent girls and young women regarding their beliefs about the benefits or advantages ("pros") of regular physical activity. Go beyond the health and fitness benefits of exercise. The social and emotional benefits will be appealing to many. Ask girls and young women to list the benefits that are most important to them at this time in their lives. The more benefits they see for being active, the more likely they are to participate in physical activity and adopt healthy lifestyles. Remember, increasing participation and promoting healthy lifestyles are the goals of fitness programming at this life stage. Some of the most common benefits or "pros" are summarized in the sidebar on the next page.

The appropriate age for a girl to begin a strength training program depends on her maturity level, skill level, and prior activity experience. It is recommended that prepubescent girls who participate in strength training seek the guidance of a qualified fitness professional in order to ensure safety and proper program design. When a strength training program is undertaken after puberty, the focus of the program should be on general motor skills and efficient movement patterns in conjunction with the strength training principles discussed in chapter 8. Adolescent girls and young women are more vulnerable than adult women to injury. Establishing a foundation of motor skills, stability, and strength is necessary for young girls as their musculoskeletal systems develop and change in order to reduce the risk

Adolescent girls and young women also have distinct barriers to physical activity. These may include lack of daily physical education in middle and high schools and lack of after-school programs that promote physical activity for nonathletes. College or educational pursuits, part-time jobs, and job and career demands may make it difficult for young women to find the time for regular physical activity. So too can family responsibilities (caring for children, preparing meals, household chores) and social activities

## Benefits or "Pros" of Regular Physical Activity During Adolescence

- ◆ Develops strong bones
- ◆ Helps avoid unwanted weight gain
- ◆ Improves posture and appearance
- ◆ Reduces stress and anxiety
- ◆ Improves self-image and confidence
- ◆ Increases energy level and reduces fatigue
- ◆ Provides opportunities for socialization and recreation
- ◆ Helps develop new skills
- ◆ Allows for creative expression
- ◆ Helps avoid negative behaviors and their consequences
- ◆ Helps avoid chronic diseases during adulthood
- ◆ Promotes overall good health (less illness and fewer absences from school or work)

# Promoting Participation in Regular Physical Activity

Title IX made sports more widely available to girls and young women. But while measured performance, winning, and aggressive behaviors appeal to some adolescent girls and young women, they don't appeal to others. Some ways to relate physical activity to the everyday lives of adolescent girls and young women are listed in the sidebar "Physical Activity in the Lives of Adolescent Girls."

Health and fitness professionals who are promoting physical activity among adolescent girls and young women should also provide

## Physical Activity in the Lives of Adolescent Girls

- ◆ Creating and playing active games with younger siblings and other children
- ◆ Dancing with friends (for socialization or creative expression)
- ◆ Physical activity for personal transportation (walking or cycling to school, to do errands, and to shop)
- ◆ Understanding energy balance ("calories in" and "calories out") and weight management
- ◆ Increasing self-awareness by monitoring thoughts, feelings, and actions
- ◆ Selecting and preparing foods to match energy needs
- ◆ Doing household chores and yard work to help with family responsibilities
- ◆ Participating in school activities that require adequate fitness (drill team, marching band, cheerleading, competitive sport)
- ◆ Managing time effectively to include physical activity with school, work, and family responsibilities
- ◆ Using physical activity for relaxation and stress management
- ◆ Learning about career opportunities in health- and fitness-related professions

Adapted from Otis and Goldingay 2000; Lutter and Jaffee 1996.

or dating. Many adolescents spend significant after-school time on their homework, typically a sedentary activity.

In addition, some girls and young women may have a dislike of vigorous, sweaty activity and feel more interested in sedentary leisure activities such as watching television, using a computer, listening to music, talking on the phone, visiting with friends, and grooming (hair, nails, clothes). Some girls and young women may experience barriers such as transportation that discourage walking or cycling and have concerns for personal safety. Others may feel at a loss due to lack of money for exercise equipment, clothing, or fitness center memberships, or may feel a lack of support from family and friends who are not active. Though many young women enjoy sport and competition, many do not, and others find that their lack of athletic skills and abilities prevents them from joining teams. Some girls engage in unhealthy practices such as smoking and alcohol use that are not conducive to regular physical activity. Finally, some young women may experience pregnancy as a major change in their lives and a barrier to regular physical activity.

for individual differences, needs, talents, and preferences. Offer choices of types of physical activity, both individual and group activities, because being able to choose from an array of options increases feelings of control. Emphasize physical activity for function and creative expression. Self-discovery and skill mastery are more important than performance for many young women. Beliefs about what they can do are the foundation of self-efficacy.

Also, explain how physical activity can help manage stress and anxiety. Help young women learn self-calming techniques and coping skills, such as deep breathing, progressive muscle relaxation, and visualization, to deal with emotional upheavals and everyday stressors.

Consider providing opportunities for girls to get involved in supportive networks. Organize physical activities in small groups with peer leaders, and encourage activity with "buddies" to provide for socialization and improve adherence to a regular exercise routine.

Because some girls and young women will need to change their behaviors, help them gain self-awareness as a first step in readiness for change. Suggest wearing a pedometer to get a baseline of physical activity and to track improvements from there. Introduce walking as a lifestyle physical activity as well as for exercise. (See the benefits of walking outlined in the sidebar.) Maximize the opportunities for positive feelings associated with physical activity by making physical activity fun and avoiding emphasis on objective measurements, competition, and aggressive actions. Instead, stress cooperation, social interaction, teamwork, and problem solving.

In addition to promoting physical activity and providing technical expertise related to program design, health and fitness professionals can serve as mentors and role models. They can provide emotional support and reliable advice for adolescent girls and young women while allowing a degree of autonomy from parents. Establishing a bond with a special adult friend, teacher, or or jogginhcoach can be significant

## Benefits of Walking for Girls and Young Women

- ◆ Requires no athletic skills
- ◆ Provides a way to be active without playing sports
- ◆ Requires no special equipment or clothing (except comfortable shoes)
- ◆ Can be done at moderate intensity (not too vigorously)
- ◆ Can be done in many places (school, shopping mall, neighborhoods)
- ◆ Has little risk of injury
- ◆ Improves fitness and helps with weight management
- ◆ Provides opportunity for socializing with friends
- ◆ Improves self-image and self-esteem

for an adolescent girl. Trusted adults may be able to steer those at risk away from negative peer friendships or environmental influences that encourage unhealthy behaviors. However, if you suspect a problem beyond your scope of professional expertise (clinical depression, eating dis-

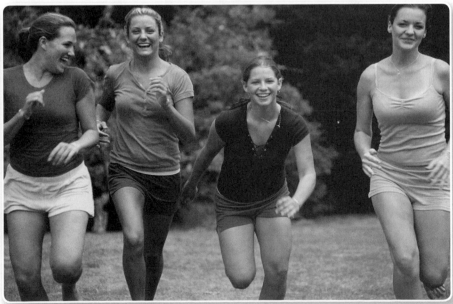

© Masterfile

Walking or jogging promotes physical activity while providing time with friends.

order, personal history of abuse), you must refer the young woman to other health professionals. Take the time to contact these professionals to learn about their qualifications, experiences, and approaches so that you feel comfortable making a referral.

# Health Issues for Adolescent Girls and Young Women

A major health issue for adolescent girls is overweight and obesity. Young women are also at risk for amenorrhea and eating disorders. When amenorrhea, osteoporosis, and disordered eating occur together, this is called the female athlete triad (Otis and Goldingay 2000). These three conditions occur together most often in competitive athletes and dancers, but each condition can occur independently in nonathletes. Amenorrhea and eating disorders are discussed in detail later in this chapter. Excessive exercising or overtraining, a means of purging calories, is also discussed.

## Overweight and Obesity

Overweight among youth has nearly tripled since the 1970s. As shown in figure 4.1, there has been a steady increase of youth who are overweight. Overweight girls often have symptoms of depression and are at risk for type 2 diabetes. Overweight adolescents are also at an increased risk of becoming overweight adults (Needham and Crosnoe 2005). And, as described in chapter 2, overweight and obesity in adult women are linked to an increased risk for cardiovascular disease, stroke, high blood pressure, high blood cholesterol and triglycerides, type 2 diabetes, and some types of cancer.

Data from the 1999 National Youth Risk Behavior Survey (a representative sample of U.S. high school students) revealed that female students were less likely than male students to be overweight, but more likely to be trying to lose weight (Lowry et al. 2002). Among females, trying to lose weight was associated with vigorous physical activity, strengthening exercises, and cigarette smoking. Only 62 percent of females trying to lose weight or to stay the same weight combined exercise with a reduced-fat and -calorie diet, while 32 percent used unhealthy weight control methods such as smoking, overtraining, fasting, diet pills, vomiting, or laxatives.

Adolescent girls and young women need to know that severe dieting doesn't work. It is impossible to stay on a severe diet over the long term for three reasons:

◆ Diets that make certain groups of foods totally off-limits are unrealistic and can lead to nutrient deficiencies. Balance and variety are keys to getting the protein, vitamins, and minerals necessary for important body functions and processes.

◆ Starvation diets cause feelings of deprivation, which increase the risk of overeating when one is feeling stressed.

◆ Severe diets alter the metabolism. The body thinks it is starving so the metabolism slows down to conserve energy. The body uses muscle as a source of energy.

Some girls overeat because of lack of knowledge and skills. They don't know how to read food labels, choose healthy foods, or control portion sizes. These girls would benefit from nutrition education or individual counseling

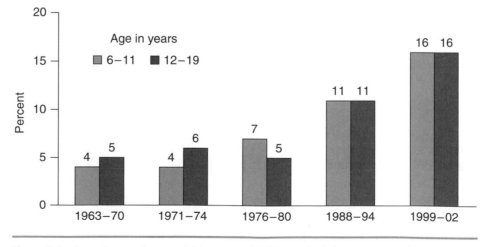

**Figure 4.1** Prevalence of overweight among children and adolescents ages 6-19 years.
From CDC/NCHS, NHES, and NHANES.

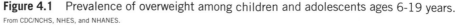

exercise alone without caloric restriction is not likely to produce sufficient weight loss. Exercise is essential to avoiding unwanted weight gain in the first place. Once a desirable weight is attained, exercise is key to keeping weight off over the long term. And, with regular physical activity, it is possible to eat more calories without gaining weight.

Reducing sedentary behaviors in adolescent girls is probably just as important for weight loss as vigorous exercise (Styne 2005). Many adolescents favor watching television, talking on the telephone, grooming, and other sedentary behaviors over physical activity. These inactive habits compound the obesity problem. Besides adding structured exercise to girls' and young women's lifestyles, we must discourage sedentary behaviors and promote lifestyle physical activity. It has also been shown that decreasing sedentary behaviors in adolescents reduces calorie intake (Epstein et al. 2005).

### Body Types, Body Image, and Weight Management

For adolescent girls, gaining height and weight is not their only concern. Their body shape begins to change. Body type is determined by genetics and begins to emerge after puberty. Though body types are easy to recognize, many people, including health and fitness professionals, do not recognize body types or understand the implications of body type on body composition and weight gain and loss.

There are three basic body types (see figure 4.2). Many young women are a blend of body types (Otis and Goldingay 2000).

- ◆ *Ectomorph*—This body type is tall and slim with long arms and legs. Young women with this body type have difficulty gaining weight and building muscle. Ballet dancers, models, and long-distance runners tend to have the ectomorph body type.

- ◆ *Mesomorph*—This body type is shorter and muscular and has stocky arms and legs. Young women with this body type are strong and gain muscle mass when they do strength training. They may have difficulty losing weight. Young women with mesomorph body types excel at power sports, such as soccer, softball, and sprinting events in track and field.

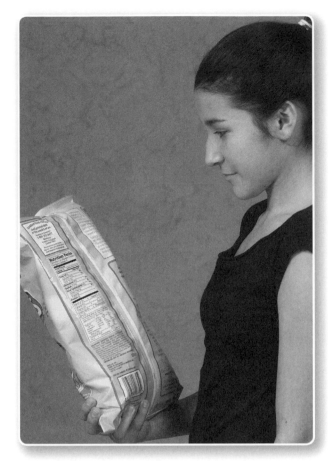

Learning to read food labels is an important weight management skill for young women.

with a registered dietitian. Share the handout on healthy eating practices for weight management that is provided in appendix B (page 219).

Other young women have difficulty managing their weight because they overeat in response to emotions rather than to hunger. Overeating is often the response to anger, sadness, joy, boredom, loneliness, or fatigue from studying or working for long hours. Encourage adolescent girls and young women who are concerned about their weight to think about what might trigger their urge to overeat when they are not really hungry. Those who are eating in response to emotional urges should be encouraged to seek professional counseling.

### Exercise in Weight Loss and Weight Management

Exercise can help with weight loss for a variety of reasons, the most basic of which is that it causes the body to expend more calories. However,

◆ *Endomorph*—This body type carries more body fat. The endomorph body type may be apple shaped or pear shaped. Young women with endomorph body types excel at distance swimming, field events, and weightlifting.

The term "body image" is used to describe the subjective attitudes and perceptions an individual holds regarding her body and appearance. It's the picture carried in the mind's eye (Lutter and Jaffee 1996). Visual, tactile, and kinesthetic (movement) impressions of one's physical self are included. In addition to reflecting how a person feels about her overall appearance, body image may focus on a specific feature or body part (hair, hips, breasts) or movement (clumsy, graceful, athletic).

A young woman's body image is influenced by many different variables, including childhood experiences, sociocultural and historical factors, and mass media (Lutter and Jaffee 1996). Girls who were overweight as children and were teased or criticized by family members or by peers may develop a negative body image early in life. Those who were a normal weight as children but began to put on weight as they entered puberty may feel embarrassed by the attention they receive as their body begins to develop (Cowlin 2002).

It is virtually impossible for young women to avoid being affected by unrealistic body images promoted through the media and other marketing venues. Young women who do not meet or match the standard of beauty as portrayed by the media may develop deeply ingrained feelings of personal inadequacy that may persist over their lifetime. It is important, however, for girls and young women to remember that the standards to which they hold themselves regarding their appearance (their body image) remain their personal choice. Body image is only one of the factors that contribute to self-esteem or self-worth. It is possible to have a positive body image and low self-esteem, or vice versa. Body image and self-esteem are both dynamic processes that can evolve and change throughout life (Otis and Goldingay 2000). Of interest, in a study of female college athletes and nonathletes, the nonathletes expressed more dissatisfaction with their bodies than athletes from a variety of sports (Robinson and Ferraro 2004).

Strength training programs can help young women develop better attitudes about their physical selves as shown in a study involving college-age women. The group of young women was enrolled in a 12-week strength training class that met twice a week (Ahmed et al. 2002). Physical fitness measurements including percent body fat, weight, circumferences, and strength were evaluated before and after the program. Questions dealing with perceptions of body image were also included. At the end of the program, strength had improved, but there was an average weight gain of 1 pound (0.45 kilograms) and an average increase in body fat of 0.9 percent. Nevertheless, the young women reported feeling healthier and more fit. And they had a better attitude about their bodies, even though they had not lost weight or body fat. It may be that a focus on what one's body can *do* rather than what it looks like can lead to a healthier body image.

More needs to be done to help adolescent girls and young women develop positive body images. Learning to develop a better match between the subjective and objective realities of body image and body type is critical. This entails an

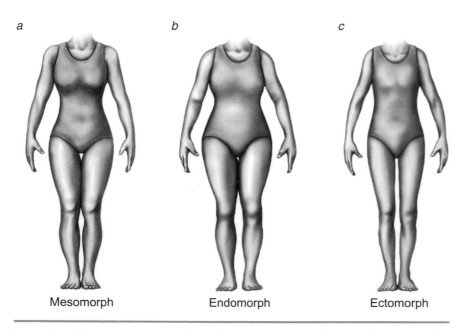

*a*     *b*     *c*

Mesomorph     Endomorph     Ectomorph

**Figure 4.2** There are three basic body types: *(a)* mesomorph, *(b)* endomorph, and *(c)* ectomorph. Many young women are a blend of body types.

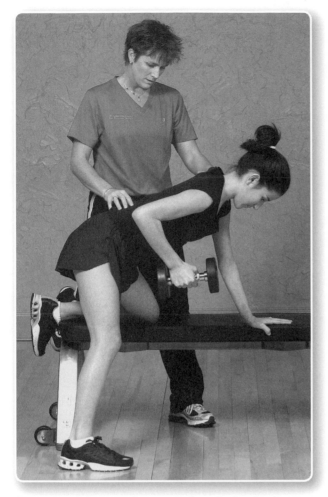

Strength training exercises are safe and effective for young women when performed under the supervision of a qualified teacher or trainer.

acceptance of the body as it is and the limits for change based on genetics. Moreover, girls and young women need to accept who they are as a whole person. A handout on improving body image is provided in appendix B (page 218). This resource, which is appropriate for women of all ages, may be especially useful with young women.

## Amenorrhea

Most healthy adolescent girls, even the most active ones, have regular menstrual cycles lasting 23 to 35 days. Stopping menstrual periods, called amenorrhea, is not normal. It is a signal that something is wrong in the body. Women with amenorrhea do not release an egg each month. They are deficient in estrogen, progesterone, and testosterone. These hormones are essential to build bone, grow hair, have glowing skin, and enjoy sex. There are two types of amenorrhea: primary amenorrhea and secondary amenorrhea.

### Primary Amenorrhea

Primary amenorrhea is the delay of menarche until after the age of 16. The chief influence on the timing of puberty is genetic. The hypothalamus controls the events of puberty. Anything that disrupts the function of the hypothalamus—restrictive diets, poor nutrition, eating disorders, and stress—can delay puberty. Increased risk is associated with extreme and prolonged exercise (particularly without adequate nutrition), body fat less than 15 to 17 percent, extreme obesity, and taking hormonal supplements. Medical problems such as diabetes, brain tumors, thyroid disorders, and other hormone problems can also delay puberty. Delayed puberty is not normal. If a girl experiences delayed puberty, all factors must be evaluated. In addition to the concern about an underlying medical condition, delayed puberty may also cause early weakening of the bones, as well as stress fractures.

Girls who have not started any breast development by age 12 or 13 should be checked for delayed puberty. The first menstrual cycle (the menarche) will come 30 to 36 months after breasts begin to develop. If a girl has not started breast development by age 14 or has not started having a period by age 16, she should be examined by a physician.

### Secondary Amenorrhea and Oligomenorrhea

Secondary amenorrhea occurs when someone who has reached menarche stops having periods for three months or more. The incidence of secondary amenorrhea (due to some cause other than pregnancy or menopause) is about 4 percent in the general population. Oligomenorrhea refers to few or irregular periods. The periods may be at irregular intervals, varying between 21 and 90 days, with usually fewer than six periods per year. Oligomenorrhea may be a precursor to amenorrhea. Like amenorrhea, oligomenorrhea is not normal. Girls or women with either secondary amenorrhea or oligomenorrhea should be checked by a physician.

If the amenorrhea or oligomenorrhea is not due to pregnancy or an underlying medical problem, it is probably due to energy drain. The hypothalamus has sensed that there is too much energy going out and not enough coming in. It turns off the reproductive system temporarily to conserve energy. Hypothalamic amenorrhea may be due to any or all of the following:

◆ Stress related—due to work demands, erratic sleep, anxiety over relationships, exams, moving, travel

◆ Exercise related—due to overexercising or overtraining

◆ Eating disordered—due to drastic weight loss or obesity

Stress is the most common cause. Periods resume when the stress is gone.

Among female athletes who are training rigorously, secondary amenorrhea is much more common. It is impossible to know exact statistics, but this type of amenorrhea can occur regardless of the physical activity or sport. Those athletes whose art or sport requires a lean appearance are the most likely to develop amenorrhea and the female athlete triad (Cowlin 2002; Otis and Goldingay 2000). Although it is more common in ballerinas and other dancers, distance runners, ice skaters, gymnasts, and cyclists, exercise-related amenorrhea is not normal. It is a warning sign for poor performance, stress fractures, and health problems. Risk factors for amenorrhea in active females are listed in the following sidebar.

## Disordered Eating

Emphasis on appearance and pressures to be thin can encourage disordered eating. Any young woman who has practiced chronic dieting and disordered eating habits is at risk for short- and long-term physiological and psychological problems, including depression, low self-esteem, stomach and digestive problems, menstrual irregularities, heart problems, and even death by heart failure or suicide.

Most girls and young women have felt pressures to be thin by the time they reach high school (Lutter and Jaffee 1996). In addition to the intense pressures from the media, pressures to be thin come from the following:

Mothers who put their daughters on diets when they reach puberty

Mothers and other women and girls who talk openly about their dissatisfaction with their own bodies

Fathers, brothers, and boyfriends who make teasing comments about the female body

Coaches, trainers, or teammates who suggest that being thin would improve performance (Cowlin 2002)

Some adolescent girls and young women follow a starvation diet in pursuit of what they see as the ideal body. When they become overwhelmed by hunger or stress, they are likely to overeat. This eating pattern could lead to an eating disorder, such as bulimia, or to weight gain due to bingeing without purging. Learning to eat right for their activity level and health can help girls and young women avoid mood swings, weight fluctuations, and serious eating problems (Otis and Goldingay 2000). See the handout on healthy eating practices for weight management in appendix B (page 219).

Dehydration is the ultimate "quick fix" weight loss program and the underlying mechanism of losing weight with most fad diets. Dehydration is also the result of purging, which is discussed later in this chapter. Because the human body is 70 percent water, it is easy to lose weight by getting rid of water. Significant water weight can be lost overnight. Diets that emphasize eating large

## Risk Factors for Amenorrhea in Active Females

◆ Never having been pregnant
◆ First menstrual cycle after age 13
◆ History of irregular menstrual cycles
◆ Low body weight
◆ Loss of more than 10 pounds (4.5 kilograms) in the past year
◆ Extreme obesity
◆ High amounts of stress
◆ Vegetarian diet
◆ Inadequate calories for amount of exercise
◆ Disordered eating, anorexia, or bulimia
◆ Overtraining

Adapted from Otis and Goldingay 2000; Lutter and Jaffee 1996.

amounts of protein (low-carb diets) also produce weight loss by dehydration. Along with the loss of water, dehydration causes loss of important and essential electrolytes that regulate the electrical and chemical balance among nerves and muscles. Dehydration can be extremely dangerous. Loss of fluids and electrolytes can lead to heart irregularities, light-headedness, fainting, muscle cramps, constipation, and poor coordination and balance. Unfortunately, weight that is lost quickly through most fad diets is usually regained. Sometimes more weight is regained than was lost.

## Anorexia Nervosa

There are two recognized subtypes of anorexia:

◆ *Restrictive anorexia*—Severe restriction in the amount and type of food eaten. This is the most common type of anorexia.

◆ *Binge–purge anorexia*—Eating (which may be considered a binge), then using a method such as vomiting or taking laxatives to attempt to get rid of the food. Binge–purge anorexia differs from bulimia. With binge–purge anorexia, overall calories are severely restricted. A distorted body image is also common with binge–purge anorexia.

Anorexia can begin with the desire to lose 5 or 10 pounds (2.3 or 4.5 kilograms). As the girl or woman loses weight, she is rewarded with positive comments from family and friends. "You look great. Have you lost weight?" Such comments reinforce her belief in the advantages of losing more weight. In the beginning, she may be happy and energetic or overactive. But over time, she becomes fixated on controlling her diet and weighing herself, and continues to lose weight. Even before the problem is noticed, subtle changes start to indicate how the lack of vital nutrition is harmful to her body. She starts to feel tired and can't concentrate. Her work habits start to suffer.

When her thinness becomes so apparent that she receives negative comments from friends, she may try to cover up her body with long sleeves and baggy pants or dresses. She will deny that there is a problem while she continues her obsession with thinness and control. Her denial of the problem makes treating anorexia very difficult (Otis and Goldingay 2000).

To be clinically diagnosed as having anorexia nervosa, the patient must meet all four of the following criteria established by the American Psychiatric Association (1994):

◆ Refusal to maintain body weight even though one is 15 percent or more below weight range expected for age and height

◆ Intense fear of gaining weight

◆ Body image distortion; feeling fat even when very underweight

◆ Absence of three or more consecutive menstrual periods

Anorexia is mostly a female disease (about 95 percent of people with anorexia are female). About 1 percent of adolescent females in the United States have anorexia (Anexoria Nervosa and Related Eating Disorders, Inc. 2004). Young women with anorexia tend to be of middle to high socioeconomic status, tend to seek "perfection" and have a desire to please others, are usually adolescents (but anorexia can occur as late as the early 30s), usually live in developed societies around the world, and typically have a distorted body image (i.e., they do not see that they are extremely thin; they truly believe they are fat, and no one can convince them otherwise). Their entire self-worth is connected to being thin. Additionally, they often have difficulty relating to others. A list of warning signs and symptoms of anorexia is presented in the sidebar on the next page.

Symptoms of anorexia are due to serious medical problems. Synthesis of vitamin A by the liver is altered. The body begins to break down muscle, which overworks the kidneys, so kidneys can fail. Electrolytes, liver function, calcium, phosphorus, and magnesium levels can be abnormal.

The resting pulse is low due to slowed metabolism because of starvation. (Do not confuse this with the low resting pulse of a highly fit woman whose heart does not have to work as hard to pump blood to her body.) Heart failure, irregular heartbeats, seizures, and possibly death can occur. Estrogen levels are low, increasing the risk for osteoporosis and serious fractures.

Anorexia is a chronic disease that can take a long time to treat. Early detection helps prevent permanent damage to the heart, brain, bones,

## Warning Signs and Symptoms of Anorexia

A young woman with anorexia may

- look ill;
- deny that she is too thin;
- say she feels fat or that she wants to lose more weight;
- have an obsession with weight, diet, and appearance;
- practice food rituals, such as dividing food into small portions and eating only certain amounts or hiding food;
- avoid social situations involving food;
- have an obsession with exercise, appear hyperactive;
- be sensitive to cold;
- wear baggy clothing to hide weight loss;
- be very fatigued;
- experience a decline in school, work, or athletic performance;
- have low muscle mass, have bones of the skeleton protruding;
- have hair that is thin on the scalp with patches of hair loss;
- develop fine baby hair (called lanugo hair) on face and body (believed to be body's attempt to keep warm)*;
- have a yellow tint to skin, palms, and soles of feet (from high levels of carotene)*;
- have dry skin and brittle nails;
- have no menstrual periods (amenorrhea);
- have slow pulse at rest, low blood pressure;
- become light-headed on standing up quickly;
- develop constipation;
- produce low amounts of urine;
- experience insomnia;
- experience depression and mood changes;
- lose bone prematurely;
- be at risk for stress fractures;
- experience delayed puberty; and
- experience temporary or permanent infertility.

(Otis and Goldingay 2000; Lutter and Jaffee 1996)

*Unique to anorexia.

and kidneys. Without treatment, some will die from heart or kidney failure or suicide. With early detection and treatment, these deaths can be prevented. Self-referral for treatment, ideally before distorted eating becomes a full-blown eating disorder, increases the likelihood of recovery. Since many young women with anorexia are concerned with high performance, their decline in performance (academic, job, or athletic) may be a way to help them recognize the toll that starvation is taking on their bodies and their lives. Treatment is best managed by a team of health professionals that may include a medical doctor, psychologist or psychiatrist, registered dietitian, and exercise professional or trainer.

### Bulimia Nervosa

While anorexia is characterized by strict control of food and body weight, bulimia is a loss of control. See the repetitive cycle that is shown as figure 4.3. The person may begin with dieting and restricting calories, which leads to hunger and stress. The hunger and stress cannot be managed, so she automatically or unconsciously overeats (binges). She feels guilty and ashamed that she has blown her diet. She feels like a failure. She turns to purging to get rid of the food and to get rid of the guilt. Some of the more common purging methods are listed in the sidebar on the next page. The feelings of relief following the purge complete the cycle. The cyclic nature of the bingeing and purging turns into a compulsion and becomes an

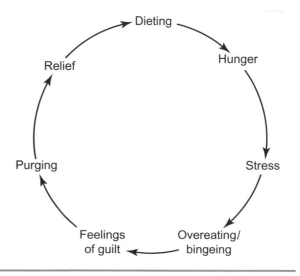

**Figure 4.3** Bingeing and purging can follow a repetitive cycle, which becomes an addictive behavior.

## Common Purging Methods

- ◆ Forced vomiting
- ◆ Laxatives
- ◆ Enemas
- ◆ Diuretics
- ◆ Overexercising

addictive behavior. The binge can also start as a response to stress (emotional eating).

According to Anorexia Nervosa and Related Eating Disorders, Inc. (ANRED), it is estimated that about 4 percent of college-aged women in the United States have bulimia. About 50 percent of people who have been anorexic develop bulimia or bulimic patterns. Ninety percent of people with bulimia are female (Anorexia Nervosa and Related Eating Disorders, Inc. 2004). Chronic dieters with low self-esteem and negative body images and people who suffer from depression and anxiety disorders are most at risk for developing bulimia. Girls and women who are victims of sexual abuse are also likely to develop bulimia. Young women with bulimia are not easily recognized. They can be normal weight or slightly overweight and be almost any age, race, or educational background. They have distorted body images and fear getting fat, but they are not as thin as people with anorexia.

The American Psychiatric Association (APA) diagnostic criteria for bulimia nervosa are as follows:

- ◆ Repeated episodes of binge eating, at least twice a week for three months
- ◆ Feeling of lack of control during eating binges
- ◆ Use of one or more purging methods: self-induced vomiting, laxatives, diuretics, or excessive exercise
- ◆ Overconcern with body shape or weight (American Psychiatric Association 1994)

Excessive exercise can take the place of other purging methods such as vomiting or using laxatives or diuretics. Exercise that is excessive is done compulsively—to burn extra calories or to undo the effects of bingeing. It is not done for fun, health, fitness, or training. Excessive exercise can lead to overuse injuries, a lack of balance with other aspects of life, depression, and low self-esteem. More information on excessive exercise (also called overtraining) is provided later in this chapter.

Most young women with bulimia are not able to stop the binge–purge cycle on their own. They are often able to hide their behavior from others until some health scare, such as severe digestive problems, requires them to seek treatment. Successful treatments deal with the eating behavior and also with the underlying psychological problems that led to self-inflicted abusive behaviors. Psychological therapy works best when it is directed at building self-esteem, developing a positive body image, overcoming depression, and recovering from a personal history of abuse.

The APA has also identified a type of eating disorder, binge eating disorder, that is broader than either anorexia or bulimia (American Psychiatric Association 1994). Women with binge eating disorder meet all the criteria for anorexia nervosa but have regular periods and, despite significant weight loss, their current weight is in the normal range. They meet all the criteria for bulimia nervosa except that purging occurs less than twice a week for less than three months. Also, women with binge eating disorder use purging behavior after eating small amounts of food, repeatedly chew and spit out but do not swallow food, and have recurrent episodes of binge eating without purging.

## Overtraining

Overtraining is the condition that results from too much exercise. The body has not had enough rest, sleep, and nutrition to recover from the strenuous workload. Overtraining is prevalent in female competitive athletes as well as recreational exercisers. While overtraining can occur at any age, it is more common in younger women. Causes of overtraining include excessive high-intensity training, inadequate recovery time, inadequate nutrition, abrupt changes in exercise load (intensity, duration, distance), stress, and insufficient sleep or rest.

Four or more of these symptoms may signal overtraining (Otis and Goldingay 2000):

- ◆ Restless sleep or insomnia
- ◆ Fatigue

- Muscle soreness that does not recover after a night's rest
- Muscle and joint pain
- Weight loss
- Frequent infections
- Mood swings and depression
- Headaches
- Lack of interest in sport training
- Injuries that do not heal
- Poor performance in school, at work, or in athletics
- Elevated pulse rate (taken before getting out of bed in the morning)
- Amenorrhea

Infertility is often associated with amenorrhea and overtraining, although a study from Harvard Medical School concluded that more ovulatory infertility among American women was due to overweight and physical inactivity than to underweight and overexertion (Rich-Edwards et al. 2002).

Treating overtraining requires stopping the energy drain and allowing the body to rest, recover, and get back in balance. For adolescent girls or young women who have been in a state of negative energy, balance can be achieved by two approaches: increasing the number of calories consumed each day or cutting back on the amount of physical activity. Often the easiest way to recover from overtraining is a combination of the two approaches.

Adequate rest is also required for recovery—at least one day a week without any vigorous activity. Rest is essential to allow the muscles to rebuild. After a few weeks without overtraining and with appropriate rest, symptoms will begin

## ◆ Conclusion ◆

Topics addressed in this chapter can help girls grow into active, healthy young women. We focused first on the immediate goal of promoting healthy lifestyles. This is challenging since puberty marks a time when physical activity among girls typically begins to decline. Developing habits of regular physical activity in childhood and adolescence and practicing them over a lifetime could result in optimal health and quality of life for many more women.

After discussing the transition of puberty and the phases of a healthy menstrual cycle, we described the role of hormones (estrogen, cortisol), nutrition (calcium, caffeine, and sodium), and exercise (especially strength training) in the development of peak bone mass (about 25 percent is developed during puberty). In an effort to make physical activity appealing to adolescent girls, we suggested ways to relate physical activity to their everyday lives. Walking for exercise is especially beneficial for girls who don't enjoy sports or athletics.

Health issues related to physical activity and exercise for adolescent girls and young women center on weight management. Increasing physical activity and reducing sedentary behaviors are important weight management strategies for young women. Helping them understand their body types and develop positive, realistic body images is also important. Unfortunately, constant dieting and emphasis on being thin can lead to amenorrhea and eating disorders. Types of risk factors for amenorrhea, anorexia nervosa, and bulimia nervosa were discussed. Exercise that is excessive (called overtraining), performed as a method of purging unwanted calories rather than for fun, fitness, or training, can be detrimental to health. Health and fitness professionals need to be aware of signs and symptoms and be prepared to refer young women with these problems to appropriate health care professionals.

In conclusion, participating in regular physical activity has the potential to help girls avoid some of the risky behaviors associated with adolescence and grow into healthy women prepared for pregnancy, should it occur. Pregnancy is the subject of the next chapter.

# CHAPTER 5

# Exercise During and After Pregnancy

## Topics in This Chapter

- Goals of fitness programs
- Physiological changes of pregnancy
- Benefits and barriers to prenatal and post-partum exercise
- Promoting participation in prenatal exercise
- Modifying exercises for the physical demands of pregnancy
- Contraindications for exercise during pregnancy
- Specialized exercises for labor and birth
- Warning signs for terminating exercise

- Nutrition guidelines for active women during pregnancy
- Exercise and special conditions—pre-eclampsia, chronic hypertension, gestational hypertension, and gestational diabetes
- At-home exercises for immediate recovery
- Exercise and the postpartum blues
- Breast-feeding and exercise
- Including the baby in postpartum exercise classes

> When we do the best that we can, we never know what miracle is wrought in our life, or in the life of another.
>
> Helen Keller

As adults, most young women interact with the health care system related to their unique issues of conception and pregnancy. The conception and childbearing years provide an excellent opportunity for health professionals to reinforce information about the role of physical activity and its benefits for lifelong health promotion and disease prevention. This is an appropriate time to encourage exercise to reduce health risks, prepare for pregnancy, and educate expectant mothers on the importance of exercise and physical activity for their children.

## Goals of Fitness Programs During and After Pregnancy

An immediate goal of fitness during pregnancy is to have a healthy baby. Putting the health of the baby first in the mother's mind helps her see her own health and fitness as a support system for a larger goal—making a healthy baby. Fitness may also prevent some of the stresses of pregnancy and birth and prevent the birth process from being viewed as an illness or procedure. In her book *Women's Fitness Program Development,* Ann Cowlin compares the birth process to exercise (Cowlin 2002). Both are perceived by the body as work. A good level of fitness can help women develop the ability to work within their own bodies during labor and make adjustments as needed, much as they would do when engaging in other strenuous physical activities.

A woman's level of fitness going into birth can play a large role in her recovery and beyond. The more fit going into the birth, the more fit she is coming out and the faster she can return to activity. Good cardiovascular fitness and metabolic function help promote tissue recovery after birth.

The long-term goal of fitness programs during and after pregnancy is to help women develop lifelong habits of physical activity for themselves and their families. Because women are often major influencers of health care decisions, fitness resources directed at women, especially during their childbearing and child-rearing years, have the potential to benefit the society as a whole.

## The Major Life Transition of Pregnancy

When a pregnancy occurs, it is a major transition in the life of a woman. Her body will change forever, never returning to its prepregnancy state. The physiological changes that occur with pregnancy put additional demands on the body, especially in relation to exercise (Cowlin 2002; Lutter and Jaffee 1996). The heart and lungs must work harder to meet the increased energy demands of pregnancy. Blood volume and resting heart rate also increase. Vein capacity increases, which helps maintain normal blood pressure, and vasodilation occurs to offset hyperthermia. Oxygen consumption is about 20 percent greater than nonpregnant levels. A feeling of breathlessness or hyperventilation can occur because of increased sensitivity to carbon dioxide (caused by increased progesterone). As the uterus grows, it pushes against the diaphragm, the lower ribs flare, and the chest expands. These changes make it more difficult to take a deep breath.

The center of gravity moves forward and upward as the baby grows and the breasts enlarge. To compensate, many women slump their shoulders and arch their backs. The resulting exaggerated low back curvature, called lumbar lordosis, can cause fatigue and lower back pain. Thoracic kyphosis (exaggerated upper back forward curvature) can also occur as the breasts enlarge. The head may tilt forward. The increased weight and shift in the center of gravity also cause a change in balance (see figure 5.1).

A study that evaluated gait kinematics during the last trimester and one year postpartum showed that women compensated for increases in body mass and changes in body mass distribution (Foti et al. 2000). They increased the use of hip extensor, hip abductor, and ankle plantar flexor muscles to keep speed, stride length, cadence, and joint angles relatively unchanged.

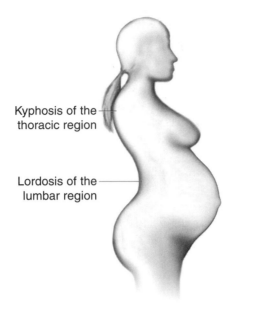

Kyphosis of the thoracic region

Lordosis of the lumbar region

**Figure 5.1** To compensate for changes in the center of gravity, many pregnant women slump their shoulders (kyphosis) and arch their backs (lordosis).

Reprinted, by permission, from W.C. Whiting and S. Rugg, 2005, *Dynatomy: Dynamic human anatomy* (Champaign, IL: Human Kinetics), 65.

The compensations resulted in overuse injuries to the muscle groups about the pelvis, hip, and ankle and contributed to low back, pelvic, and hip pain; calf cramps; and other painful lower extremity musculoskeletal conditions. An appropriate exercise and conditioning program during and after pregnancy can help to avoid these overuse injuries. See chapters 8, 9, and 10 for more information about exercises to deal with these problems.

Increased levels of the hormone relaxin cause connective tissues (ligaments and cartilage) to soften and stretch so the pelvic outlet will accommodate the baby during birth. It is easier to turn an ankle or twist a knee during and after pregnancy because joints are able to stretch farther than normal. Some women experience pain in one or both sides of their lower abdomen due to stretching of the round ligaments that support the uterus.

During pregnancy, more heat is generated by the mother and the baby. More blood is pumped to the skin, and more sweat is produced by the sweat glands. It is easy for overheating to occur, especially during activity in hot and humid environments. Thermoregulation is very important, especially during the first trimester. The major organ systems that are developing in the fetus at this time are sensitive to overheating. Maternal hyperthermia is known to be related to neural tube defects. A study of temperature and oxygen saturation responses to low-impact aerobic exercise in healthy pregnant women showed that exercise at about 70 percent of maximum heart rate was safe in terms of risk of maternal hyperthermia (Larsson and Lindqvist 2005). None of the pregnant women in the study were even close to approaching a dangerous body temperature, and no measurement was below 95 percent in oxygen saturation at maximum exercise or after exercise.

The remainder of this section deals with current research findings related to exercise and birth outcomes, mood, and body image, as well as beliefs about exercise and exercise behaviors.

## Exercise and Birth Outcomes

Because having a healthy baby is the foremost goal, it is important to consider the effects of physical activity on birth outcomes. Physical activity during pregnancy appears to have no deleterious effects on birth outcomes and may, in fact, reduce the risk of low birth weight. A study of 9,089 women from the 1988 National Maternal and Infant Health Study (NMIHS) assessed the effect of regular leisure physical activity on two different adverse birth outcomes: timeliness (preterm/postterm) of delivery and low birth weight (Leiferman and Evenson 2003). Regular leisure physical activity, as determined by responses to questionnaires, was defined as exercising or playing sports at least three times a week. Women who failed to engage in regular leisure physical activity before and during their pregnancy were more likely to give birth to a very low birth weight baby compared with women who remained active before and during pregnancy. Moreover, previously active women who stopped physical activity during pregnancy were more likely to give birth to a low birth weight or very low birth weight baby than women who remained active before and during pregnancy. There was no significant relationship between participation in regular leisure physical activity and timeliness of delivery.

Another study, comparing women who exercised three times per week during the second half of pregnancy with a control group, showed no significant difference in neonatal weight or length of pregnancy (Garshasbi and Faghih 2005). Whether exercise during pregnancy affects gestation length is unclear.

In a study by Clapp and colleagues (2000), previously sedentary low-risk women had heavier, longer, leaner babies when moderate-intensity weight-bearing exercise was started at eight to nine weeks gestation and continued until delivery. The exercise group in this study exercised on a treadmill or stair stepper or did step aerobics to 55 to 60 percent of maximal heart rate three to five times a week for 20 minutes per session.

Generally, a heavier baby is a healthier baby. But, for women at risk for overgrown babies, such as women with diabetes, these results are a concern. Interestingly, an earlier study by the same lead author showed that vigorous exercise (running and dancing) in late pregnancy resulted in lighter, leaner babies (Clapp and Capeless 1990).

It is not clear whether exercise has any direct effect on labor and delivery. There is no guarantee that being physically and psychologically fit leads to a perfect and easy delivery. However, it is realistic to expect that women who are fit and prepared for the work of birth will tolerate the process more easily and with greater confidence.

## Exercise and Mood

While studies have confirmed elevated stress and depressed mood during pregnancy, few have examined exercise in relation to psychosocial outcomes during pregnancy (Da Costa et al. 2003). A study of 180 pregnant women collected data monthly, beginning in the third month, on a variety of psychosocial inventories, including depressed mood, anxiety, pregnancy-specific stress, and daily hassles. Information on frequency, form, and duration of leisure-time physical activity was collected through structured interviews. Compared to nonexercisers, women participating in leisure-time physical activity reported less depressed mood, daily hassles, anxiety, and pregnancy-specific stress in the first and second trimesters. Women who exercised in the third trimester reported less anxiety in that trimester compared to nonexercisers. As discussed later in this chapter, physical activity is also recommended to improve symptoms of the "postpartum blues."

## Exercise and Body Image

Adjusting to physical changes in their bodies and associated changes in body image is a challenge for pregnant women. A prospective study compared ratings of body image satisfaction from six months prepregnancy to 23 to 30 weeks gestation for high-exercising (40 women) and low-exercising (31 women) healthy pregnant women (Boscaglia et al. 2003). The criterion for assignment to the high exercise group was at least 90 minutes per week of moderate-intensity activity. Women reporting no or minimal amounts of exercise were considered low exercisers. The authors also compared expectations of body image satisfaction for the postpartum period in the two exercise groups. At 15 to 22 weeks gestation, high exercisers demonstrated significantly higher levels of body image satisfaction compared to low exercisers. No other significant differences were noted between groups. Of interest, however, was within-group differences among high exercisers. They were

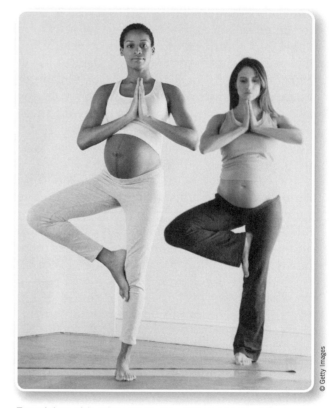

Exercising with other pregnant women can provide security, build confidence, and bring about a positive sense of self.

significantly more satisfied with their bodies at 15 to 22 weeks gestation compared to six months prepregnancy. Low exercisers demonstrated no significant changes over time. The findings suggest that women are able to assimilate the bodily changes of pregnancy with a positive shift in body image satisfaction.

### Beliefs About Exercise and Exercise Behaviors

Limited research has addressed women's beliefs about the value of exercise and their actual exercise behaviors during pregnancy and postpartum. A retrospective study of postpartum women was conducted to examine women's most salient beliefs about exercise (Symons Downs and Hausenblas 2004). The most common beliefs during pregnancy were that exercise improves mood and that physical limitations (such as nausea) obstructed exercise participation. The most common exercise beliefs during the postpartum period were that exercise controls weight gain and that lack of time obstructed exercise participation. Women's husbands or partners and family members most strongly influenced their pregnancy and postpartum exercise behavior, a finding confirmed in other studies (Blum et al. 2004).

# Benefits and Barriers to Physical Activity During and After Pregnancy

Understanding women's beliefs about exercise during and after pregnancy is useful when one is designing programs and strategies to increase participation in physical activity and exercise. Potential benefits or advantages ("pros") of prenatal exercise are listed next along with some of the common barriers or disadvantages ("cons"). Each woman will weigh her individual "pros" and "cons" when making a decision about exercising during pregnancy. A positive decision results from increasing the "pros," eliminating or overcoming the "cons," or both.

Most of the barriers to prenatal exercise are also present after the baby arrives. Finding ways to overcome the barriers before the birth increases the likelihood that a regular exercise

## Benefits and Barriers to Prenatal Exercise

Benefits ("pros") of prenatal exercise:

- ◆ Improves mood and self-esteem
- ◆ Provides relief of discomfort such as nausea, fatigue, and back pain
- ◆ Promotes health of the baby
- ◆ Helps control weight gain
- ◆ Develops skills for labor and birth
- ◆ Speeds recovery from labor and delivery
- ◆ Helps the woman assimilate bodily changes without negative impact on body image
- ◆ Provides opportunities to be with other pregnant women
- ◆ Provides a source of information and reassurance

Barriers ("cons") to prenatal exercise:

- ◆ Physical limitations (nausea, fatigue, back pain)
- ◆ Lack of support from family and friends
- ◆ Lack of child care
- ◆ Lack of time
- ◆ Lack of access to appropriate exercise programs
- ◆ Lack of education about healthy behaviors
- ◆ Lack of safe exercise environments
- ◆ Lack of transportation.

program will be part of the postpartum experience. In fact, a prenatal exercise program can be the introduction to lifelong physical activity and fitness.

## Promoting Participation in Prenatal Exercise Programs

Research has shown that a woman without significant health problems can participate in regular, low- to moderate-intensity activity during an uncomplicated pregnancy. There are, however, some conditions that preclude exercise during pregnancy. Absolute contraindications to aerobic exercise include the following:

◆ Significant cardiac disease

◆ Restrictive lung disease

◆ Cervical incompetence

◆ Multiple gestation at risk for premature labor

◆ Placental abruption (separation of the placenta from the uterus)

◆ Placenta previa (low-lying placenta)

◆ Persistent bleeding

◆ Premature labor

◆ Ruptured fetal membranes

◆ Preeclampsia (hypertension diagnosed after 20 weeks gestation with protein in the urine)

Relative contraindications include the following:

◆ Severe anemia

◆ Unevaluated arrhythmia

◆ Chronic bronchitis

◆ Poorly controlled diabetes, hypertension, seizure disorder, or thyroid disease

◆ Extreme obesity or underweight

◆ Very sedentary lifestyle

◆ Fetal growth restriction

◆ Heavy smoking

Adapted, by permission, from ACOG, 2002, "ACOG committee opinion number 267," *Obstetrics and Gynecology* 99: 171.

While the development and delivery of prenatal exercise programs should be individualized for each woman, here are a few general guidelines that are especially important in work with this special population (Cowlin 2002):

◆ Conduct a comprehensive initial screening. Any medical conditions that preclude exercise must be identified by the obstetrician, and clearance from the doctor must be obtained.

◆ Develop the initial exercise prescription based on the woman's age, level of fitness and prior experience with exercise, heart disease risk factors, orthopedic issues, current medications, other significant medical problems, prior obstetric history, and stage of pregnancy.

◆ Monitor and modify exercise programs based on the individual woman's tolerance and experience.

◆ Encourage women to keep an exercise log. Having precise information about each exercise component will help pinpoint areas where adjustments are needed.

◆ Encourage women to review their exercise programs with their health care providers at their regular prenatal checkups. This review becomes a means for the provider to advise if any changes in activity are needed.

◆ Provide an exercise setting that is safe and that encourages skill mastery, cooperation, and companionship.

◆ Integrate education and support into prenatal exercise classes. Bring reliable sources of information into class and arrange displays for review before and after class. Organize talks by local birth educators, medical professionals, lactation consultants, and parenting experts. Invite husbands or partners, family members, and close friends to participate in the group educational activities.

◆ Help the woman stay focused on the goal of having a healthy baby. Resist the tendency to commiserate with women about how pregnancy is debilitating to the body. Women who are concerned about giving up their usual fitness routine should be encouraged to remember that making a healthy baby is goal number one. Remind them that the restrictions on their fitness program due to pregnancy are short-lived. Pregnancy is the time for them to be present in their new body and focus on the possible rather than the impossible.

◆ Suggest that experienced exercisers take up a new activity, such as swimming laps. Sports that require complicated equipment (such as scuba diving) or a potentially hazardous environment (such as soccer or squash) are unsafe during pregnancy. See "Exercises to Completely Avoid During Pregnancy" in the sidebar on page 80. For women who participated in competitive athletics, a safe alternative is to perform the movements of the sport or activity in a safe setting, without equipment or other players.

◆ Encourage women to seek support for physical activity from their husbands or partners, family members, and friends. Women need to learn how to ask specifically for the type of support they want. People can give support directly by serving as a walking partner or attending a prenatal class, or indirectly by providing care for children or help with chores so the woman can attend an exercise class. Praise for initiating and maintaining physical activity is also meaningful.

◆ Avoid making diagnoses of discomforts that might be medical conditions. However, many common discomforts can be relieved by simple noninvasive methods. Share the handout on tips for dealing with discomforts of pregnancy that is provided in appendix B (page 226).

# Prenatal Exercise

The physical demands described earlier require that modifications be made to various aspects of the exercise routine, especially for women who have medical or obstetrical complications. A clinical evaluation should be done by an obstetrician or gynecologist before any pregnant woman embarks on a fitness program.

## Frequency, Intensity, Time, and Type

To assist women in planning for exercise during pregnancy, the type of exercise, as well as the intensity, frequency, and durations, should be reviewed. Frequency can be daily. Weight-bearing aerobic sessions should be from 20 minutes (for the less fit woman) to a maximum of 45 minutes (for the highly fit woman). Women need also be aware that as the pregnancy progresses, exercise becomes more difficult and may need to be modified in intensity, type, or duration.

Because of changes in the cardiovascular system during pregnancy, heart rate is not always a good indicator of how hard a woman is exercising. A subjective measure of effort, such as the Borg scale (rating of perceived exertion or RPE; see table 7.1 on page 114), is useful, especially during the second and third trimesters. "Fairly light" to "hard" (10 to 14 on the scale) is a safe, moderate range that is effective for reducing discomforts, promoting placenta development, and improving cardiovascular conditioning in preparation for labor and delivery. Lower ratings ("fairly light"—10 to 11) are appropriate when the woman is experiencing sleeplessness or nausea. Women who desire to work at a high subjective level ("very hard"—16 or above) must have written instructions from their health care provider stating that this range is appropriate for them.

Swimming is probably the safest and most relaxing physical activity during pregnancy. It has the added advantage of weightlessness and allows for cooling, which is important to

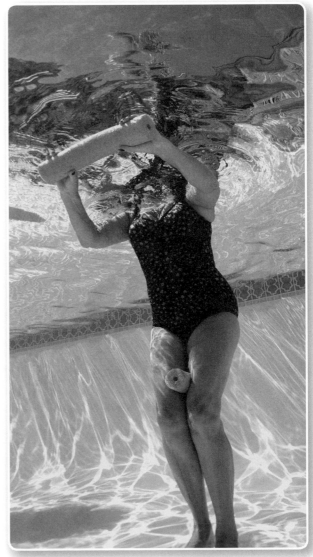

Advise pregnant swimmers to avoid crowded pools to reduce the risk of getting kicked.

## Exercises to Completely Avoid During Pregnancy

- ◆ Contact sports
- ◆ Scuba diving
- ◆ Supine exercise (after the first trimester)
- ◆ High-altitude exercise
- ◆ Any activity that increases risk for abdominal trauma or falls, such as water skiing, skateboarding, or squash

Adapted, by permission, from ACOG, 2002, "ACOG committee opinion number 267," *Obstetrics and Gynecology* 99: 171

avoid heat stress. Jogging, on the other hand, is a higher-risk activity during pregnancy. But women who have participated in jogging or running prepregnancy often elect to continue and can do so safely. Share the handouts in appendix B with women who want to swim or jog during pregnancy (pages 224 and 225).

### Positions and Biomechanical Adjustments

After the first trimester, lying in the supine position (on the back) is not advised because it can cause orthostatic hypotensive syndrome. Orthostatic hypotensive syndrome refers to a very low blood pressure due to body position. Standing still for long periods of time may also cause this problem. In the second and third trimesters, exercises normally done on the back should be done on the side, while seated, or on the hands and knees.

The changes in body alignment shown in figure 5.1 increase the risk for injury. The spine and the pelvis are the most critical areas to address in maintaining near-normal alignment during pregnancy. Improved alignment can be achieved through posture awareness, education, and corrective exercises.

### Special Strength and Flexibility Exercises

Exercises to strengthen weak muscles and stretch tight muscles are needed. The musculoskeletal system has to adjust to the changes as the pregnancy progresses. Always be aware of the muscle groups that are becoming increasingly shortened and lengthened and adjust the exercise

program accordingly. The strengthening parts of a prenatal exercise program should emphasize the following:

◆ Strengthening the gluteals, hamstrings, hips, and quadriceps for lower body strength—Pregnant women can do most standard exercises for these muscles unless a specific exercise causes discomfort or is not recommended due to another underlying issue, such as orthopedic injuries or lumbo-pelvic-hip complex issues. Examples of exercises include the following:

- – Seated hamstring machine or standing leg curls.
- – Standing hip extension using a cable system or resistance bands.
- – Side-lying hip abduction with or without resistance (bands).
- – Basic body squats to strengthen the whole leg. Body squats performed with wide foot positioning and outwardly rotated hips can prepare for the birth squat, which is shown in figure 5.2.

◆ Strengthening the deep abdominal muscles and pelvic floor—Abdominal exercises can be done in a seated position, crawling position (on hands and knees), and while lying on the side.

- – Pelvic tilts can be done either supine, standing, or in the crawling position (shown in figure 5.3).
- – Anterior-posterior pelvic tilts can be combined with lateral pelvic tilts to produce a rotation action of the pelvis on the spine and legs.

◆ Strengthening the pelvic floor (Kegels)—It is important that women learn to relax, as well as contract, these muscles. Kegels and other exercises for the pelvic floor can help prevent and reduce urinary incontinence (Chiarelli and Cockburn 2002; Morkved et al. 2003) Three muscular actions are recommended.

- – Closing and opening the pelvic outlet by contracting the ischiocavernous, transverse perineal, and gluteal muscles, pulling the ischia, pubis, and coccyx together to make the pelvic outlet smaller.
- – Lifting and lowering and preparation for pushing (called elevator Kegels) by lifting the pelvic floor and holding the internal organs in position, then exhaling and compressing the transverse muscle, pushing (bearing down) the diaphragm toward the vaginal

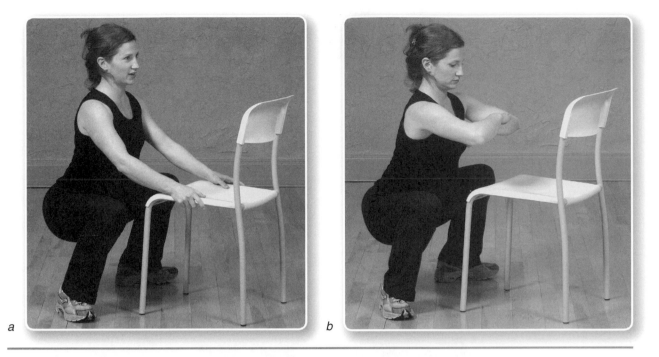

**Figure 5.2** Birth squats may help prepare for delivery. The woman may use a chair for support *(a)* when first attempting the birth squat; with practice she progresses to the unsupported squat *(b)*.

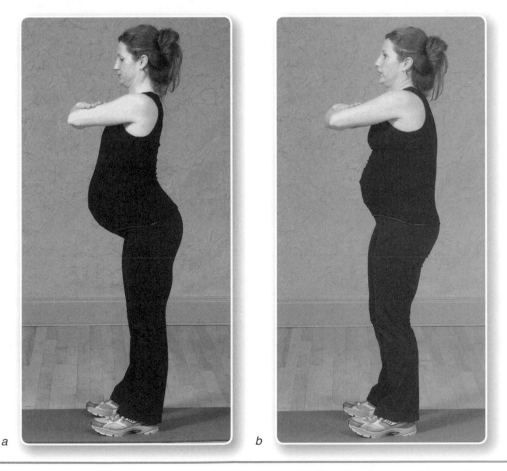

**Figure 5.3** Anterior-posterior pelvic tilt: *(a)* anterior tilt; *(b)* posterior tilt. These motions, combined with lateral pelvic tilts, help strengthen the muscles that control the pelvis.

opening (women can gently practice this exercise once a month during a relaxation session, but should not do this pushing action regularly or with any force until pushing in labor).

- Contracting the sphincter muscles by closing the orifices of the vagina and urethra, and the anus, respectively, then relaxing (called wave Kegels). To test the strength of the sphincter that controls the vaginal and urethral openings, women can urinate until the bladder is about two-thirds empty, then squeeze and stop the flow of urine. They hold for a few seconds, then relax and empty completely. Include these exercises as part of a workout and instruct women to evaluate improvements in strength periodically with the urine test.

◆ Strengthening the upper back and posterior aspects of shoulders—Machines, bands, hand weights, and cables can be used for these exercises.

- Scapula retraction and depression (see the seated row exercise in figure 5.4).
- Rear deltoid (reverse fly).
- Extension of the thoracic spine (see figure 5.5).

◆ Strengthening chest, shoulders, and arms

- Keep in mind the chest and anterior aspects of the shoulder may already be shortened.

Strength training can continue during pregnancy if the proper guidelines are followed. Advise women to avoid the Valsalva maneuver.

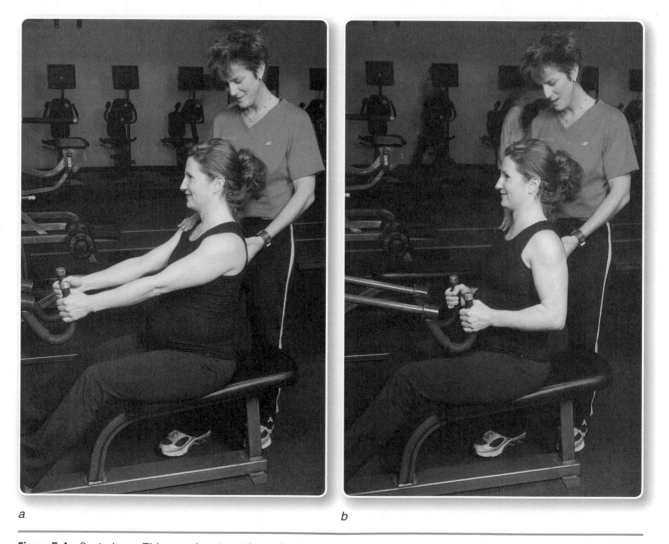

*a*　　　　　　　　　　　　　　　　　　*b*

**Figure 5.4** Seated row. This exercise strengthens the back and improves posture. Be sure to keep the back straight and the head upright at the start *(a)* and end *(b)* of exercise.

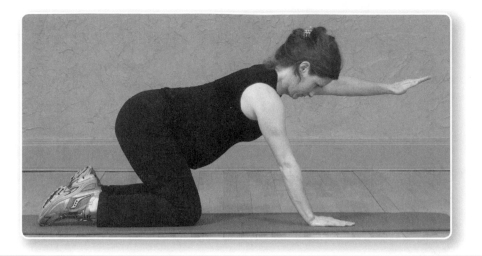

**Figure 5.5** Modified quadraplex with single arm raise. This exercise increases strength in the erector spinae.

They should exhale through the most difficult part of the exercise and inhale during the less stressful phase of the exercise. When putting together strength programs for pregnant women, be sure to use free weights with caution; use machines at low resistance; and use bands, tubes, or the body's own weight for resistance. Whenever feasible, pregnant women should perform strength exercises from a seated rather than a standing position; and again, they should avoid the supine position after the first trimester. Low to moderate resistance, medium to high repetitions, and many sets, sometimes spread out or in a circuit training technique, most closely mimic the physical demands of pregnancy (Cowlin 2002).

The flexibility parts of the prenatal exercise program should emphasize the following:

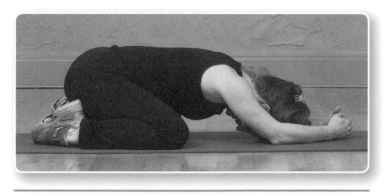

**Figure 5.6** Rest pose. Resting in this position provides an opportunity for muscles governing the spine and trunk to relax and for the low back to stretch gently. As the pregnancy progresses, a woman will find that opening the knees wider creates more space for the baby.

- ◆ Stretching the low back (see the rest pose in figure 5.6).
- ◆ Stretching the hip flexors, adductors, IT band, and tensor fascia latae.
- ◆ Stretching the chest and anterior aspects of the shoulder (see figure 5.7).
- ◆ Centering activities such as yoga or tai chi (physical balance and mental calm) to promote efficient alignment and motion should also be included. Yoga-based prenatal exercises and Pilates movements can be especially helpful and enjoyable during pregnancy (see figure 5.8, modified reverse plank).

Rolling exercises should be omitted, however, and abdominal exercises should be limited during and after the second trimester. Pilates stretches, modified bridges, side leg kicks, and modified push-ups can be continued through the third trimester.

There are a few specific recommendations for stretching during pregnancy. Advise women to move slowly and use good form, identifying the line of stretch. They should breathe deeply and remain static for 15 to 30 seconds, focusing on lengthening the line of stretch and letting go of tension or tightness. The downward dog maneuver, shown in Figure 5.9, is one example. Make sure pregnant women avoid overstretching, ballistic movements and extreme ranges of joint motions. They should avoid

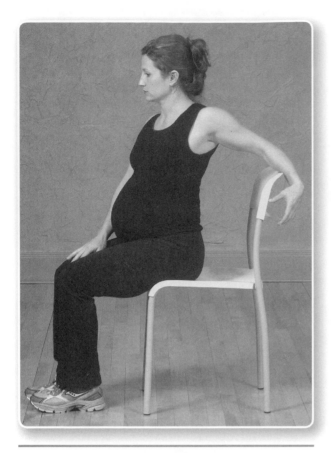

**Figure 5.7** Chest stretch. The woman sits in a comfortable position with the neck and back straight. Perform the stretch by placing one arm over the back of a chair, creating slight tension in the chest and shoulder.

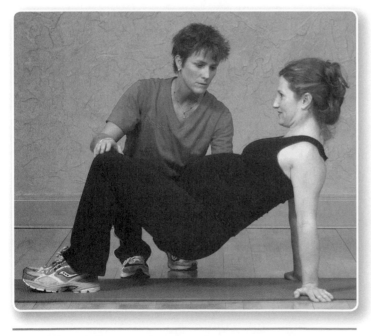

**Figure 5.8** Modified reverse plank. This maneuver increases core strength.

*overstretching* the hamstring and adductor muscles, which may increase pelvic girdle instability or hypermobility. More information about general stretching programs is provided in chapter 9. Information about postural imbalances during pregnancy is provided in chapter 10.

## Breathing, Fatigue, and Hydration

The hormone progesterone causes pregnant women to have a tendency to hyperventilate. To avoid hyperventilation and breathlessness, the woman should breathe slowly and deeply through all phases of exercise. If necessary, she should slow down for a moment. Slow, deep breathing during aerobic exercise approximates the breathing associated with labor. It helps the woman learn to stay focused and remain calm and relaxed during a challenging activity. Slowly inhaling and exhaling during strength and flexibility exercises is also important.

During pregnancy, less blood glucose is available for exercise, causing fatigue. Women should stop exercising when feeling fatigued. Sometimes a small carbohydrate snack and water or juice will provide enough sugar to allow them to continue exercising. Adequate protein in the overall diet is important to maintain energy over the course of the day.

Adequate water is needed for the cooling process and to ensure adequate blood volume. Before exercising, pregnant women should drink 4 to 8 ounces (118 to 237 milliliters) of water. They should drink an additional 2 to 4 ounces (59 to 118 milliliters) every 20 to 30 minutes during exercise. Total consumption of water should equal 2 quarts (8 cups or about 2 liters) over the course of the day, more if needed. Very active women should be encouraged to drink water until their urine is light yellow, since thirst is not a reliable predictor of dehydration. During hot, humid weather, exercise should take place only in a cooled or air-conditioned environment.

## Terminating Exercise

A well-designed prenatal exercise program is safe for most women. However, if a woman experiences any of the warning signs listed in the sidebar, she should stop exercising and seek immediate evaluation by an obstetrician. Fortunately, for the majority of women, these warnings are unlikely to occur.

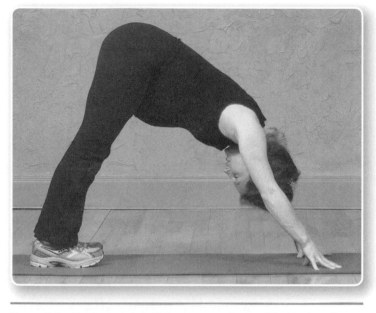

**Figure 5.9** Downward dog. This pose may be modified by bending the knees. Note that she uses her fingertips instead of her palms; this helps reduce wrist pain and risk of carpal tunnel syndrome.

## Warning Signs for Terminating Exercise

- ◆ Vaginal bleeding
- ◆ Dyspnea (shortness of breath) prior to exertion
- ◆ Light-headedness
- ◆ Headache
- ◆ Chest pain
- ◆ Muscle weakness
- ◆ Signs of thrombophlebitis (swollen, tender leg veins)
- ◆ Uterine contractions
- ◆ Decreased fetal movement
- ◆ Leakage of amniotic fluid

Adapted from ACOG Committee Opinion Number 267, January 2002. *Obstet Gynecol* 2002;99:171.
Source: © 2005 *UpToDate* ® www.uptodate.com

## Nutrition Guidelines for Active Women During Pregnancy

After the first trimester, women require an additional 300 calories per day during pregnancy. They should choose a wide variety of foods with approximately 60 to 90 grams of protein per day for a single baby (or an additional 10 grams per baby per day above their nonpregnancy needs) spread among the various meals and snacks (Cowlin 2002). Pregnant women should consume diets high in complex carbohydrates but avoid intake of large quantities of concentrated carbohydrates over brief time periods. When eating fats, they should choose high-quality vegetable oils such as olive or canola oils, avocados, nuts, and seeds and avoid saturated and trans fats. They should eat 200 to 300 calories every 2 to 3 hours, depending on gestational stage, body weight, and level of activity. To avoid hypoglycemia, exercise time should be limited to 45 minutes. The recommended weight gain during pregnancy is 25 to 35 pounds (11.3 to 15.9 kilograms) if the woman's prepregnancy weight is normal. Overweight women should gain 15 to 25 pounds (6.8 to 11.3 kilograms), and obese women should gain less than 15 pounds.

## Special Conditions and Circumstances

Pregnancy and birth are normal processes for women, and most have a successful experience. Discomforts such as nausea, fatigue, constipation, backache, and leg cramps are common and can usually be managed. Share the tips for dealing with these and other discomforts during pregnancy (see handout in appendix B on page 226). Also, encourage women who are thinking about having a baby to assess their health and make lifestyle changes that can benefit their health (and the health of their baby) before becoming pregnant. Participating in regular physical activity, eating a healthy diet, and losing weight if they are overweight can help them avoid complications during their pregnancy. Serious conditions that may be improved or affected by physical activity include preeclampsia and gestational diabetes.

### Preeclampsia, Chronic Hypertension, and Gestational Hypertension

Hypertensive disorders are among the most common medical complications in pregnancy.

There are several major hypertensive disorders of pregnancy: preeclampsia, chronic hypertension, and gestational hypertension. Preeclampsia occurs in 6 to 8 percent of all pregnancies in the United States. About 70 percent of preeclampsia cases occur with first-time pregnancies (National Heart, Lung, and Blood Institute 2005). Preeclampsia is characterized by the development of high blood pressure and protein in the urine after the 20th week of pregnancy. It is unknown why first pregnancies are at higher risk for preeclampsia. Chronic hypertension refers to the condition in women who have been diagnosed with high blood pressure prior to pregnancy. Preeclampsia can be superimposed on chronic hypertension. Gestational hypertension usually develops late in pregnancy, is mild, and does not feature proteinuria (as preeclampsia does). Although many pregnant women with high blood pressure have healthy babies without serious problems, high blood pressure can be dangerous for both the mother and the fetus.

Risk factors for preeclampsia are listed in the following sidebar. Regular prenatal care includes monitoring blood pressure and protein in the urine. Even though high blood pressure and related disorders during pregnancy can be serious, most women with high blood pressure and those who develop preeclampsia have successful pregnancies.

According to the National High Blood Pressure Education Program (National Heart, Lung, and Blood Institute 2005), preeclampsia does not in general increase a woman's risk for developing chronic hypertension or other heart-related problems. The National High Blood Pressure Education Program (NHBPEP) also reports that for women with normal blood pressure who develop preeclampsia after the 20th week of their first pregnancy, short-term complications—including increased blood pressure—usually go away within about six weeks after delivery.

Specific problems associated with preeclampsia are outlined in the sidebar "Preeclampsia—Problems for the Mother and the Fetus."

## Risk Factors for Preeclampsia

- First pregnancy
- Chronic high blood pressure before pregnancy
- Preeclampsia during a previous pregnancy
- Obesity prior to pregnancy
- Pregnancy before age of 20 or after age of 35
- African American or Hispanic ethnicity
- Family history of preeclampsia
- Pregnancy with more than one baby
- Presence of diabetes, kidney disease, rheumatoid arthritis, lupus, or scleroderma

## Preeclampsia—Problems for the Mother and the Fetus

For the mother:

- Pulmonary edema (fluid in the lungs)
- Decreased kidney function
- Liver damage
- Seizures (called eclampsia)
- Headache, blurry vision, cerebral hemorrhage
- Death

For the fetus:

- Growth restriction
- Placental abruption
- Hypoxia
- Premature birth (necessitated by maternal or fetal complications)
- Stillbirth

Epidemiologic studies show that occupational and leisure-time physical activity is associated with a reduced incidence of preeclampsia (Weissgerber et al. 2004). The protective effect of exercise could result from one or more of the following mechanisms:

- Stimulation of placental growth and vascularity
- Reduction of oxidative stress
- Exercise-induced reversal of maternal endothelial dysfunction

Because the pathologic mechanisms in preeclampsia are similar to those in cardiovascular disease, for which physical activity is shown to be protective, studying the potential benefits of physical activity on preeclampsia risk has significant merit.

The effects of work and regular leisure-time physical activity during early pregnancy on risk of preeclampsia and gestational hypertension were studied in women recruited from 13 obstetric practices (Saftlas et al. 2004). Information on time at work spent sitting, standing, and walking, and on leisure-time physical activity before and during pregnancy, was collected via face-to-face interviews. Findings suggested that women who engaged in any regular leisure-time physical activity (regardless of caloric expenditure), were unemployed, or had nonsedentary jobs were at a decreased risk of preeclampsia. No protective effect of physical activity was shown for gestational hypertension.

Another study assessed the potential benefits and risks of recreational physical activity before and during pregnancy in 201 preeclamptic and 383 normotensive women (Sorensen et al. 2003). Using a case control design, the authors collected information about the type, intensity, frequency, and duration of physical activity performed during the first 20 weeks of pregnancy and during the year before pregnancy. Overall, women who engaged in any regular physical activity during early pregnancy, compared with inactive women, experienced a 35 percent reduced risk of preeclampsia. Compared with inactive women, those engaged in light or moderate activities experienced a 24 percent reduced risk of preeclampsia. Women participating in vigorous activities during early pregnancy experienced a 54 percent reduction in risk. Recreational physical activity performed during the year before pregnancy was associated with similar reductions in preeclampsia risk.

## Gestational Diabetes

Gestational diabetes is a condition characterized by high blood glucose levels that begin during pregnancy and disappear following delivery. About 3 to 5 percent of all pregnant women in the United States are diagnosed with gestational diabetes.

Unlike type 1 or type 2 diabetes, gestational diabetes does not cause birth defects. Birth defects typically originate during the first trimester (before week 13) of pregnancy in women with diabetes whose blood glucose levels are not well controlled. Gestational diabetes usually does not occur until approximately the 24th week. Women who develop gestational diabetes generally have normal blood glucose levels during the critical first trimester of their pregnancies.

Children of mothers who had gestational diabetes have a greater than normal risk of developing obesity and diabetes in late adolescence and young adulthood. Women with gestational diabetes have a 60 percent increased risk of developing a permanent form of diabetes later in life (American Diabetes Association 2002). In addition, women who have had gestational diabetes during one pregnancy have a 40 to 50 percent chance of developing gestational diabetes in the next pregnancy.

With gestational diabetes, the problem does not occur because the pancreas is not producing enough insulin (as is the case with type I diabetes). Women with gestational diabetes produce plenty of insulin. In fact, they usually have more insulin in their blood than women who are not pregnant. The problem is in the placenta. During pregnancy, the placenta provides the baby with nourishment. The placenta also produces a number of hormones that have a blocking effect on insulin, making the cells of the body resistant to insulin. The larger the placenta grows, the more these hormones are produced and the greater the insulin resistance becomes (Touchette 2002).

Because the pancreas works to produce extra quantities of insulin to compensate for insulin resistance, most pregnant women do not suffer from gestational diabetes. When the pancreas makes all the insulin it can and there still isn't enough to overcome the effect of the placenta's hormones, gestational diabetes results. The blocking effect on insulin usually begins about midway (20 to 24 weeks) through pregnancy and stops after delivery when the placenta is no longer releasing hormones into the mother's blood (Touchette 2002).

Most women with gestational diabetes have no recognizable symptoms of diabetes. Women with gestational diabetes may be more likely to develop high blood pressure during their pregnancy. Undiagnosed and untreated gestational diabetes is risky to the developing child. Without treatment, the mother's blood glucose levels will be consistently too high.

A common problem among babies of women with gestational diabetes is a condition called macrosomia, or excessive fetal birth weight. If the mother's blood has too much glucose, the excess glucose will cross the placenta and pour into the baby's system through the umbilical cord. The unborn baby's pancreas will respond to the high level of glucose by producing larger amounts of insulin. The insulin will allow the baby's cells to take in the glucose, where it will be converted to fat and stored. Babies of mothers with gestational diabetes can be abnormally large.

Babies who are abnormally large cause more difficult deliveries. The mother may also develop too much amniotic fluid, which can cause the baby to be born too soon. High blood glucose levels in the mother may be associated with increased risk of fetal demise during the last four to eight weeks of pregnancy.

Because gestational diabetes can exist with no symptoms and because it puts the developing baby at an increased risk, risk assessment and testing for the condition are a routine part of pregnancy care. Testing for gestational diabetes is usually done between the 24th and 28th week of pregnancy. By this time, the hormones from the placenta have reached a level sufficient to cause insulin resistance.

Women who are at high risk for gestational diabetes (see sidebar) will usually undergo glucose testing as soon as possible. Women of high risk who do not have gestational diabetes at the initial screening will be tested again between the 24th and 28th week of their pregnancy. Women of average risk will be tested at 24 to 28 weeks. Women with low risk of developing gestational diabetes do not require glucose testing, but this category is limited to women who possess none of the risk factors listed.

In an article aptly titled "No need for a pregnant pause..." Dempsey and colleagues review the literature regarding the role of physical activity in prevention and control of gestational diabetes mellitus (2005). Their review of observational studies and clinical trials suggested that roughly 30 minutes per day of moderate-intensity activity during pregnancy may substantially decrease the risk of developing gestational diabetes. Sixty minutes per day of moderate-intensity activity

## Risk Factors for Gestational Diabetes

◆ Overweight (20 percent or more over ideal body weight before pregnancy)
◆ Family history of diabetes (parents or siblings have diabetes)
◆ Having previously given birth to a very large, very heavy baby (over 9 pounds or 4 kilograms)
◆ Having previously had a baby who was stillborn or was born with a birth defect
◆ Excess amount of amniotic fluid (the cushioning fluid within the uterus that surrounds the developing child)
◆ Over 25 years of age
◆ Member of an ethnic group known to experience higher rates of gestational diabetes (in the United States, these groups include Mexican Americans, American Indians, and African Americans, as well as individuals from Asia, India, or the Pacific Islands)
◆ Previous history of gestational diabetes during a pregnancy

for those already diagnosed with gestational diabetes may result in better glycemic control. Another small study of women with gestational diabetes showed that resistance training may help overweight women delay the need for insulin or reduce the amount of insulin needed for diabetes control during pregnancy (Brankston 2004).

Women with gestational diabetes who are unable to control their blood glucose levels by following a meal plan and exercising regularly may need to take insulin by injections. Women who use insulin are at risk for a low blood glucose reaction or hypoglycemia if they do not eat enough food, if they skip a meal, if they do not eat at the right time of day, or if they exercise more than usual. Hypoglycemia is a serious problem that needs to be treated right away. Symptoms of hypoglycemia include the following:

◆ Confusion
◆ Dizziness
◆ Feeling shaky

◆ Headaches

◆ Sudden hunger

◆ Sweating

◆ Weakness

After pregnancy, women with gestational diabetes should follow a meal plan and regular exercise program to manage their weight and reduce their risk of developing gestational diabetes with a future pregnancy or type 2 diabetes in the future. They should encourage healthy eating and regular exercise among their children to prevent them from developing type 2 diabetes later in life. While lifestyle changes are recommended for women with gestational diabetes, one study showed that, even though the majority of women with gestational diabetes were concerned about developing overt diabetes, only a few made changes in their lifestyles and lost weight after pregnancy (Stage et al. 2004).

# Postpartum Exercise

Technically, the postpartum period refers only to the first six weeks following birth. During this time, the woman's reproductive tract returns to its nonpregnant condition. Even after birth, many of the physiological characteristics of the pregnancy remain, such as enlarged feet and stressed knees and hips; soft abdomen; possibly hemorrhoids and varicosities; enlarged waist circumference due to expansion of the rib cage; and swollen breasts. Stress incontinence, periods of heavy sweating and skin blotches, and sleeplessness may also persist after pregnancy. Some of the musculoskeletal conditions resulting from pregnancy and birth are listed in the sidebar.

There are also several common muscle imbalances that a woman may experience after pregnancy. Because of shifts during pregnancy, muscles can be improperly aligned, causing the following alterations in muscle action:

◆ Shortening and tightening of low back and iliopsoas (hip flexors)

◆ Shortening of thoracic spinal flexors and pectoral muscles

◆ Overstretching and weakening of gluteals and hamstrings

## Musculoskeletal Conditions Resulting From Pregnancy and Birth

◆ *Diastasis recti*—the separation or tearing of abdominal muscles away from the linea alba or a plastic stretching of the linea alba that results in a widening or deepening (or both) of the trough between the recti abdominal muscles

◆ *Separation of the symphysis pubis*—damage to the connective tissue of the symphysis pubis to the extent that the two pubic rami move independently

◆ *Sacroiliac dysfunction/sciatica*—sacroiliac slippage, spasm in the medial gluteal, or spasm in the piriformis muscle

◆ *Fractured coccyx*—occurs when the coccyx bones are severely pushed back during delivery, enough to cause a fracture

◆ *Upper back pain*—can be caused by the positioning of the baby during nursing or from extreme shoulder tension during the pushing phase of labor

◆ *Low and mid-back pain*—results from poor biomechanics, decreased abdominal strength, and postepidural discomfort

◆ *Lower limb problems*—circulation problems, as well as problems due to joint laxity

◆ Overstretching and weakening of abdominal muscles and pelvic floor

◆ Overstretching and weakening of upper back muscles

The postpartum period allows for healing of tissues, realigning the body toward a normal posture, and learning to manage the stresses associated with meeting the baby's needs. Balancing the demands of a new baby with the desire to get back in shape takes some planning. Although the baby takes number-one priority in the mother's life, she needs to care for her own body so it will recover and function normally. Postpartum women can restart an exercise program as soon as they feel able. For some, this is as early as a few days after delivery. Be sure the

## Exercise Safety in the Postpartum Period

◆ Conduct an assessment to check for complications.

◆ Develop an individualized program that includes basic core body exercises and walking.

◆ Avoid quick abduction of the legs for about 8 to 10 weeks.

◆ Avoid percussive, ballistic, or high-impact movements until core body strength is restored and joint laxity or soreness has disappeared.

◆ Advise women to maintain a healthy diet and adequate fluid intake, especially if breast-feeding (see the handout "Tips for Physically Active Nursing Mothers" on page 227 in appendix B).

woman has obtained clearance from her health care provider before beginning any postpartum exercise program. Guidelines for exercise safety in the postpartum period are outlined in the sidebar above.

### At-Home Exercises for Immediate Recovery

It is beneficial for the new mother to set aside a few minutes several times during the day—perhaps while the baby is sleeping—to focus on these recovery activities. Appropriate at-home exercises for immediate recovery include Kegels or pelvic floor exercises. Strengthening and stretching exercises to correct muscle imbalances are critical. Use the information in chapters 8, 9, and 10 to recommend exercises to correct the muscle imbalances listed earlier. Walking or other nonimpact aerobic activity is also recommended.

As soon as the woman feels able, she can do abdominal exercises to correct minor cases of diastasis recti. For a defect greater than 0.8 inches (2 centimeters) or very deep defects, consultation with a physical therapist is helpful. For women who undergo cesarean section, abdominal exercises should be delayed until six to eight weeks postpartum.

### Exercise and the Postpartum Blues

Rapid hormonal changes, shifting attention of family and friends, and a sense of loss after pregnancy may produce a mild depressive state. Called the "postpartum blues," these feelings often occur around the third to fifth day following birth. A positive environment and caregiving from family and friends can help minimize these feelings and their effects. It is important, however, to distinguish between the blues and true postpartum depression. If a woman demonstrates ongoing negative emotions, extreme fatigue, or an inability to deal with her infant, encourage her to see her obstetrician or a mental health professional.

Exercise in the postpartum period is recommended to improve mood, decrease anxiety, and facilitate weight loss. One study addressed maternal well-being on the basis of sport or exercise activity participation during prepregnancy and through the postpartum period (Blum et al. 2004). Women who maintained or increased sport or exercise activity showed better well-being compared to women who reported no sport or exercise activity or decreased activity from prepregnancy to postpartum. As reported previously, support from husband or partner, family, and friends was a significant factor in maintaining or increasing exercise activity.

### Breast-Feeding and Exercise

Women who are breast-feeding worry that exercise may affect milk production. A study by Dr. Kathryn Dewey showed that exercise doesn't decrease milk production in humans (Dewey et al. 1994). Exercise does increase the content of lactic acid in breast milk, especially if exercise is vigorous and if the breasts are not emptied prior to exercise. However, in Dewey's study this didn't lead to rejection of nursing by infants of mothers who exercised vigorously. The exercise also had no effect on infant weight gain. If an infant does reject milk postexercise, then advise the mother to collect milk pre-exercise and pump and discard milk postexercise. For other sound advice about hydration, clothing, and ways to relieve the discomforts of nursing, share the handout "Tips for Physically Active Nursing Mothers" on page 227 in appendix B with women who exercise while nursing.

## Including the Baby in Postpartum Exercise Classes

When they are ready, an exercise class is an excellent opportunity for mom and baby to do something together outside of the house. Babies usually begin attending exercise classes with mom after about six weeks, although this time frame probably depends more on the mother than the baby's age. In the beginning, just managing to get to the class with the baby and all the associated supplies is a major accomplishment. Group exercise instructors must be tolerant of late arrivers and provide a setting in which mothers and babies feel relaxed. Expect that it may take one or two sessions for newcomers (mom and baby) to adjust to the surroundings and the stimulation of the class.

As the mothers are able to become more involved in their own exercise routines, they can include exercises that allow them to interact with their babies, such as abdominal muscle or other floor exercises. Moms should not hold their infants in a wrap or sling device while doing standing exercises (too much biomechanical stress). The instructor should also advise about the risk of shaken baby syndrome during any upright movement while a baby is being held or carried. Older babies and toddlers enjoy stroller workouts (see www.strollerfit.com for locations of programs).

During the exercise classes for baby and mother, babies benefit from receiving extra stimulation from the other mothers and babies and from the exercise instructor. Moms can also help their babies work on developmental tasks, such as grabbing for an object, holding their heads up, or crawling (Cowlin 2002).

# Nutrition and Weight Loss After Pregnancy

Achieving prepregnancy weight is a major concern for most women in the postpartum period. One of the most important pieces of advice a health care professional can give a woman is to avoid excessive weight gain during pregnancy. Excess weight gained during pregnancy and failure to lose weight by six months postpartum is associated with long-term obesity (Rooney and Schauberger 2002).

If the woman has eaten a healthy diet during pregnancy and continues to follow an appropriate eating plan in the postpartum period, her body weight should return to a healthy, nonpregnant weight. How long this takes depends upon genetics, diet, physical activity, and breastfeeding. Women who are breast-feeding generally require an additional 300 to 500 calories a day during this time. However, it is easy for women to fall into the habit of eating for comfort because this is something that is providing for the baby. If a woman is not breast-feeding, the metabolic rate slows, reducing the need to eat as much or as often. Restarting regular exercise will assist women in achieving their weight

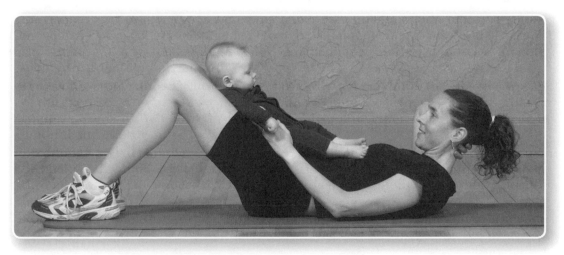

A mother can work on her abdominal strength while interacting with her baby.

loss goal, usually over 6 to 12 months. Women should consider all these factors and be realistic when setting expectations for losing weight after pregnancy.

Health and fitness professionals should strongly encourage postpartum women to enroll in a structured diet and exercise program. A study addressed the impact of an individualized, structured diet and physical activity program on weight loss in overweight women during the first year postpartum (O'Toole et al. 2003). Forty overweight postpartum women were randomized to either a structured or a self-directed intervention. Women in the structured program received individualized diet and physical activity prescriptions derived from baseline measure-

ments. They met weekly for the first 12 weeks and kept daily food and activity diaries. Women in the self-directed program received a 1-hour educational session on diet and activity. Of the 40 participants, only 23 remained in the study after one year postpartum. Of those remaining, women in the structured intervention showed a significant weight loss and decrease in body fat. There were no significant changes in the women in the self-directed group. The women who committed to one class per week for 12 weeks had a high likelihood of successful weight loss that persisted at one year. Women who were overweight before pregnancy were unlikely to lose the pregnancy-related weight without the help of a formal intervention.

## ◆ Conclusion ◆

We began this chapter with an overview of the physical changes occurring in the pregnant woman's body that relate to physical activity. Shifts in the center of gravity affect posture and balance and create opportunities for overuse injuries. Increases in levels of the hormone relaxin also increase the risk of injury. Because of the additional heat generated by the mother and baby, thermoregulation during physical activity is a concern.

A review of current research studies indicates that appropriate physical activity during pregnancy appears to have no deleterious effects on birth outcomes. Physical activity may reduce the risk of low birth weight. It is not clear whether exercise has any direct effect on labor and delivery. Compared to nonexercisers, women participating in leisure-time physical activity reported less depressed mood, fewer daily hassles, and less pregnancy-specific stress. High exercisers demonstrated higher levels of body image satisfaction compared to lower exercisers.

A well-designed prenatal exercise program is safe for most women. However, fitness professionals need to be aware of the absolute and relative contraindications to exercise, exercises to completely avoid during pregnancy, and signs for terminating exercise. Suggestions for appropriate modifications to aerobic exercise, strength training, and flexibility programs were given, with specific illustrations for correcting posture and muscle imbalances and preparing for delivery. We also discussed serious conditions that may be improved or affected by physical activity, including preeclampsia and gestational diabetes.

Exercise in the postpartum period is recommended to improve mood, decrease anxiety, and facilitate weight loss. We provided guidelines for exercise safety, at-home exercises for immediate recovery, ways to include the baby in postpartum exercise classes, and tips for active nursing mothers.

In conclusion, physical activity can help women achieve a sense of general well-being and health as they experience the childbearing years and transition to menopause. Menopause is the subject of the next chapter of this book.

# CHAPTER 6

# Exercise During and After Menopause

## Topics in This Chapter

- ◆ Goals of fitness programs
- ◆ Phases and characteristics of menopause
- ◆ Benefits and barriers to activity after menopause
- ◆ Promoting participation in regular physical activity
- ◆ Essential exercise components
- ◆ Frailty and its consequences
- ◆ Functional fitness
- ◆ Fitness programming in retirement communities and care facilities

Keep in mind that exercising after forty is no longer about competition or looking cute in a leotard. This isn't about the buns of steel or a six-pack abdomen. This is about using exercise as a way to destress your daily mental wear and tear, decrease your perimenopausal symptoms, get fit and firm, and guarantee high-quality living into the twenty-first century.

Pamela Peeke, MD, MPH, author of *Fight Fat After Forty*

Life expectancy of women in the United States is approximately 80 years, which means that menopause occurs at a time when women have yet to experience more than one-third of their total life span. With the population aging, an estimated 40 million American women will experience menopause during the next 20 years. There is a growing need to address the health issues of women in the menopause years. Their quality of life depends on it.

When discussing menopause, it is important to remember that it is a normal event in a woman's life, not a disease. Some women view menopause as a positive and liberating experience. Others think of it as a negative event. Menopause offers health and fitness professionals an opportunity to encourage physical activity and fitness as a way to prevent disease, optimize health, and improve quality of life.

## Goals of Fitness Programs for Women During and After Menopause

Women who are approaching menopause and those who have recently completed the menopausal transition are among the leading edge of the "baby boomers." They are more likely than older women to have been involved in some type of performance-based fitness program in past years. At this time, however, the goal of their fitness programs may need to shift from performance to disease prevention and management.

Older women who have never participated in a traditional exercise program have much to gain from being active in their later years of life—70s, 80s, and even 90s. It is important for older women to know that it is never too late to get started with a fitness program and enjoy the benefits.

Maintaining or improving physical function is, of course, the short-term goal of fitness for women after menopause. Midlife is a good time to begin to focus on the goal of building the strength and coordination that may have been neglected in the younger years. Adequate strength is necessary for good balance and can help prevent falls and fractures in future years. Improving posture also appeals to a woman's desire to look good. Some women in this age group may have or develop limitations and may need special attention or rehabilitation. The long-term goal for older women is to promote independent living and quality of life for as long as possible.

## The Major Life Transition of Menopause

Western medicine defines three phases of change associated with menopause: perimenopause, menopause, and postmenopause.

◆ *Perimenopause* is about a three- to six-year period before menopause. During this time, women and their health care providers begin to identify changes. Fewer follicles (in the ovaries) lead to anovulatory cycles and elongated periods. Estrogen and progesterone decrease, the luteal phase shortens, and other menstrual irregularities increase. Levels of follicle stimulating hormone and luteinizing hormone remain high. Gonadotropin production is no longer inhibited. There is usually a lessening of menstrual flow. But frequent or heavier periods may be experienced for a while by some women. Eventually menses stops.

◆ *Menopause* is the time after 12 months of amenorrhea (cessation of menses). When a woman has stopped having periods for a full year, she is considered to have reached menopause. The average age when women stop menstruating is 51 years. However, some women attain menopause as early as the late 30s or as late as the early 60s. Menopause occurs earlier in women who smoke, have a family history of early menopause, or have never been pregnant. Menopause occurs later in women with multiparity and in those who are obese. The term "surgical menopause" is used when a woman has both ovaries removed. Menopause may also be induced by chemotherapy or pelvic radiation.

◆ *Postmenopause* is the time after menopause. Changes continue to occur. Increased rates of heart disease, osteoporosis, type 2 diabetes, Alzheimer's, obesity, high blood pressure, high cholesterol, and other conditions are noted in the postmenopausal years.

Bone loss with age disproportionately affects women. Women have smaller, lighter bones than men. As shown in figure 6.1, with menopause women experience a period of rapid bone loss over several years. Starting perhaps as early as their 30s, women lose bone every year. At menopause, this effect is exaggerated and women experience more rapid bone loss for several years. After this period of rapid bone loss, bone density continues to decrease, but at a much slower rate, typically less than 1 percent bone loss per year (Kohrt et al. 2004). As shown in figure 6.2, with cumulative bone loss, fracture risk increases.

Some of the changes associated with menopause are due to lower levels of estrogen. In fact, hormone replacement therapy (estrogen and progesterone given together) has been shown to lower risk of osteoporotic fracture and colon cancer. Unfortunately, hormone therapy has also been shown to increase risk of heart attack, stroke, blood clot, and breast cancer (Rossouw et

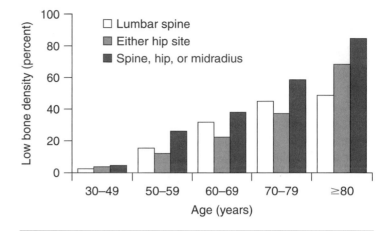

**Figure 6.1** The incidence of low bone density increases rapidly above age 50 in the spine, hip, and midradius.

Reproduced with permission from: Rosen, HN, Basow, DS. Screening for osteoporosis. In: UpToDate, Rose, BD (Ed), UpToDate, Waltham, MA, 2006. Copyright 2006 UpToDate, Inc. For more information visit www.uptodate.com.

al. 2002). In women who take estrogen without progesterone (usually women who have had their uterus removed), stroke risk and blood clot risk were increased, but not heart attack and breast cancer risk (Anderson et al. 2004).

Many studies have demonstrated that menopause has no significant effect on age-related weight gain. The weight gain that occurs after age 50 may be associated more with decreases in resting metabolic rate than with hormonal shifts. Unless women make adjustments in calorie intake and physical activity, they can expect to gain about 1 pound (0.45 kilograms) per year (Sternfeld et al. 2004). A handout with tips for healthy eating practices and weight management

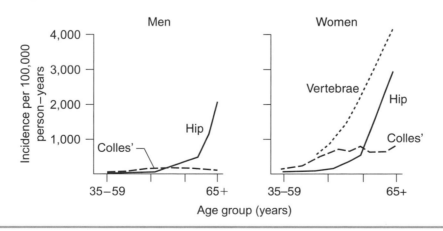

**Figure 6.2** Incidence rates for the three common osteoporotic fractures in men and women, plotted according to patient age at the time of fracture. The overall fracture rate is increased approximately threefold in women. Information on vertebral fracture incidence in men was not included in the study.

Reprinted, by permission, from B.L. Riggs and L.J. Melton III, 1986, "Medical progress: Involutional osteoporosis," *New England Journal of Medicine* 314: 1676-1686. Copyright © 1986 Massachusetts Medical Society. All rights reserved.

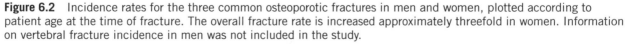

is provided in appendix B on page 219. The handout on calcium supplementation in appendix B (page 222) is also appropriate for women after menopause.

Menopause is associated with modest increases in total fatness and accelerated accumulation of abdominal body fat. High levels of body fat are a predictor of kyphosis, one of the major postural deformities seen in older women. Abdominal fat gain is also associated with increases in cholesterol levels, blood pressure, cardiovascular disease, type 2 diabetes, breast cancer, and arthritis.

### Characteristics of Menopause

Family history, genetics, and lifestyle determine how women experience menopause. Although there is no one universal pattern, there are a number of identifiable characteristics that many women experience in response to hormonal changes. Only vasomotor symptoms (hot flashes), disordered sleep, and some vulvovaginal symptoms have shown more favorable relief after hormone replacement therapy than placebo and can therefore be convincingly attributed to changing hormone levels and menopause.

Symptoms directly or indirectly related to the menopause transition include the following:

Vasomotor symptoms (hot flashes and night sweats)

Sleep-related symptoms

Mood changes

Sexual dysfunction

Problems with concentration and memory

Irregular menses

Urogenital symptoms

Vasomotor symptoms are the most common characteristic of menopause. Over 80 percent of women report these symptoms at some time. These conditions are real and are aggravated by stress. Avoiding hot spicy foods and beverages, reducing caffeine, and avoiding alcohol help manage vasomotor symptoms. Wearing layered clothing that can be removed or added as necessary is another way to deal with hot flashes. Any use of medications or supplements to relieve these symptoms should be directed by a qualified health care provider after consideration of the individual woman's health status, risk factors for certain diseases, and preferences.

### Exercise and Symptoms of Menopause

There is conflicting evidence as to whether exercise improves menopausal vasomotor symptoms. One study by Li and colleagues (1999) sums up the literature best. This study of 214 perimenopausal women showed no differences in vasomotor and menstrual symptoms with regard to activity level. Interestingly, though, more-active women reported fewer psychosomatic symptoms such as irritability, forgetfulness, and headache, as well as fewer sexual symptoms such as vaginal dryness and decreased sex drive. The important message from this study, and others like it, is that exercise helps to reduce some menopausal symptoms and therefore may make hot flashes more tolerable. Fortunately, vasomotor symptoms eventually go away after menopause.

Vaginal thinning contributes to a reduction in mucus production that may cause discomfort during sexual intercourse. Intravaginal estrogen cream, tablets, or vaginal lubricants may be helpful in relieving symptoms. Changes in the vagina may also mean that women are more inclined to contract vaginal or urinary tract infections.

Urogenital problems, such as bladder thinning and bladder or uterine prolapse, are more common after menopause. Bladder thinning can cause urinary urgency and incontinence. Most incontinence can be treated with medications, Kegel exercises, or behavior modification techniques. Exercises to strengthen the pelvic floor muscles may also help reduce symptoms from bladder or uterine prolapse. High-impact weight-bearing physical activity may not be advised for postmenopausal women with significant prolapse.

## Benefits and Barriers to Physical Activity in Menopausal Women

Physical activity has the potential to reduce the negative impact of menopause and prevent or delay some conditions associated with aging. Specifically, there is significant evidence that physical activity and exercise can improve health outcomes (lower the risk of cardiovascular disease, stroke, some cancers, obesity, type 2 diabetes, osteoporosis, and other conditions)—all more common, but not inevitable, with age. Fitness has an important role to play in reducing almost every risk factor for chronic disease that women face. There is nothing, however, known to medical science that will stop normal aging.

In addition to benefits to physical health, physical activity may help relieve stress. Stresses in midlife are significant. Many women in their 50s often have responsibility for parenting their own children while at the same time serving as caregivers for aging parents. That's why they are sometimes called the "sandwich generation." Add the demands of a full-time job outside the home and the body and identity changes associated with menopause and aging, and it's no wonder that some women feel stressed.

Promote regular physical activity as an effective stress management technique and a way to achieve balance among major life areas (family responsibilities, job responsibilities, and personal care). Stretching, deep breathing, and progressive muscle relaxation are other ways to promote relaxation. Encourage women to select a strategy and practice it several times a week for at least 15 minutes at a time. As with other types of exercise, these strategies must be practiced regularly to yield the desired results.

As just mentioned, one particular stress that this age group of women often has to deal with is caring for an elderly parent. Providing care for an elderly or disabled adult requires a great deal of energy, patience, time, and love. All too often, women who are caregivers don't take care of themselves. And sometimes caregivers are hesitant to ask for help or support from others. If you know a woman who is a caregiver, listen carefully for indicators that she needs help. Remind her that she can't help others if she doesn't take care of herself first. Encourage her to identify whether she is having any of the following problems.

- Difficulty taking care of her personal needs—eating, exercising, grooming
- Not getting enough rest
- Feeling overwhelmed, fearful, or angry as a result of being a caregiver
- Feeling negative toward the person she is caring for
- Receiving abuse from the person she is caring for
- Experiencing financial constraints
- Experiencing difficulties dealing with her spouse or other family members

If so, then suggest that she turn to whatever support systems she has developed or recommend professional help.

Having a positive body image also has definite advantages for women as they grow older and begin to encounter the unique image problems related to aging. In a society that defines feminine beauty with reference to a teenage movie star, older women are at a distinct disadvantage. And many older women lack positive examples of active women in their age group. The challenge for the older woman is to adjust her self-image as her body changes and to congratulate herself for who she is at the particular time in her life (Lutter and Jaffee 1996). Being physically active is one of the best ways for older women to improve and maintain a positive self-image. Other tips for helping women improve their body image are provided as a handout on page 218 in appendix B.

Clearly there are numerous benefits for older women who participate in regular physical

## Barriers ("Cons") to Physical Activity

- Pain of osteoarthritis
- Poor health and functional capacity
- Fears of injury
- Urinary incontinence
- Lack of knowledge about the benefits of being active
- Lack of skills
- Bad weather
- Time constraints due to work, family, or caregiving responsibilities
- Financial constraints
- Lack of transportation
- Embarrassment in wearing exercise clothes
- Feeling uncomfortable in exercise facilities
- Lack of an exercise partner
- Lack of social support
- Travel or vacation plans

activity. Still, there are barriers to overcome. Consider the barriers unique for this age group as listed in the sidebar on the previous page. Handouts are provided in appendix B for women dealing with osteoarthritis and incontinence, which are common barriers to physical activity for older women. The handout on osteoarthritis gives tips related to medications, exercise, hot/cold treatments and topical pain relievers, joint protection, good posture, weight control, and coping skills. The handout on urinary incontinence explains how the body makes, stores, and releases urine. Types of urinary incontinence are defined, and diagnostic and treatment options are explained.

Encourage women to weigh their personal "pros" and "cons." Focus on helping them see more advantages to being active and engage in problem-solving exercises to overcome the barriers or disadvantages. It's all a matter of decisional balance. Until women see more "pros" than "cons" for physical activity, they will resist participating in regular physical activity or have difficulty maintaining a fitness program.

# Promoting Participation in Regular Physical Activity

When developing programs to promote physical activity and fitness among older women, give consideration to the following:

◆ *Place for exercise:* Some women are comfortable in a traditional fitness center or gym, while others prefer a women's gym. Some are more likely to attend fitness programs in places where they go for other functions, such as a church or community center. Others prefer the advantages of exercising at home, perhaps with an exercise video, or walking in their neighborhood with a friend. For women who choose to exercise at a fitness facility, the physical characteristics of the space are important. Cleanliness, attractiveness, temperature control and comfort, access to bathrooms, and comfortable floor surfaces are features that older women say influence their decisions about a specific exercise facility.

◆ *Opportunity for socialization:* Enjoyment is a critical factor in long-term adherence to physical activity. Women enjoy exercising with other women. Social support and networking—hallmarks of the female life cycle—are critical to a

woman's wellness during midlife and beyond. By this time in life, most women have already developed skills for adjusting or acquiring an appropriate social network. Women benefit from the opportunities to share their experiences of stressful life events (death of family member, divorce, relationship issues, job change) with other women.

◆ *Education:* Including education along with time for exercising, socializing, and networking appeals to many women. Organizing rehabilitative exercise groups for older women around lifestyle or disease management issues, such as heart disease, breast cancer, diabetes, or osteoporosis, may attract women with special needs.

◆ *Sport programs:* Masters sport programs (softball and basketball leagues and track, field, and swim meets) provide competitive outlets for those women so inclined.

◆ *Pool training:* Water exercise is safe and effective and adds variety to the exercise program. It is especially effective for women with mobility challenges and chronic joint conditions or those recovering from surgery.

◆ *Flexible schedules:* A revolving-door approach to fitness programming for postmenopausal women is best. Attendance may vary with the seasons. Don't require or expect commitment for classes or programs of more than about eight weeks in duration.

◆ *Lifestyle physical activity:* Because lack of time is a major barrier to physical activity for some postmenopausal women, be sure to promote lifestyle physical activity. Help women figure out for themselves how they can fit physical activity into their daily lives. Housework, gardening, playing with and caring for grandchildren, and walking to do errands are examples of ways to include physical activity with other routines or tasks.

◆ *Screenings and assessments:* A variety of information is needed to help develop individualized exercise plans for women in this age group. Try to use an intake survey that collects information about the woman's prior as well as current physical capabilities. Build on experiences from her youth to encourage present-day physical activity.

◆ *Program evaluation techniques:* Participant satisfaction and subjective appraisals of participants' experience are better indicators of program success than objective measures of clinical outcomes. Attendance and adherence are also useful evalu-

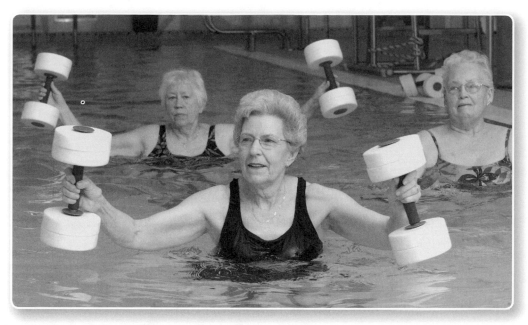

Exercising in water is especially appealing to women with osteoarthritis.

ation tools. Asking clients to evaluate personal outcomes and program elements on a rating scale can be helpful.

## Essential Exercise Components for Balanced Fitness

While the aerobic component may be given highest priority in younger women, the other exercise components (strength, stability, flexibility) should have increasing emphasis after menopause. This section presents general guidelines that are appropriate for a balanced fitness program for postmenopausal women. More information about specific components of fitness is provided in chapters 7, 8, and 9.

### Aerobic Activity

As shown in figure 6.3, one-fourth of women between 65 and 74, and 40 percent of women over 75, do not engage in regular physical activity. With age and lack of activity, women experience a decline in $\dot{V}O_2max$. The decline in $\dot{V}O_2max$ is multifactorial, but largely due to decrease in maximal heart rate, stroke volume, and cardiac output (Wiebe et al. 1999). A study by Fleg and colleagues (2005) showed that the decline in $\dot{V}O_2max$ in healthy women is not

steady with age, but accelerates markedly with each age decade. However, the level of fitness of exercisers will be far better than in those who are inactive, at any age. As compared to inactive women, exercising women will likely have five or more years of life and less disability. It can be difficult to motivate older women to exercise more, but we must convey to them that if they give up doing things that are hard, inevitably things that once were easy become hard.

More detailed information about aerobic activity for women is provided in chapter 7. The guidelines in the sidebar on the following page are useful in work with older women.

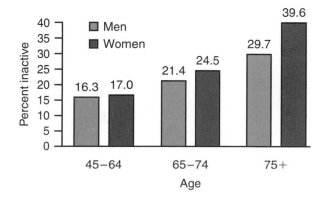

**Figure 6.3** Many older women do not engage in regular physical activity.

From U.S. Department of Health and Human Services, Centers for Disease Control and Prevention, National Center for Chronic Disease Prevention and Health Promotion.

# Aerobic Exercise Guidelines for Older Women

General principles of exercise prescription apply to adults of all ages. Elderly people should be encouraged to meet the population-wide recommendations to accumulate at least 30 minutes of moderate-intensity physical activity on most and preferably all days of the week. This can be accomplished with activities such as brisk walking, gardening, yard work, housework, climbing stairs, and active recreational pursuits (Whaley 2006). Guidelines are as follows:

◆ *Frequency:* Three to five days per week.

◆ *Intensity:* 40/50 percent to 85 percent $\dot{V}O_2R$ (inactive elderly people should start low and individually progress according to tolerance and preference).

◆ *Mode:* Walking is excellent. Aquatic and stationary cycling are advantageous for those with reduced ability to tolerate weight-bearing activity. (Exercise modality should not impose excessive orthopedic stress.)

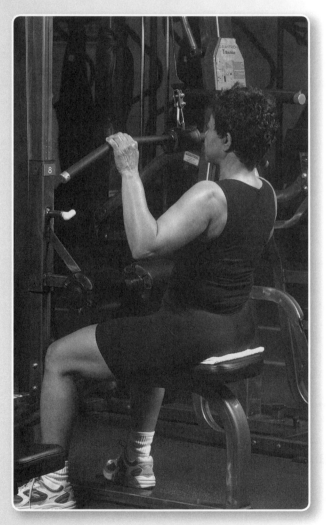

◆ *Duration:* 20 to 60 minutes. Those who have difficulty sustaining exercise for 30 minutes or prefer shorter bouts can be advised to exercise for 10-minute periods at different times throughout the day. Exercise duration need not be continuous to produce benefits. To avoid injury and ensure safety, older individuals should initially increase duration rather than intensity.

◆ Warm-up and cool-down periods ranging from 5 to 10 minutes are typically recommended. Older women may feel more comfortable with warm-up and cool-down periods of 7 to 10 minutes.

More tips:

◆ Suggest using a pedometer to assess or monitor lifestyle activity.

◆ Offer water exercise programs year-round (if an indoor pool is available) or seasonally in warm climates.

◆ Be aware of medications (especially beta-blockers) that alter the heart rate when considering intensity of aerobic activities.

◆ For beginners, be sure they know the signs of exertion (breathing changes, feeling warm, fatigue), how to take their pulse, and subjective ways to assess their level of exertion.

Women who are already fit may be challenged with circuit training, which combines aerobic exercise and strength training.

◆ Share the handout on hydration tips provided on page 220 in appendix B.

◆ Recognize that the already fit woman may prefer to exercise at a higher intensity.

## Strength Training

As shown in figure 6.4, only about 12 percent of adults 65 to 74 years of age and about 10 percent of adults 75 years of age and older meet current strength training recommendations. Several physical changes attributed to normal aging include decrease in number and size of muscle fibers and cells, decreased circulation (increases injury healing time), increased recovery time, and decreased neural function (reduction in motor response). However, with regular strength training, these changes can be delayed or their effects can be minimized (Reichel 1989).

In addition to the specific strength training guidelines provided in chapter 8, keep the points in the sidebar in mind when developing strength training programs for older women.

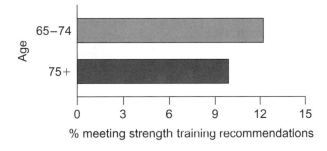

**Figure 6.4** Few older adults meet the recommendations for strength training.

From U.S. Department of Health and Human Services, Centers for Disease Control and Prevention, National Center for Chronic Disease Prevention and Health Promotion.

## Balance and Stabilization

Balance and stabilization training are crucial for older women, especially in the prevention of falls. A study of older men and women compared physical function and activity, falling history, and fear of falling (Gardner and Montgomery 2004). Older women had reduced amounts of physical function, expended fewer calories daily, and experienced a higher prevalence of falling and fear of falling than older men. Tai chi training is an effective activity for diminishing fear of falling in older adults (Harmer et al. 2002). Tai chi is also beneficial for developing better joint **proprioception** and static and dynamic balance.

Details for developing stabilization programs are provided in chapters 8 and 9. Women can

## Strength Training Guidelines for Older Women

- ◆ Focus on functional performance rather than specific sport or athletic performance.

- ◆ Include strength training on two days per week, then progress to three days per week.

- ◆ Strength training sessions should last from 20 to 45 minutes. Longer durations of strength training sessions are not necessarily better and may even cause extreme fatigue.

- ◆ Include exercises that safely load the spine, pelvis, and femurs to help minimize bone and muscle loss.

- ◆ Strength in the hips, trunk, and legs is essential for balance and coordination.

- ◆ When possible, focus on multijoint exercises and activities (such as holding a static squat position while performing a row), rather than single-joint exercises, to work more than one muscle group per exercise.

- ◆ Begin with one set of exercises and progress to no more than three sets. Increasing the number of repetitions may be a better way to progress than increasing the load. (Maximum strength testing is not recommended for older women.)

- ◆ Allow muscles to rest for a day between strength training sessions. Each woman will need to make adjustments to prevent inflammation and soreness.

learn the sensations of core body stabilization through centering techniques, tai chi, Pilates, dance, yoga, and the use of exercise balls. Include exercises to manage or correct poor posture, if needed. Conclude exercise programs with a period of relaxation and other stress management techniques. Share the handout for reducing risks for falls and fractures that is provided on pages 231-332 in appendix B. The handout presents tips for preventing falls, ways to reduce the risk of falls at home, and recommendations for what to do if a fall occurs.

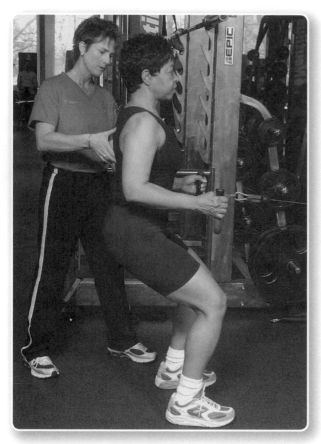

When possible, focus on multijoint exercises that safely load the spine, pelvis, and femurs such as a static squat while performing a row.

## Flexibility

Loss of flexibility and reductions in joint range of motion are the result of lack of activity as much as the aging process. Flexibility training in older adults can delay soft tissue dehydration, improve range of motion, and reduce tissue damage and injury (Clark 2001). Options for flexibility training include stretching, Pilates, yoga, tai chi, and water exercises. Women who have arthritic conditions, fibromyalgia, or who have had joint replacement should be encouraged to participate in water activities, especially on days of increased pain and discomfort.

Several physical changes affecting flexibility are attributed to normal aging (Clark 2001):

◆ Muscle atrophy
◆ Neural (nerve) atrophy
◆ Tissue dehydration
◆ Increase of tissue stiffness (tendons, ligaments, fascia)

## Stretching Guidelines for Older Women

Include stretching as a part of every group fitness program or personal training session. For women who exercise on their own, encourage them to include five to seven sessions each week. Ideally, stretching should be done every day. Remind them to

◆ perform slow, static stretches to the point of end range of motion tightness (no pain);
◆ hold stretches for 15 to 30 seconds; and
◆ perform a minimum of two to four repetitions of stretches for each of the major muscle or tendon groups (or both) (Whaley 2006).

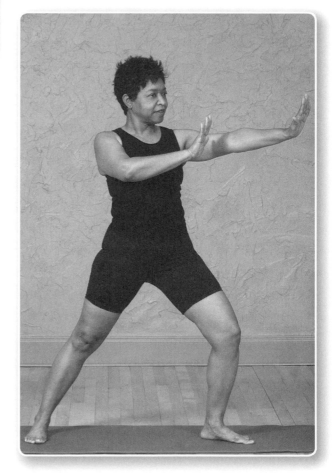

Tai chi helps improve balance in older women, which is important in preventing falls and fractures.

Stretching guidelines for older adults are similar to those for the general population (Whaley 2006; see the sidebar). For more specific information about flexibility programs, see chapter 9.

# Exercise to Forestall Frailty

Keeping women physically active may forestall frailty. After age 65, women are more likely to be affected by frailty than men. Because elderly women outnumber elderly men in the population, frailty is an especially important issue for women and their health care providers. The definition of frailty isn't perfectly clear, but women who meet three or more of the criteria listed in the sidebar below are likely to be frail (Fried et al. 2001). Having any of these warning signs of frailty may lead to development of other signs and more serious consequences.

And for women who already meet these criteria, regular exercise can help reverse frailty. A 2002 randomized controlled trial showed that a supervised exercise program can significantly improve $\dot{V}O_2$peak and strength in frail individuals aged 78 or older (Binder et al. 2002). The

nine-month exercise program in this study was administered in three 3-month parts. The first part addressed stretching, balance, and mild strength training. The second part of the program built on this foundation by adding a more strenuous weightlifting component. The final three months focused on endurance exercise, but also continued exercises from the first two parts. The rate of injury in the study was quite low, likely due to the progressive nature of the program. This was the first study of its kind to show that the losses seniors experience with frailty can be reversed with a supervised, progressive exercise program.

Even the frailest of elderly women should perform regular weight-bearing and strength training activities to maintain bone health and reduce risk of falls. Reducing falls is critical to reducing fractures in the elderly. A home-based exercise program for strength and balance retraining of women aged 80 and older reduced falls and injuries and was initiated with just four home visits by a physical therapist (Campbell et al. 1997). This study was replicated using a trained nurse instead of a physical therapist and again, falls and injuries were reduced in elderly women (Robertson 2001). A review article examining 12 different studies of fall prevention in the elderly showed that falls were successfully reduced in studies that used strength and balance retraining, endurance training, or tai chi (Gardner 2000). Of course, extra attention to safety during exercise is warranted for those with frailty.

Stronger back muscles are associated with reduced risk of vertebral fracture, as shown in a study by Sinaki and colleagues (2002). In this study, postmenopausal women were reexamined eight years after completing a randomized controlled trial of resistive back-strengthening exercises. Eight years after the study, the women who completed the exercise program still had stronger muscles than the control (nonexercising) women. The relative risk of compression fracture of the spine was 2.7 times greater in the control (nonexercising) women.

Depression is a consequence of frailty and this may also be improved with exercise. In a small study of depressed elders, supervised progressive resistance training three times a week not only elevated mood, but also improved strength, morale, and quality of life (Singh 1997a). This same study of depressed elders also showed that a supervised weight-training program

## Warning Signs and Consequences of Frailty

Warning signs of frailty

- ◆ Unintentional loss of 10 pounds (4.5 kilograms) or more in the previous year
- ◆ Exhaustion
- ◆ Ranking in the weakest 20 percent for one's age on measure of grip strength
- ◆ Ranking in the slowest 20 percent for one's age on walking speed
- ◆ Expending less than 270 calories per week on physical activity

Consequences of frailty

- ◆ Infections
- ◆ Fractures from falls
- ◆ Depression
- ◆ Loss of independence
- ◆ Premature death

improved subjective sleep quality (Singh 1997b). Since exhaustion is a sign of frailty, improving sleep through increasing physical activity is appropriate.

# Functional Fitness in Older Women

One of the key aspects of aging successfully is maintaining functional fitness. Functional fitness is the ability to independently perform basic activities of daily living. A study by Nelson and colleagues (2004) showed that women aged 70 and older improved their function as measured on a physical performance test after participating in a six-month program of progressive strength, balance, and general physical activity exercises.

All older women, particularly the very old or frail, can improve mobility and function with regular physical activity, even if they have problems such as arthritis. The ability to perform these movements enables older women to live independently and enjoy the best possible quality of life. In addition to the personal benefits of staying independent, there are significant economic benefits. Staying active reduces the cost of health care and medications as shown in figure 6.5. Note the sharp increase in costs beginning after age 65. It also costs less to live independently than to live in an assisted-living facility. And it costs less to live in an assisted-living facility than in a nursing home.

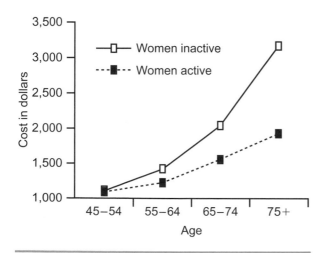

**Figure 6.5** Staying active reduces the cost of health care and medications.

From U.S. Department of Health and Human Services, Centers for Disease Control and Prevention, National Center for Chronic Disease Prevention and Health Promotion.

## Promoting Programs for Functional Fitness

As you design and deliver programs to help older women improve their functional abilities, don't just teach them to perform the exercises. Also educate them about the role of function in performing activities of daily living. A 12-week weight training study confirmed the benefit of education along with exercise. One group was educated about training-related strength gains and performing activities of daily living. The second group received instructions on proper weight training technique only. At the end of the study, group 1 had greater self-efficacy for performing activities of daily living in the lab than group 2 (Vincent et al. 2002).

Here are more tips for promoting programs to improve functional fitness:

◆ Conduct a needs assessment. Ask the participants about their medical conditions and limitations. Consult with family members, physical therapists, or other health care providers as needed.

◆ Perform tests to assess functional fitness and identify risk for loss of functional mobility. (See information on *Senior Fitness Test Manual* by Rikli and Jones, 2001, later in this section.)

◆ Select exercises geared to the specific muscle groups needing attention. (See information on *Functional Fitness for Older Adults* by Brill, 2004, later in this section.)

◆ During the class, explain how the specific exercise relates to an activity of daily living (something the participant wants to be able to do) and improves quality of life.

◆ Start slowly and gradually increase activity time and intensity. Once a participant achieves a maintenance level of fitness, vary the regimen to enhance compliance.

## Recruiting Participants in Retirement Communities and Care Facilities

Retirement and assisted-living communities, nursing homes, and Alzheimer's care facilities can also benefit from offering physical activity programs for their residents. Residents who participate in regular physical activity are usually happier and healthier. Active and independent residents mean less work for overburdened aides, also reducing the costs associated with turnover of residents (residents moving to nursing homes). In addition, a physical activity program is a great marketing tool for attracting new residents.

It may seem that older women, especially those who live in retirement or assisted-living communities, would be motivated to participate in group exercise programs. (They enjoy socializing and lack of time is not generally a barrier at this time in life.) However, as for all age groups, there are unique barriers to participating in physical activity. You will have to work just as hard to get older women to participate in your classes as with any other age group. Here are a few tips to help increase participation in group activity programs in retirement and assisted-living communities:

- Enlist the help of others—friends, caregivers, aides.
- Offer classes in areas where people naturally congregate—cafeteria, arts and crafts room.
- Schedule the class before or after another popular activity, such as crafts classes or sing-alongs.
- Don't call it an exercise class. Instead use words such as "activity," "club," or "games."
- Extend personal invitations to join the activity.
- Introduce a new participant to the group. Assign a "buddy" to make her feel welcome.
- Let participants who miss classes know they are missed.
- Invite nonparticipants to observe the class.
- Ask participants to demonstrate some of the movements and give personal testimony about how they have benefited.
- Play music. Let participants make the selections.
- Have a theme class, such as a luau, country-western, belly dancing, or Halloween.
- Take photos and post them on a bulletin board.
- Track attendance. Develop a recognition program or honor roll. Give small door prizes or certificates.
- Note improvement. As appropriate, lead participants in applause or a cheer.
- Report progress to family members and health care providers. Encourage them to praise the participant's effort and progress.

## Functional Fitness Resources

With the number of older adults, especially women, increasing dramatically, health and fitness professionals need more resources on functional fitness. Here are two recent references you should consider for your professional library:

*Functional Fitness for Older Adults* is an illustrated guide for activity professionals working with adults over the age of 65—especially those who are unable to complete activities of daily living because of poor functional fitness levels. The book includes a variety of specialized activity programs developed to meet the specific needs of older adults. They are designed to improve upper- and lower-body strength, balance, range of motion, and functional performance. The exercise programs are approximately 20 to 30 minutes each and fit easily into busy schedules, a variety of participants' needs, and institutional budgets. Extensive research has verified that the guidelines and programs are safe and will result in significant functional gains for most participants, improving their health-related quality of life. Specific guidelines are included for working with older adults with chronic conditions. A Program Finder helps match the program's functional purpose to the participant's characteristics. The following program guides are provided:

Lift to Function

Squeeze to Function

Strengthen to Function

Balance to Function

Walk 'n' Wheel to Function

Step Up to Function

Hold It to Function

Move to Function

Remember to Function

The *Senior Fitness Test Manual* provides simple tests to assess the functional fitness of older adults and identify people who are at risk for loss of functional mobility. An accompanying video demonstrates the seven individual fitness tests involving common activities such as getting up from a chair, walking, lifting, bending, and stretching. It also explains what equipment is needed to conduct the tests, provides safety tips, and demonstrates how to score each item. Test items include the following:

Chair stand test (lower-body strength)

Arm curl test (upper-body strength)

Six-minute walk test (aerobic endurance)

Two-minute step test (alternate measure of aerobic endurance)

Chair sit-and-reach test (lower-body flexibility)

Back scratch test (upper-body flexibility)

Eight-foot up-and-go test (agility/dynamic balance) (see figure 6.6)

Height and weight (body composition)

The Senior Fitness Test (SFT) produces continuous-scale scores on all test items across a broad range of ability levels from the borderline frail to the highly fit. Another especially important feature of the SFT is that it has accompanying performance standards for use in evaluating test results. Specifically, the SFT has five-year age-group percentile norms for independent-living men and women, ages 60 to 94, on all test items. The tests have been proven safe and enjoyable for older adults. Many exercise leaders say that taking the test is a motivating experience for this

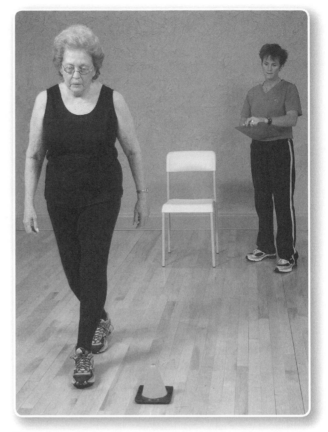

**Figure 6.6** Conduct ongoing assessments of functional fitness to determine improvements and to make any necessary changes to the program.

population. Test results can be used to set appropriate and realistic goals for fitness programs and evaluate progress.

## ◆ Conclusion ◆

With the population aging, an estimated 40 million American women will experience menopause during the next 20 years. Menopause offers health and fitness professionals an opportunity to encourage physical activity and fitness as a way to help women prevent disease, optimize heath, and improve quality of life.

This chapter began with an overview of the phases and changes associated with menopause. With menopause, women experience a period of rapid bone loss, weight gain, and vasomotor symptoms over several years. The weight gain that occurs after age 50 may be associated more with decreases in resting metabolic rate than with hormonal shifts. There is conflicting evidence as to whether exercise improves menopausal vasomotor symptoms. In one study, more-active women reported fewer psychosomatic symptoms, such as irritability, forgetfulness, headache, vaginal dryness, and decreased sex drive. Urogenital problems, such as bladder or uterine prolapse, may be reduced by exercises to strengthen the pelvic floor muscles. There is significant evidence that physical activity and exercise can improve health outcomes (lower the risk of cardiovascular disease, stroke, some cancers, obesity, type 2 diabetes, osteoporosis, and other conditions)—all more common, but not inevitable, with age.

We gave practical suggestions for promoting participation in regular physical activity among older women, as well as guidelines that are appropriate for a balanced fitness program. The strength/stability and flexibility components of fitness programming deserve added emphasis after menopause. Balance and stability are crucial for older women, especially in the prevention of falls. Keeping women physically active may forestall or reverse frailty. All older women, particularly the very old or frail, can improve mobility and function (ability to independently perform basic activities of daily living) with regular physical activity. We provide tips and resources for promoting and conducting programs to improve functional fitness, including programs for women living in retirement communities and care facilities.

In conclusion, maintaining fitness is a must for older women. No doubt, exercise routines may change, or require supervision, but it is reassuring to note that even in the oldest at-risk population, exercise can be done safely and effectively.

The three chapters in this section have looked at life events and transitions—puberty, pregnancy, menopause and the senior years—as each relates to participation in physical activity and exercise. Each transition presents unique challenges that affect health outcomes. In every case, physical activity has the potential to improve health and quality of life. Of course, it is better to adopt an active lifestyle earlier, rather than later, in life. But an important message for older women is that it is never too late to get started on an active way of life and reap benefits.

# PART III

# Exercise Prescription for Women

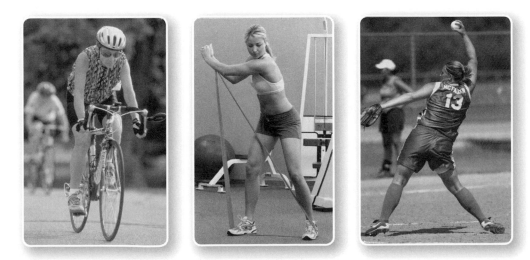

# CHAPTER 7

# Aerobic Exercise for Women

## Topics in This Chapter

- **Principles of aerobic exercise**
- **Commonly used versus customized target heart rate range**
- **Tests to determine maximum heart rate**
- **Classifications of exercise intensity**
- **Energy metabolism—burning fats and carbohydrates**
- **Intermittent versus continuous exercise**
- **Structured exercise versus lifestyle physical activity**
- **Cross and interval training**
- **How to quantify fitness levels in women**
- **Traditional aerobic exercise choices**
- **Weight-bearing versus non-weight-bearing exercising**
- **Injury prevention**

Through running, I found athleticism, but I've realized that, more important, I found strength. My body is lean, toned, and healthy. I can feel the power in my muscles, heart, and lungs. I have more energy and endurance for all things, and this is true mentally as well.

Claire Kowalchik, author of *Running for Women*

In the preceding chapters we discussed the reasons that women need exercise throughout the life span. Now it's time to talk specifically about types of exercise and how women can develop a balanced exercise program. A balanced program should have an aerobic component; a strength, power, and stability component; and a flexibility component. The relative importance of each of these components differs based on a woman's age, stage of life, medical issues, personal goals, and resources. In this chapter, we'll discuss aerobic exercise. As we covered at length in chapters 2 and 3, there are many health benefits to regular aerobic exercise.

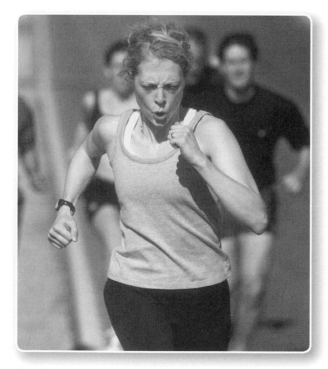

Running is just one of many aerobic exercises.

The term "aerobics" was coined by Kenneth Cooper, MD, MPH, with the publication of his book by that name in 1968. The book is often credited with spawning a "jogging craze" that encouraged millions to begin regular exercise. Dr. Cooper received countless letters in response to his book, and many were from women who wanted to know more, especially about issues unique to female exercisers. *Aerobics for Women* was published in 1972 by Dr. Cooper and his wife, Millie, to address these issues (Cooper and Cooper 1972). To this day, it contains basic information about exercise that holds true. But thousands of books and studies on exercise have been published since Dr. Cooper's original book. To better understand the relevance of new data, we must first review some basic principles of exercise. Some of these principles have stood the test of time; others have been discarded or modified based on current literature.

## Principles of Aerobic Exercise

Aerobic exercise is defined as a system of physical conditioning designed to improve respiratory and circulatory function by exercises (as running, walking, or swimming) that increase oxygen consumption. The principles of aerobic exercise are frequency, intensity, time (duration), and type, otherwise known as FITT. Most coaches, trainers, or others in fitness professions know these principles. How are they used to help women meet their goals?

### Exercise Recommendations

Using these principles, several respected groups have made exercise recommendations, including the Institute of Medicine (IOM), Centers for Disease Control (CDC), and American College of Sports Medicine (ACSM). The CDC and ACSM issued a position statement in 1995 recommending at least 30 minutes of moderate-intensity exercise (such as brisk walking) on most days of the week (Pate et al. 1995). There were ample scientific data to support this recommendation, especially for cardiovascular disease risk reduction.

In 2002, the IOM built on this recommendation by addressing weight control (Institute of Medicine 2002). Its recommendation for 60 minutes of daily moderate intensity was also backed by solid literature and was especially relevant given the obesity epidemic in the United States. The most recent exercise guidelines published jointly by the Departments of Health and Human Services and Agriculture (2005) state that adults who've lost significant weight may need up to 90 minutes of daily moderate-intensity exercise to sustain that loss. This publication also emphasizes the importance of reducing sedentary behaviors, such as television viewing, in favor of more active leisure-time activities.

## Exercise Intensity

The duration and frequency of exercise are simple to track. It is more difficult to understand exercise intensity. Brisk walking is often described as moderate intensity, but how do we objectively define brisk or moderate? This is one area of the exercise recommendation that has become more precise. Calculating target heart rate range to gauge exercise intensity merits further review.

### Commonly Used Target Heart Rate Range

What is target heart rate range and how do we calculate it? Fitness professionals should realize that target heart rate range varies between individuals and is dependent on type of exercise and current level of fitness. Therefore, it must be calculated for each individual and customized by activity. The most commonly used (and least accurate) range is derived by taking a person's age, subtracting it from 220, and then multiplying by anywhere from 50 percent to 85 percent to develop a range. For example, let's say a 50-year-old fairly fit woman wants to know her target heart rate. She plans to start a walking program.

220 – 50 (her age) = 170

170 × 0.60 (for 60 percent) = 102

170 × 0.70 (for 70 percent) = 119

So her target heart range is 102 to 119 beats per minute.

The problem with this formula is that it means every 50-year-old fairly fit woman (and man!) will have the same target heart rate. That doesn't seem right, does it? It is true that age can be used to generally predict maximum heart rate. But it is probably more accurate to say that maximum heart rate decreases with age. This is the premise behind the formula: It presumes that maximum

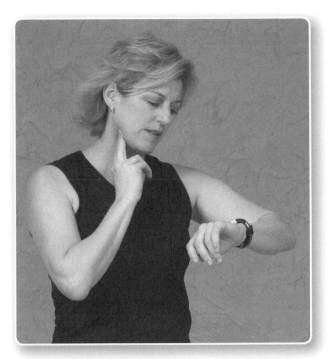

Women can learn to take their heart rate while exercising to make sure they're in an appropriate range.

heart rate at birth is 220 and that we lose one beat per year with age. Keep in mind that the formula 220 minus age was derived from a non-random sample of men in the 1960s and was not intended to be used as a general formula for all exercisers. Nonetheless, it is widely used, programmed into virtually all exercise machines that measure heart rate, and a source of concern for the large percentage of women (and men) for whom it is not accurate. Other formulas have been proposed to calculate maximal heart rate, but they all have the same problem. They just aren't accurate enough.

In this situation, it certainly is reasonable to tell a woman that checking her heart rate is not essential. For a sedentary woman, attention to frequency and duration of exercise is simply more important. For beginners, emphasize the importance of being physically active every day for at least 30 minutes without regard to heart rate. Using a subjective rating of exercise intensity, as outlined next, is useful in this situation.

### Subjective Rating of Exercise Intensity

Using Dr. Gunnar Borg's scale to rate perceived exertion (RPE) during exercise is recommended for beginning exercisers (table 7.1). This scale is

◆ **TABLE 7.1** ◆

## Borg Scale (Rating of Perceived Exertion)

| 6 | |
|---|---|
| 7 | Very, very light |
| 8 | |
| 9 | Very light |
| 10 | |
| 11 | Fairly light |
| 12 | |
| 13 | Somewhat hard |
| 14 | |
| 15 | Hard |
| 16 | |
| 17 | Very hard |
| 18 | |
| 19 | |
| 20 | Very, very hard |

Reprinted, by permission, from G. Borg, *Borg's perceived exertion and pain scales* (Champaign, IL: Human Kinetics), 47.

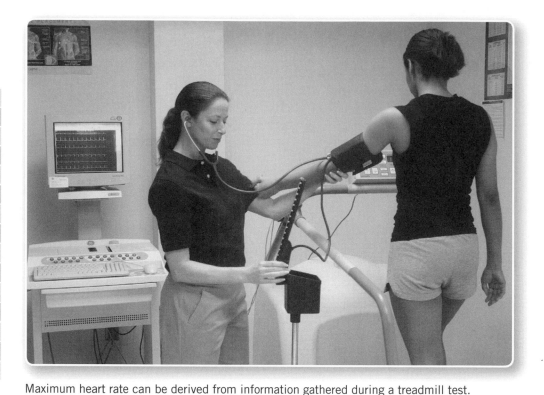

Maximum heart rate can be derived from information gathered during a treadmill test.

also useful for pregnant women or patients on beta-blockers. Of course, anyone can use this scale; advise healthy nonpregnant women to work at an intensity between 12 and 16. Sedentary women can start at lower intensity, and of course competitive athletes may train at higher levels of intensity.

Another even simpler test of exercise intensity is the "talk test." Instruct women that they should be able to carry on a conversation while exercising. If they can't talk, they should slow down. If they can sing, they could probably work a little harder. This is a convenient test that has science to support its usefulness, especially in young women (Persinger et al. 2004).

### Customized Target Heart Rate Range

For women with specific goals and those beyond the beginner level, a more precise target heart range is useful. To customize target heart rate, we need more information about a given woman. First, we need to account for resting heart rate. To determine resting heart rate, the woman takes her resting pulse three mornings in a row, just after waking up. She adds all three together and divides by three to get the average. The more conditioned a woman becomes, the lower her

resting heart rate, so it is important not to forget to recheck resting heart rate periodically.

The second piece of information needed to calculate a customized training heart rate is a true maximum heart rate, not a predicted maximum based solely on age. There are a number of ways to determine a woman's maximum heart rate. A maximum stress test can be done in a doctor's office. Treadmill stress tests are commonly done to screen for heart disease, but are also an excellent way to assess fitness, heart rate, and blood

## Calculating Resting Heart Rate

- ◆ Take the pulse for three consecutive mornings before getting out of bed.
- ◆ Morning 1 = 67.
- ◆ Morning 2 = 71.
- ◆ Morning 3 = 72.
- ◆ Divide the total by 3 to obtain the average: 210/3.
- ◆ Resting heart rate = 70 beats per minute.

pressure. It is important to keep in mind that maximum heart rates derived from treadmill tests are most applicable to walking, running, and treadmill exercise.

Because maximum heart rate varies by activity (due to the number and size of muscles involved), many clinics offer cycling stress tests so as to customize the training heart rate by individual and activity. For example, the maximum heart rate achieved during swimming is less than during running by 12 to 15 beats per minute (Cooper Institute 2005). Cyclists generally have a slightly lower (three to five beats) maximum heart rate during exercise on the bike as compared to the treadmill.

Also, the maximum heart rate achieved on a test may not be a true maximum if the test was limited by symptoms other than from a woman's cardiovascular limit, such as leg cramps or other orthopedic issues.

A maximum stress test can also be done without a doctor's help for healthy girls and healthy women under age 40. Doing a maximum stress test requires one to work as hard as possible. If there is any doubt about performing the test without medical supervision, then don't hesitate to schedule a treadmill test with a doctor.

Next are two examples of running tests to determine maximum heart rate. Before having anyone do either of these tests, a proper warm-up is essential. *These tests should be done only on a girl or woman who has been exercising regularly, is injury free, hasn't raced in the past few weeks, isn't sick with any illness, and has done only light workouts in the week preceding this test.* Using a heart rate monitor, preferably one that records and is capable of giving readings every second, is preferred.

For female athletes, doing this test even once can provide valuable information for calculating target heart rate. For women and girls just starting an exercise program, it is helpful to repeat the test periodically as their fitness and confidence improve. Of course, resting and maximal heart rate will change with conditioning. This is another reason to repeat the test periodically for all women.

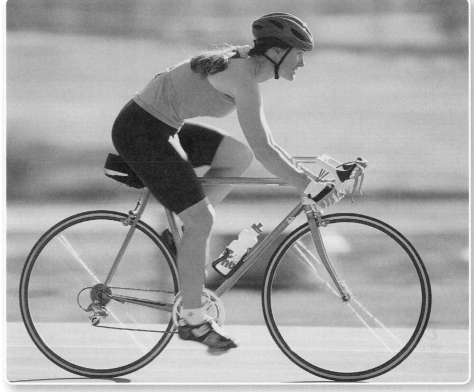

A woman's maximum heart rate for cycling is different than for running.

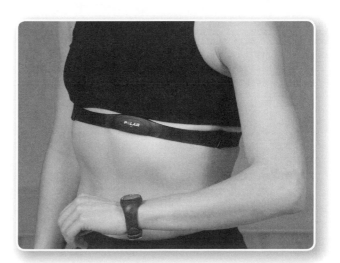

Heart rate monitors are available at a variety of price points and levels of technology. Some women find them very useful for monitoring exercise intensity.

## Running Test #1

Location: a hill that takes about 2 minutes to run up or is a distance of about 200 to 300 yards (183 to 274 meters)
Procedures:

◆ A warm-up run of 2 to 4 miles (3.2 to 6.4 kilometers) is recommended.

◆ Have the runner perform a series of sprints of gradually increasing intensity up the hill.

◆ After each sprint, have the runner jog back down the hill.

◆ Repeat the sprints about four to six times, with the last sprint being an all-out effort to the top.

◆ Record the maximal heart rate from the last sprint.

Once you have accurate numbers for resting and maximum heart rates, you can calculate training heart rate range. The Karvonen formula is very useful for this purpose:

target heart rate = (heart rate reserve) (% training range) + resting heart rate

heart rate reserve = maximal heart rate – resting heart rate

Also, keep in mind that training heart rate recommendations depend on current level of fitness, so see table 7.2 to determine what percentage range to use in the formula.

Minor modifications in the maximal heart rate should be made for non-weight-bearing or arm

## Running Test #2

Location: a flat surface or track
Procedures:

◆ After warming up for 2 to 4 miles, the runner performs an 875-yard (800-meter) sprint. For the first 437 yards (400 meters), she gradually increases speed, and for the second half puts forth an all-out effort.

◆ Repeat the sprints two to three times.

◆ Record the maximal heart rate from the last sprint.

## Determining Target Heart Rate Range

Example: A fairly fit 50-year-old woman plans to exercise on a treadmill. Because her fitness is "fair," a training range of 60 to 70 percent is recommended (table 7.2).

resting heart rate = 70 beats per minute

maximal heart rate from treadmill test = 175 beats per minute

heart rate reserve = 175 – 70 = 105

105 × (60 to 70 percent) + 70 = target heart rate

105 × 0.6 (60 percent training percentage) = 63 + 70 = 133

105 × 0.7 (70 percent training percentage) = 74 + 70 = 144

target heart rate range = 133 to 144 beats per minute*

*Note the difference between this range and the one based solely on age.

◆ TABLE 7.2 ◆

### Recommended Cardiovascular Training Program Using Heart Rate

| Factor | Very poor & poor, low fitness level | Fair & good, average fitness level | Excellent & superior, high fitness level |
|---|---|---|---|
| Frequency (days/week) | 3 | 3 or 4 | 5 |
| Duration* (minutes at target heart rate) | 10-30 | 15-45 | 30-60 |
| Intensity (% HR reserve) | 50-60 | 60-70 | 70-85 |
| Mode** (type of exercise) | Walk, swim, cycle | Walk, jog, run, swim, cycle | Jog, run, swim, cycle |

*Duration can be accumulated by performing shorter multiple bouts if desired.

**Other activities such as cross-country skiing, in-line skating, and stair climbing may also be used.

exercise modes. For swimming, subtract 10 to 15 beats from the maximal heart rate before calculating the training range. For cycling or rowing, subtract 3 to 5 beats.

The easiest way to keep track of one's heart rate while exercising is with a heart rate monitor. But women can also periodically check their pulse manually, which is usually done by counting heartbeats for 15 seconds. So to get a 15-second target, divide each number in a woman's target range by 4. For the woman in the example, that would be 33 to 36 beats over 15 seconds. When counting heartbeats, start with zero for the first beat.

### Scientific Classifications of Cardiorespiratory Fitness and Exercise Intensity

When health care professionals discuss fitness or exercise intensity, they often use the term "$\dot{V}O_2$max." **$\dot{V}O_2$max** is defined as the maximal amount of oxygen a body can consume during exertion before becoming anaerobic. For most women, measurement of $\dot{V}O_2$max isn't necessary because exercise intensity can be prescribed using the guidelines outlined previously. For competitive or elite athletes who desire more precise exercise prescription, measuring $\dot{V}O_2$max is appropriate.

Of interest, in 1998, ACSM revised its exercise prescription guidelines (Pollock et al. 1998). In the past, it was proposed that $\dot{V}O_2$max and heart rate reserve (HRR) were directly correlated. But now it appears more accurate to say that oxygen reserve uptake ($\dot{V}O_2$R) and HRR are better correlated. The difference is that HRR and $\dot{V}O_2$R are related to a level of metabolism that starts at rest, not at zero. This is illustrated in the formula presented on page 116 for calculating training heart rate based on the Karvonen method. By incorporating resting heart rate into the formula, the Karvonen method assumes a certain "resting" level of energy expenditure, as opposed to using zero for energy expenditure at rest. This makes sense because even when the body isn't exercising, it is using energy to maintain bodily functions (such as breathing). If a resting level of energy expenditure is not accounted for, the main error in calculating heart rate for exercise intensity will occur at low levels of exertion. For example, if the 220 – age formula is used to calculate exercise intensity for a 55-year-old beginning walker, the heart

rate obtained may be lower than the individual's resting heart rate.

In an editorial, Franklin and Swain (2003) further elaborate that exercise intensities as low as 30 percent $\dot{V}O_2$R are sufficient to realize cardiovascular benefit in sedentary individuals. This means that "light" exercise, such as walking 2 miles (3.2 kilometers) in an hour, may still be an adequate intensity for health and fitness improvement in deconditioned women. Table 7.3 shows more detail on this concept.

◆ **TABLE 7.3** ◆

### Classification of Exercise Intensity, Based on Physical Activity Lasting Up to 60 Minutes[*]

**ENDURANCE-TYPE ACTIVITY (RELATIVE INTENSITY)**

| Intensity | $\dot{V}O_2$R(%) | HR reserve(%) | RPE[†] |
|---|---|---|---|
| Very light | <20 | <20 | <10 |
| Light | 20-39 | 20-39 | 10-11 |
| Moderate | 40-59 | 40-59 | 12-13 |
| Hard | 60-84 | 60-84 | 14-16 |
| Very Hard | ≥85 | ≥85 | 17-19 |
| Maximal[‡] | 100 | 100 | 20 |

HR = heart rate.

[*]Adapted from the 1998 ACSM position stand; [†]rating of perceived exertion 6-20 scale, Borg; [‡]maximal values are mean values achieved during maximal exercise by healthy adults.

Reproduced with permission Franklin, B et al. New Insights on the Threshold Intensity for Improving Cardiorespiratory Fitness. *Prev. Cardio.* 2003; 6:3: 118-121. Copyright 2003 by CHF, Inc.

### Energy Metabolism

It is important to address the oft-cited "fat-burning" zone. Women have been told that if they exercise at a lower intensity they will burn more calories from fat. Intensity of exercise is one of the factors that determine the number of calories burned. A 130-pound (59-kilogram) woman who runs for 30 minutes at her usual 10 minute per mile pace will burn about 300 calories. Because running is a higher-intensity activity, let's estimate that about 70 percent of calories burned will be from carbohydrate sources (210 calories) and 30 percent of calories burned will come from fat (90 calories). The same woman walking for 35 minutes at a 20 minute per mile pace will burn about 150 calories—about 50

## Key Principles of Aerobic Exercise Intensity

◆ Encourage women to be active on most days of the week for at least 30 minutes, more if they want to lose weight.

◆ Calculate a training heart rate for women. To derive the best target heart range, perform actual measurements of resting and maximal heart rate and then use the Karvonen formula.

◆ If it is not possible to calculate maximal heart rate, use the Borg scale to rate exercise intensity.

◆ Keep in mind that for sedentary individuals, intensity levels as low as 30 percent confer cardiovascular benefit.

**Examples of activities that use 150 calories**

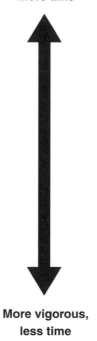

Washing and waxing a car for 45–60 minutes
Washing windows or floors for 45–60 minutes
Playing volleyball for 45 minutes
Playing touch football for 30–45 minutes
Gardening for 30–45 minutes
Wheeling self in wheelchair for 30–40 minutes
Walking 1-3/4 miles in 35 minutes (20 min/mile)
Basketball (shooting baskets) for 30 minutes
Bicycling 5 miles in 30 minutes
Dancing fast (social) for 30 minutes
Pushing a stroller 1.5 miles in 30 minutes
Raking leaves for 30 minutes
Walking 2 miles in 30 minutes (15 min/mile)
Water aerobics for 30 minutes
Swimming laps for 20 minutes
Wheelchair basketball for 20 minutes
Basketball (playing a game) for 15–20 minutes
Bicycling 4 miles for 15 minutes
Jumping rope for 15 minutes
Running 1.5 miles in 15 minutes (10 min/mile)
Shoveling snow for 15 minutes
Stairwalking for 15 minutes

**Less vigorous, more time**

**More vigorous, less time**

**Figure 7.1** A moderate amount of physical activity is roughly equivalent to physical activity that uses approximately 150 calories (kcal) of energy per day, or 1,000 calories per week. Some activities can be performed at various intensities; the suggested durations correspond to the expected intensity of effort.

percent of calories burned will be from carbohydrate (75 calories) and 50 percent from fat (75 calories). If a woman is trying only to maintain her current weight and fitness, then regular walking may be adequate exercise. But for a woman who wants to lose weight, the more calories burned, the sooner her goal is achieved. In this example, data from figure 7.1 provided information on total calories burned, and data from figure 7.2b provide information on the relative percentage of calories burned from fat or carbohydrate sources.

Keep in mind that a woman who pushes her heart rate higher, exercises more frequently, or exercises for longer durations will burn more calories. From the example just cited, it is apparent that at lower-intensity exercise, a higher percentage of calories burned come from fat. But the bottom line is that the runner in the example burned more fat calories than the walker because she burned more total calories (90 vs. 75 and 300 vs. 150, respectively). Encourage women, therefore, to focus on total calories burned, not on a "fat-burning" zone. Beginning low-intensity exercisers can match total calories burned by high-intensity exercisers through longer duration of activity. For beginners, lower-intensity exercise may be easier to adhere to and likely confers a lower risk of injury.

Remember, running and walking aren't the only activities that apply here. Any exercise done at lower intensity favors calorie metabolism from lipolysis. When exercise intensity is higher, energy metabolism shifts to carbohydrate sources (Hawley 1998). Women generally have higher maximal fat oxidation than men, and women reach maximal fat oxidation at a higher $\dot{V}O_2$max than men as shown in figure 7.2 (Venables et al. 2005). These are general rules. Energy metabolism varies from person to person, with fitness level, as well as with meal composition and timing. So, again, focus more on total calories burned and far less on concern about fat versus carbohydrate metabolism.

One final thought to remember about energy metabolism is that it is altered

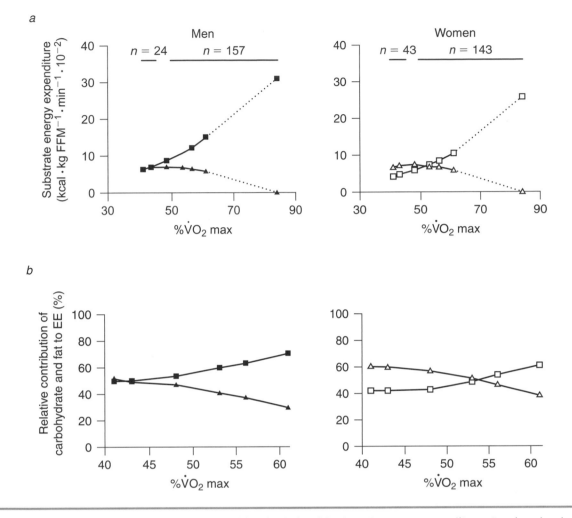

**Figure 7.2** Gender differences in mean absolute *(a)* and relative *(b)* substrate energy expenditure at various levels of $\dot{V}O_2$max. △, women fat; ▲, men fat; □, women carbohydrate; ■, men carbohydrate. Values are means ± standard error; *n* = 157 men, *n* = 143 women.

Reprinted, by permission, from M.C. Venables, J. Achten, and A.E. Jeukendrup, 2005, "Determinants of fat oxidation during exercise in healthy men and women: A cross-sectional study," *Journal of Applied Physiology* 98: 160-167.

only during exercise, not after. Some sources may suggest that there is a sustained increase in metabolism after exercise or a significant increase in resting metabolism from regular exercise. This simply isn't true (Poehlman et al. 2002). There is a small increase in resting metabolism of 7 to 10 kcal per day per pound of fat-free mass gained. Even with a regular vigorous resistance program, women will gain only a few pounds of fat-free mass in a year. So, at most, resting metabolism may increase 30 kcal per day. Therefore, women should count the calories burned during exercise and not expect any significant calorie-burning effect after aerobic exercise.

## Duration and Types of Aerobic Exercise

Over the years, we've learned a lot about how much and how intense exercise should be to yield benefits. We used to believe that exercise had to be vigorous to confer benefits, but we've learned through research that moderate and light exercise, such as walking, is very beneficial. We've also learned that exercise can be accumulated throughout the day, instead of completed in a single 30-minute session. Exercise also doesn't necessarily have to be "structured." Many women are very active without ever stepping on a treadmill or going out for a jog. Finally, it is important to note that women can and should do many different activities for aerobic exercise; cross and interval training are ways women can further benefit from regular activity.

### *Intermittent Versus Continuous Exercise*

The original study showing that exercise can be broken down into 10-minute bouts was done at Stanford University and included only men (DeBusk et al. 1990). In this study, two groups of 18 men (average age 51) did moderate-intensity exercise (65 to 75 percent of peak treadmill heart rate) either for one 30-minute session per day or three 10-minute sessions per day. Both groups significantly improved their $\dot{V}O_2max$ over the eight-week study period. This was a very exciting finding that changed exercise prescription. Unfortunately, the resulting exercise prescriptions often overlook the fact that women were not included in the study. Also, note that the exercise intensity was moderate, not light. Finally, the men exercised every day. Keep these parameters in mind if you recommend shorter bouts of exercise instead of one long session.

For many women, shorter bouts of exercise can be a much more practical approach to exercise. It is often easier to find an extra 10 minutes three times a day than 30 minutes all at one time. Women may find that stationary cycling for 10 minutes in the morning, walking for 10 minutes at lunch, and playing kickball with the kids after dinner for 15 minutes are easy, fun ways to integrate activity into the day. So, don't dismiss this as a viable option, especially for women who have been sedentary. Any physical activity is better than none.

### *Structured Exercise Versus Lifestyle Physical Activity*

We've also learned that exercise doesn't have to be a structured, traditional activity. Many activi-

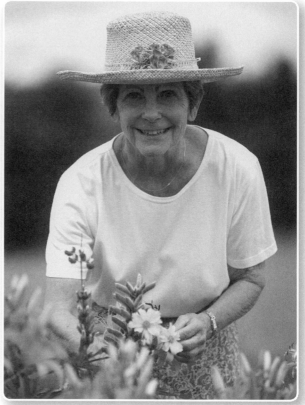

Daily life activities such as gardening can be demanding enough to qualify as physical activity.

ties that women and girls perform elevate the heart rate and therefore qualify as physical activity. Chores around the house, gardening, chasing kids around, playing games, and, of course, work-related activity all contribute to health. By the end of the day, if a woman performs at least three moderate-intensity activities in bursts of at least 10 minutes, she can accumulate enough activity to be considered physically active.

### *Cross Training and Interval Training*

The more a particular exercise is performed, the more efficient the body becomes at performing it. In one way, this is good. Less energy is used to perform the same task once it is mastered. For competitive athletes, this means they can go faster or farther and use less energy. However, if a woman's main goal is to burn calories (to lose weight, for example), then she doesn't want to burn fewer calories while doing the same amount of exercise. This is one of the reasons cross training and interval training are so important! To keep burning the same amount of calories during

## Recommendations for Shorter Bouts of Exercise

- ◆ Exercise for at least 10 minutes at a time, for a daily total of at least 30 minutes.
- ◆ Exercise at moderate intensity, not light.
- ◆ Exercise every day.

workouts, the workouts have to vary in some way.

Cross training means doing different activities instead of the same exercise over and over again. There is the potential to burn more calories when using cross training, even though exercise duration is unchanged. The reason is usually that the body is not as familiar with the new activity and the activity therefore requires more effort, whether through the use of different or more muscles.

Cross training also helps to prevent injury by resting specific muscles that would otherwise be overused. Athletes who are injured can use cross training. For example, a cyclist with a knee problem may add strength training and swimming to compensate. Cross training can also reduce repetitive joint movements by changing the aerobic routine from primarily sagittal plane motions (standard cardiovascular equipment: bike, elliptical, and treadmill) to any activities that train the transverse and frontal planes (basketball, soccer, racquetball). Cross training helps to strengthen the entire body; runners and walkers benefit by adding upper-body activities. Finally, cross training provides a mental break. It can be tedious to do the same exercise over and over again. Cross training provides a much needed break in routine, thereby promoting physical and mental well-being.

Interval training is another important exercise principle. Women can do interval training with any aerobic activity. When one places bursts of sprint effort activity throughout the workout,

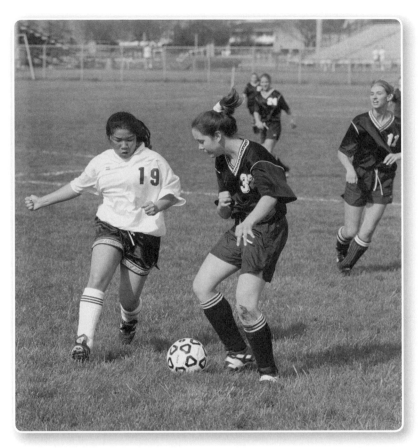

Soccer is an activity that trains the body in all three planes of motion: transverse, frontal, and sagittal.

more calories are burned, monotony is avoided, and power is improved. Power is not just about how strong women are, but about how strong and fast they are. Interval training increases power by forcing women to pay attention to speed.

## Benefits of Cross Training

- ◆ Reduces the risk of overuse injuries
- ◆ Provides an alternative exercise when an injury occurs
- ◆ Reduces repetitive joint movements by changing the plane of motion
- ◆ Strengthens the entire body
- ◆ Provides a mental break
- ◆ Relieves boredom

## Sample Interval Training Routine

- ◆ Do a usual warm-up.
- ◆ Start the aerobic activity.
- ◆ After 5 minutes, take the exertion level up to a higher intensity, or sprint effort. Remain at this level for 1 to 2 minutes maximum.
- ◆ Taper back down to moderate exertion. Remain at this level for 3 to 5 minutes.
- ◆ Repeat the intervals.

# Quantifying Activity and Fitness Levels

Some women feel they are active enough doing their daily activities that they don't need structured exercise. Many times women are right about this. It is helpful to prove it, though! Using a pedometer to assess a woman's level of activity is useful to determine if she needs to add structured aerobic exercise. There are also ways to assess fitness level by doing simple running tests, as outlined further on.

## Using a Pedometer to Assess Activity

Pedometers are beeper-sized units that are worn at the waistline and count every step a woman takes. We prefer the pedometers that are most simple. A woman shouldn't have to calculate her stride length or expect to learn how many calories are burned. Rather, a simple pedometer that counts every single step is preferred. These can be purchased at any sporting goods store.

To test the pedometer, walk around briskly counting out 100 steps while wearing the

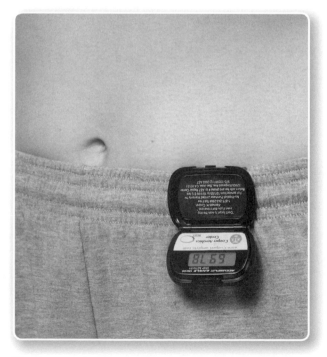

Wearing a pedometer is an easy way to monitor daily activity.

pedometer. Check the pedometer to be sure it is within five steps of being correct. We recommend wearing the pedometer every day. The goal is to achieve 10,000 steps a day. If a woman can achieve 10,000 steps in a day, then she doesn't need to do "structured" aerobic exercise that day. At least one study has shown that women who accumulate at least 10,000 steps have normal body mass index (Thompson et al. 2004). If a woman falls short, she can add structured exercise to reach 10,000 steps. Pedometers work on treadmills and elliptical trainers, and (sometimes) on cycles.

## Cooper Institute Tests to Quantify Fitness Levels in Women

The Cooper Institute has researched two cardiorespiratory fitness tests for quantifying fitness levels for women. After warm-up, have a woman run as far as she can in 12 minutes. Alternatively, time a woman during a 1.5-mile (2.4-kilometer) run. To quantify fitness level as S (superior), E (excellent), G (good), F (fair), P (poor), or VP (very poor), see the figures in appendix A (pp. 200-202). For example, to achieve a good category of fitness, a 40-year-old woman must run at least 1.29 miles (2 kilometers) in 12 minutes or run 1.5 miles (2.4 kilometers) in 15 minutes 17 seconds or faster.

Also, any woman can perform a maximal exercise treadmill test to determine her level of fitness. This should be done under a doctor's supervision. The Cooper Institute published fitness levels based on treadmill testing, and these are included in appendix A as well (pp. 200-202). For example, for a 50-year-old woman to qualify for the "good" category of fitness, she should be able to walk on the treadmill (without holding on) for at least 11 minutes and 23 seconds using a modified Balke protocol. The modified Balke protocol is a pace of 3.3 miles (5.3 kilometers) per hour with progressive incline. During the test, the incline rises 2 percent after the first minute and 1 percent each minute thereafter. If a woman reaches 25 minutes, the speed starts to increase 0.3 miles (0.48 kilometers) per hour per minute, and the incline remains at 26 percent. Women who are unable to achieve a "good" level of fitness on any of these tests generally need to add more structured activity to their lifestyles.

# Traditional Aerobic Exercise Choices

Before getting started with aerobic exercise, women should make sure they're physically ready to do so. The Physical Activity Readiness Questionnaire is one of several popular screening tools that are available to help determine who may benefit from a medical exam before increasing their activity. A copy is provided in appendix A on page 198. Called the PAR-Q, it was developed by Canadian public health and exercise experts. Ask your client to complete it as the first step in preparing to become more physically active. The PAR-Q is designed for people up to age 69. A companion form can be given to the client's personal doctor if an exam is needed to obtain medical clearance.

A stress test may be recommended for women planning to start an exercise program, especially if they are over 45 or have a family history of heart disease or a personal history of diabetes, high blood pressure, abnormal cholesterol, smoking, or overweight.

In this section we'll cover walking, running, cycling, swimming, exercise machines, and aerobics classes.

## Walking

The most popular form of aerobic exercise in the United States is walking. Walking has numerous advantages over other forms of aerobic exercise. Virtually everyone can do it, since no special skill is required. Also, it is convenient for most women. Walking can usually be done in a neighborhood or on a home treadmill. Since it can be done at home, mothers with children don't have to worry about getting someone to watch the kids or using a day care at a gym. No special equipment is required except a comfortable pair of walking shoes. People can walk while listening to music or watching television. Importantly, walking has a low risk for injury. In fact, walking is used as a rehabilitative exercise for many athletes who've been injured in various sports.

Walking can also be a family or social event. For parents and kids, walking can be therapeutic,

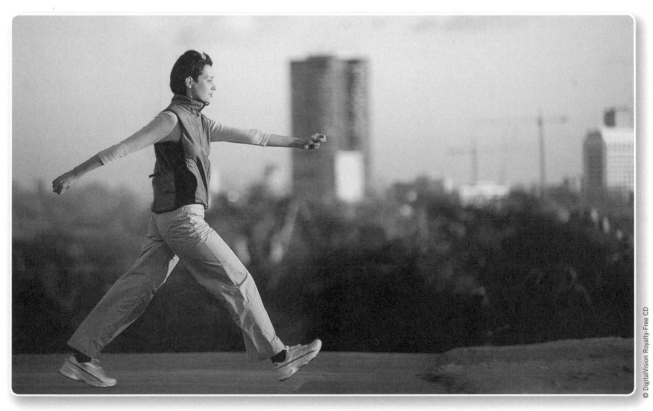

Walking remains one of the easiest and most versatile forms of exercise.

allowing time for discussion without direct confrontation. Friends can get together for a walk and catch up on happenings in each other's lives. Many charitable events are focused on walks. The number of walking and jogging weekend events has mushroomed over the years.

People can adjust walking to increase intensity by swinging the arms, walking faster, going up hills, pushing a stroller, or even adding short spurts (intervals!) of jogging. It's easy to incorporate more walking into daily activities. For years, health advocates have recommended taking the stairs instead of the escalator or elevator, parking farther away from one's destination, and walking for errands instead of driving. For women who wear pedometers, it becomes clear very quickly that every extra step adds up to get them to that recommended 10,000 steps per day.

## Jogging or Running

Jogging or running is a very efficient form of exercise. There are few exercises that surpass running in calories burned per minute. That's why so many runners swear by it and decline other exercises. Running requires the body to use its largest muscles, elevating the heart rate to higher levels than other aerobic activities. The difference between jogging and running is simply speed. In fact, many new exercisers enjoy starting out as walkers and eventually progressing to jogging and running.

For women who are just starting an exercise program, running may seem impossible. That's why emphasizing progression is important. A woman should start with walking, then slowly add in some jogging intervals. When jogging becomes comfortable, she can do it continuously. Then she can add in some faster jogging or running intervals. If desired, she can progress to running continuously and eventually adding sprint intervals.

### Running Form and Stride

Many women probably don't give a second thought to how they run. They just do it. But there are some basic elements of running form to consider. Good posture is essential: Runners should look straight ahead, not down; hold shoulders back and down, not slumped forward or hunched up; keep arms and hands relaxed, not tensed or clenched; and swing the arms close to the body and bend elbows to about 90 degrees.

A woman shouldn't worry about changing her running form dramatically, since most of the form comes naturally. Addressing corrective flexibility and strength issues, as well as trunk stability, is always a must when training runners.

## Case Study—55-Year-Old Woman

◆ Physical capabilities: She has not been active for 20 years. She used to jog when she was younger.

◆ Limitations: She is overweight and experiences periodic knee pain with no diagnosis.

◆ Goal: New Year's resolution is to "get back in shape" by starting to jog again.

◆ Recommendations: Because of her extra weight, increased stress to the joints, decreased muscle endurance and strength due to aging, and overall low fitness level, this woman must start out slowly. Walking, rather than jogging, is recommended in the beginning. Many joint and muscle injuries can occur when someone progresses too quickly or exercises outside her physiological capabilities. Also, encourage cross training, such as stationary cycling or the elliptical trainer, to decrease joint stress. Don't discourage jogging as a long-term goal, but help her understand that it will take patience and hard work. Address the issues (weight loss, endurance, strength, knee/hip stability, core stability) before sending her out to the track for higher intensity exercise like jogging. Her weight loss goal as well as her needs for increased strength and stability should be addressed through addition of a strength training component to her program as well. Many women think that aerobic exercise is all they need to do through their lifetime to remain fit. As most health professionals know, a balanced program includes strength/stability and flexibility work. In fact, after age 50 these components become increasingly important; they will be reviewed in chapters 8 and 9.

These topics are discussed further in the strength, flexibility, and program design chapters.

Running form also improves with strength and speed. Women who work on strength training, especially improving their trunk muscle strength, will naturally improve their posture. Running faster generally improves form too, so working on speed sessions with a coach is helpful.

Stride has several components, including length and rate. Stride length is something that changes naturally. Stride length may increase as a girl grows or as a woman becomes faster and stronger. Trying to artificially change stride isn't recommended. According to Claire Kowalchik in *The Complete Book of Running for Women* (1999), runners should strive to take 180 steps per minute. Focus on this stride rate as opposed to stride length. It is easy enough to count the number of strides per minute with a watch that has a stopwatch function or a second hand. Increasing stride rate is a matter of picking the feet up more quickly. This change will shorten the stride slightly, which limits the time the feet are in the air. The force of the foot strike is reduced, which may lessen risk of injury.

### Breathing

Breathing is another thing that runners don't think about much because it comes naturally. Exhaling is naturally more forceful and faster than inhaling. It doesn't matter whether breathing is through the nose or the mouth. Most runners breathe through their nose and mouth at the same time.

For elite or long-distance runners, giving a little attention to breathing may pay off in reduced injuries. Coaches generally recommend inhaling over two to three steps and exhaling over one to two steps. The advantage to having an odd number of steps over which inhalation and exhalation occur is as follows: The foot hits the ground with the most force at the beginning of exhalation. Always exhaling when the same foot is striking may increase risk for injury on that side (Kowalchik 1999). Slower runs should have a 3:2 pattern of inhalation to exhalation (inhale for three foot strikes and exhale for two foot strikes; see figure 7.3). Faster runs will naturally have a 2:1 ratio of inhalation to exhalation.

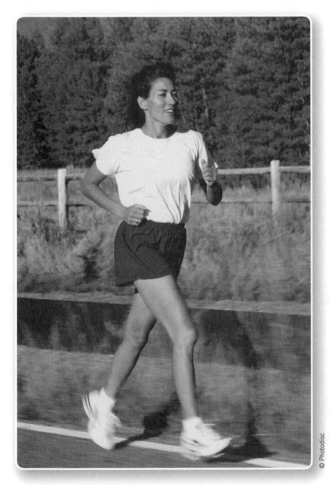

Good running posture is an important part of running form.

© Photodisc

| Foot-strike | Breathing |
|---|---|
| Left<br>Right<br>Left | Inhale |
| Right<br>Left | Exhale |
| Right<br>Left<br>Right | Inhale |
| Left<br>Right | Exhale |

**Figure 7.3** Foot strikes and breathing. This is a 3:2 inhalation-to-exhalation pattern.

Encourage women to set goals, run a race if they never have, or run a longer race than they've done before. Many women have no idea what they can achieve until they try. Races aren't just for "elite" runners, and they don't necessarily require hard training. Many racing events are combined with walks or fun runs, so just about anyone can participate.

## Cycling

Cycling is an excellent aerobic exercise women can enjoy. Of course, outdoor cycling requires more equipment and more attention to safety than walking or running. A biking helmet must always be worn. Women must pay close attention to cars, road conditions, and street signs. With the advent of spinning classes as an indoor cycling option, women can enjoy safe cycling year-round. For women with limited cycling experience, starting with indoor classes is a safe way to get comfortable with a bike before heading outdoors. Beginners can also practice in safe places, such as cul de sacs or cycling trails.

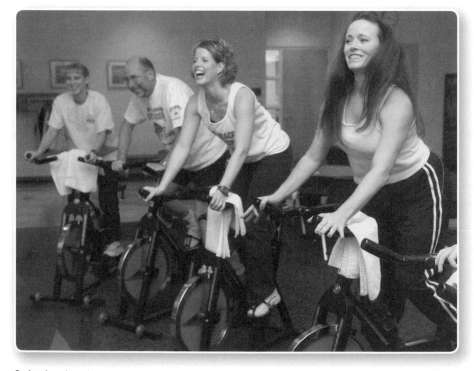

Spinning has become a popular choice for women looking for a challenging aerobic workout.

### Cycling Outdoors

Different types of bicycles are available for outdoor use, with four basic models: mountain, touring, hybrid, and racing. The type of bike a woman chooses should be based on where and how she plans to use it. Mountain bikes are made for use on rugged, off-road terrain but can function on any surface. Mountain bikes are very stable and durable, with thick knobby tires. Touring bikes have thinner wheels than mountain bikes and dropped handlebars designed for longer rides. Touring bikes are great for casual riding. A hybrid bike is a cross between a mountain bike and a touring bike. The hybrid has tires that are fat enough for mountain biking, but smooth enough for on-road use. Racing bikes have narrow tires and are designed for speed and responsiveness. Newer lightweight materials are used for high-end racing bikes. Some bikes are specifically designed for women, with a modified frame (the top bar angles downward) and extra padding in the seat. The type of bike a woman chooses will depend on the terrain and type of cycling she plans to do. This is one reason hybrid bikes are popular; they can be used on varying terrain. For racing, though, women will need a true racing bike to be competitive.

Another change in bike design is updated pedal systems. Pedals can be "clipless," meaning that bikers snap their shoes into a cleat. This allows for more power with pedaling. Newer "floating" clipless pedals aren't as rigid as earlier models. For women who have no experience with clipless pedals, trying them out on a stationary cycle first is appropriate.

Bicycle fit is important for comfort, injury prevention, and performance. There are four components to bicycle fit: frame size, seat height, seat fore–aft position, and foot placement. Fit actually varies depending on the type of bike and the type of activity. Cycle shop employees and spinning instructors can be a tremendous help in determining proper fit.

## *Cycling Indoors*

Spinning classes were invented by Johnny Goldberg in an effort to make indoor cycling more appealing. Most fitness facilities offer Spinning classes. Each participant is seated on a cycle made specifically for spinning. An instructor leads the class through a ride. The participant controls her own speed and resistance to simulate an outdoor ride. Participants often wear heart rate monitors to determine how hard they are working. Spinning offers most of the advantages of cycling and offers the bonus of being much safer than riding outdoors. It is a great option for women who can't run or walk because of injuries. For women with little cycling experience, recommend beginner classes; instructors in these classes will review the basics, and the class will start at a slower pace.

## Swimming and Water Exercise

Some women turn to swimming as an exercise after injury has forced them to find a non-weight-bearing activity. Other women use swimming as the basis for their aerobic exercise program. Swimming is one of the most popular forms of aerobic exercise for women of all ages. Another advantage of swimming is that it can be enjoyed by the entire family. Swimming requires minimal equipment: a bathing suit, goggles, and cap. For adults who didn't learn to swim as kids, lessons are strongly recommended.

For leisure swimmers, injury risk is low, but competitive swimmers have an increased risk of injury. Breaststroke swimmers are more likely to experience knee problems (due to kicking mechanics), and butterfly swimmers are prone to shoulder problems.

Most pools have large time clocks nearby, making it easy to stop and quickly check heart rate. But remember, swimming usually doesn't elevate the heart rate as much as running or cycling. Swimming, however, is excellent cross training for any other exercise. Women can compensate for the lower heart rate during this activity by increasing the length of time they are in the pool to burn an equivalent amount of calories.

Swimmers often focus exclusively on leg or arm work by using kickboards or pull buoys. Breaking up a swimming routine by changing from freestyle, to another stroke, to kicking, to

## Advantages of Swimming

- ◆ The risk of injury during leisure swimming is low.
- ◆ Swimming requires minimal equipment.
- ◆ Swimming is an excellent cross-training exercise.
- ◆ Decreases joint and muscle tissue stress.

pulling makes a workout more interesting and challenging. Other ways to add variety, increase intensity, or compensate for injuries are to use fins on the feet or gloves during swimming.

## Disadvantages of Swimming

- ◆ Swimming doesn't elevate the heart rate as much as some other aerobic exercises.
- ◆ Swimming doesn't benefit bone density.
- ◆ Compared to another exercise, it may take more time to burn an equivalent amount of calories with swimming.
- ◆ There may be a cost to use a pool.
- ◆ Some skill is required. Lessons may be needed.
- ◆ Swimming in open water can be dangerous.
- ◆ Competitive swimmers are at risk for overuse injuries.

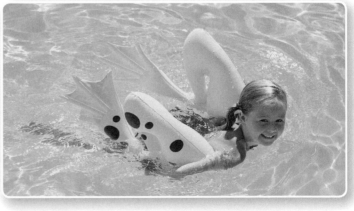

© Eyewire/Photodisc/Getty Images

Simply playing in the pool is good exercise, especially for younger girls who may not be interested in swimming laps.

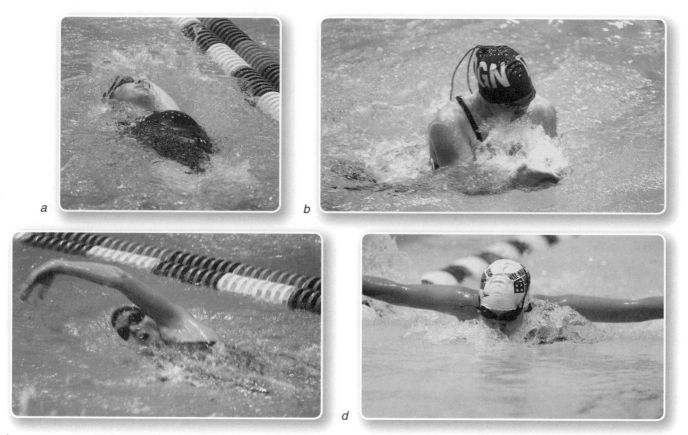

Swimmers can vary their workouts by using all four strokes. *(a)* Backstroke, *(b)* breaststroke, *(c)* freestyle or "the crawl," and *(d)* butterfly.

Women should also keep in mind that exercising in the pool isn't limited to traditional swimming strokes. Water aerobics classes are increasingly available. Jogging in the pool, which is often used in rehabilitation for runners, is also a great exercise for nonrunners.

### Cardiovascular Machines and Aerobic Exercise Classes

The treadmill and stationary cycle were the mainstays of exercise machines for years. Now other choices are available. Elliptical trainers have become very popular. Elliptical trainers are appealing because they mimic running without the foot strike, causing less impact on joints than jogging or running. Women with various injuries, especially knee pain, often try the elliptical trainer as a substitute for high-impact activities.

Most fitness centers offer a variety of aerobic exercise classes. The instructor, lively music, and the opportunity to exercise with others can make

## Triathlons

Every year, more women enter triathlons, which combine swimming, biking, and running in one event. Event distances range from supersprint distance (375-meter swim; 10-kilometer bike; 2.5-kilometer run) to iron man distance (2.4-mile swim; 112-mile bike; 26.2-mile run). For more information on triathlons, check www.triathlon.org, Web site of the International Triathlon Union (ITU).

the experience motivational and fun. During the class, participants are encouraged to check target heart rate to gauge effort, making the class both enjoyable and effective. Some women are more motivated and consistent in their attendance of exercise classes because such classes give them an appointed time to add exercise to their daily schedule. Classes can be a nice break from the

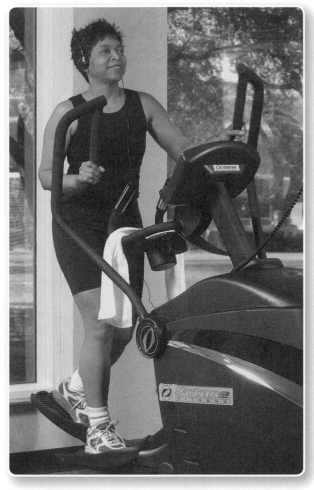

Many women choose the elliptical trainer for their aerobic workouts.

monotony of standard cardiovascular equipment. Encourage women to try a variety of classes to find one that suits their ability and that they will enjoy.

### Weight-Bearing Versus Non-Weight-Bearing Activities

When we discuss aerobic exercise, we often make a distinction between weight-bearing and non-weight-bearing activities. The reason is that the benefits differ for exercise depending on whether weight bearing occurs. For example, to benefit bone health, exercise must be weight bearing. This means that activities like walking, jogging, and using a treadmill are beneficial to the bone, whereas swimming is not. The main goal of aerobic exercise is to keep the heart healthy, so any exercise, whether weight bearing or not,

will achieve that goal. But if a woman has other goals, particularly relating to bone health, then weight-bearing aerobic activity should be her dominant activity.

Don't forget that strength training also benefits bone health. So, if for whatever reason a woman can't do weight-bearing activity but wants to maintain bone health, she can benefit from strength training. Women who have difficulty with both weight-bearing and strength training exercises present a real challenge to the health and fitness professional in regard to bone health. If a woman's limitations for weight-bearing and strength training exercises are temporary, as with a leg fracture, no major loss of bone will occur. But if limitations are permanent, as with severe rheumatoid arthritis, then consultation with a physician specializing in rehabilitation may be appropriate.

### Other Aerobic Choices

There are lots of aerobic activities to choose from. Be sure women are aware that outdoor activities such as hiking, in-line skating, and skiing all count as exercise. The same guidelines regarding frequency, intensity, and duration of exercise all apply. There are always new concepts for aerobic exercise, such as "boot camp" classes to try. By having variety in their workout and incorporating already enjoyable activities, most women can find exercise they can continue and enjoy for a lifetime.

## Injury Prevention

There are basic rules for injury prevention that every fitness specialist should recommend in the areas of footwear, surfaces, progression, warm-up and cool-down, and rest. Also, see the information on common injuries in chapter 11.

Women should wear the appropriate shoe for the activity they are pursuing. Runners should wear running shoes. Tennis players should wear tennis shoes because of the added support for the multiplanar movements of tennis. Shoes should be replaced at the first signs of wear. Rotating shoes is one way to always have an appropriate pair available. For running in particular, having feet and gait evaluated at a running store is very helpful in finding the right shoe.

Choose exercise surfaces wisely. Running and walking on asphalt streets are fine for most women. As much as possible, it is wise to avoid running on concrete. Trails, cinder paths, and cross country routes generally provide a softer surface and better views than roads or sidewalks, but people need to beware of ruts, roots, rocks, and other obstacles. Using a track at a local school is a great change from other surfaces, especially for speed work.

To prevent injury, women should increase the duration of exercise gradually. Although this principle is sport specific, in general we recommend increasing total mileage no more than 10 to 15 percent a week. Also, after increasing total mileage for two weeks straight, a woman should consider dropping back to the previous level for one week before increasing again.

Warming up prior to exercise is important to help prevent injury. Walking comfortably for a few minutes before picking up the intensity is recommended. Walking or jogging while swinging the arms is a good warm-up prior to strength training.

Adequate hydration is a must. See the "Hydration Hints" handout on page 220 in appendix B. Endurance athletes should calculate their unique "sweat rate" to determine total fluid needed to replace exercise losses.

Cooling down is necessary after exercise and is recommended. To cool down, one reduces the intensity of the activity, such as to a slow walk, or lowers the resistance level on a bike or elliptical trainer. Details on warm-up and cool-down are provided in the chapter on flexibility.

Rest days are critical for best performance and injury prevention. Most women will benefit by having one day off per week. For athletes who cross train, cross-training days may be considered rest days. Also, the day after a challenging workout, doing the same exercise but going easy can feel like a day off.

## ◆ Conclusion ◆

This chapter dealt with aerobic exercise. Health and fitness professionals should assist women in designing appropriate programs that address frequency, intensity, type, and duration of exercise based on the information in this chapter. But aerobics is only one part of a balanced fitness program. Chapter 8 addresses strength training. Incorporating strength training into a woman's routine will help to maintain muscle; improve strength, balance, and stability; and reduce injury. By strengthening muscles, women can offset muscle imbalance. Strength training, in particular core strengthening, encourages proper posture, which in turn improves function and reduces injury risk. The final component of a balanced exercise program includes flexibility work, which is reviewed in chapter 9.

# CHAPTER 8

# Strength Training for Women

## Topics in This Chapter

- ◆ Traditional versus functional strength training
- ◆ Free weights
- ◆ Resistance bands and cable equipment
- ◆ Stability balls
- ◆ Body mechanics and spinal alignment
- ◆ Training principles and variables
- ◆ Periodization
- ◆ Core training
- ◆ Balance and neuromuscular stability training
- ◆ Fitness clubs versus home training

If you've lost strength, you can regain it. If your energy has sagged, you can raise it. If you've lost muscle and gained fat, you can reverse it. If you've become flabby, you can get trim. If you feel older than you like, you can feel younger, stronger, and more vigorous— perhaps better than you've ever felt in your entire life. Strength training, we have learned, is a fountain of youth.

Miriam E. Nelson, PhD, author of *Strong Women Stay Young*

Strength training provides significant health and functional benefits for women. Strength training can increase lean muscle mass, decrease body fat, increase metabolic efficiency, decrease risk of injury, reduce the risk of certain diseases, and improve functional abilities. But the benefits of strength training go beyond just physiological and performance rewards. Increased strength can improve body image at any age.

The need for strength training becomes more urgent as women age. As part of aging we experience sarcopenia, or decreased muscle mass. To prevent or treat sarcopenia, and preserve or improve function, strength training is not only necessary, but also just as important as aerobic exercise in women. The earlier women begin to strength train, the greater the possible long-term benefits. Studies have shown that women of all ages can improve in strength and enhance daily function through a training program.

Strength training has evolved, especially in the past few years. The emphasis has shifted from "pumping iron" for pure strength or for a toned aesthetic look to performing "functional" exercises to keep women strong, capable, and independent. There are, of course, general principles of strength training that any fitness professional should be familiar with, and we'll review these. Core strength, balance, and stability are vital concepts we explore in detail in this chapter.

## Types of Strength Training

Traditional strength training programs focus on developing strength by isolating muscle groups as well as moving the joint(s) through a single plane of motion (mainly **sagittal:** flexion and extension). While this type of training has merit for the woman interested in building absolute strength, bodybuilding, or meeting specific rehabilitation needs, it has limitations for most women. Traditional strength training may not adequately prepare women for the activities they perform at home, at work, or in leisure pursuits. Functional strength training possesses many benefits over traditional strength training.

### Traditional Strength Training

Women who exclusively perform traditional, single-planar or single-joint exercises (or both) do not get maximum benefit from their training. Because of the way muscles are attached at joints, they do not move in straight lines in most life activities and sports. However, most standard machines (fixed machines), such as leg extension, hamstring curl, or tricep extension machines, force the body to move in straight lines. Fixed machines allow for single-joint or single-plane movement and impose low neuromuscular demand. If absolute strength or hypertrophy is the goal, then standard machines are appropriate. However, for most women, these machines should not be the only pieces of equipment they use in the weight room. Any exercise or strength equipment consistently used in this traditional training approach will not achieve optimal or functional training benefit.

It is easy for women to be attracted to fixed machines because they seem safer and easier to use than free weights, stability balls, or cable machines and they reinforce proper mechanics. Standard machines provide external stabilization (pads, seats, belts, or a combination of these), so they require limited effort for postural and joint control. An example is a standard chest press machine (figure 8.1). After a woman has been shown a standard machine once or twice, she usually needs little or no further instruction or education to proceed with her program. The limitations of this training method is that it will not provide continual and functional progression.

Even though traditional strength training machines are beneficial for improving general muscle strength, they minimize the use of stabilizing muscles and reduce the opportunity for natural joint range of motion and **functional**

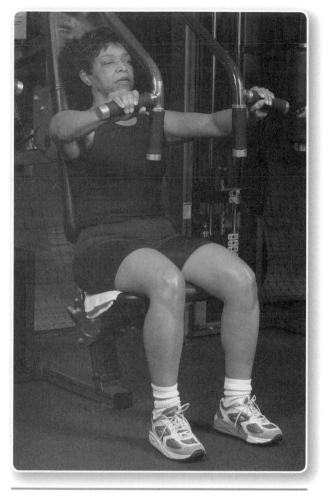

**Figure 8.1** Standard (fixed) chest press exercise.

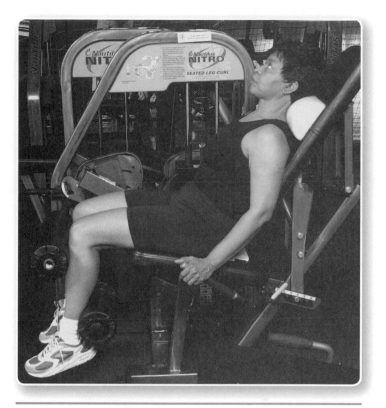

**Figure 8.2** The traditional hamstring curl exercise is used to isolate the hamstrings.

**strength** movement patterns. For example, knee flexion exercises are typically prescribed to strengthen the hamstrings (figure 8.2). But are the hamstrings most often used in a flexed-knee position in daily activities? Not usually. The hamstrings are mostly used eccentrically in the deceleration of knee extension and hip flexion, and as hip extensors and rotators. For example, the hamstrings are active prior to the heel strike during walking or running. The hamstrings also extend the femur during standing hip extension activities, such as squatting or leaning over to pick something up. It is important to train the hamstrings for the daily movements they usually perform (squatting, leaning over, extending the leg; figures 8.3 and 8.4). Does this mean that standard hamstring flexion machines are of little or no value? Absolutely not. However, a standard hamstring exercise should not be the only form of hamstring strengthening incorporated into an exercise program.

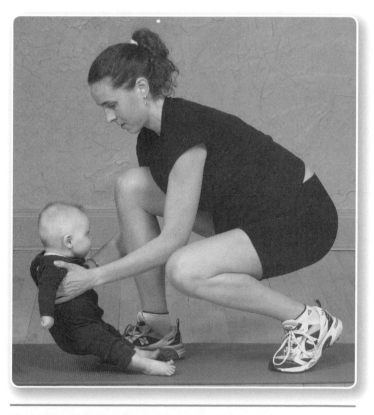

**Figure 8.3** The hamstrings are engaged in daily life such as squatting or lifting.

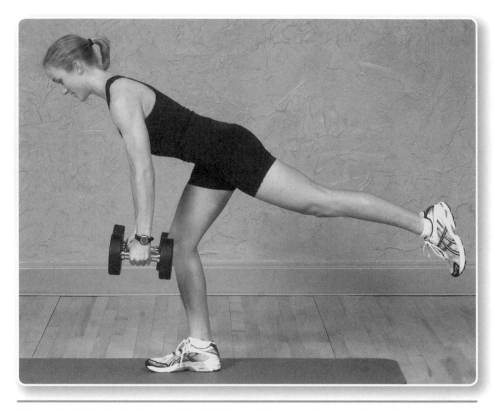

**Figure 8.4** The single-leg dumbbell 45-degree hip extension exercise helps to prepare a woman for daily-life activity.

## Functional Strength Training

The emphasis on functional training is relatively new in the fitness industry. It has been embraced by personal trainers, coaches, athletic trainers, and physical therapists. Functional training promotes exercise that is applicable to real-life movements and activities, such as getting groceries out of the trunk of the car, getting the baby in and out of the stroller, moving furniture, digging in the garden. Functional movements require the use of the **kinetic chain** during **multijoint** and **multiplanar** movements.

Efficient movement depends upon proper function of the kinetic chain. The kinetic chain is made up of the muscular (soft tissue), neural, and articular systems of the body. These systems work together as a unit in order to perform specific movement patterns. Dysfunction in even one of these components can cause compromise and imbalance throughout the kinetic chain. More information about **kinetic chain dysfunction** and muscle balance is provided in chapters 9 and 10.

Functional training involves strength, endurance, flexibility, **stabilization,** speed, power,

and neuromuscular control (balance) in both static (no movement) and dynamic (movement) positions, as well as including multiplanar movements (sagittal, **frontal, transverse**). Functional training should include force production (**concentric** contractions), force reduction (**eccentric** contractions), and stabilization (**isometric** contractions) (Clark 2001).

Functional training can be done with a variety of equipment and tools. As in any exercise program, the specific exercise and tool chosen should coincide with the level and ability of the individual. In this chapter we focus on a few common tools used in training. More information on common exercise tools is provided in chapter 10. Free weights, resistance bands, stability balls, and cable machines are excellent types of equipment that can be utilized to enhance function and improve stability. Depending on budget for equipment, all of these are appropriate for home use.

### Free Weights

Free weights have been used for joint stability and balance training for decades. In the past, women thought free weights were men's equipment. They may have heard that free weights were more difficult to use correctly and therefore increased the risk of injury. Or they may have resisted using free weights because they believed the result would be bulky muscles.

With appropriate education, today's active women are becoming more comfortable with free weights. Free weights can develop balance and strength in stabilizing muscles and also allow natural (free) joint movement. When a given exercise is performed with dumbbells, the movement pattern may seem exactly the same as with a fixed weight machine, but there are differences. With free weights, the muscle recruitment patterns may be different on every repetition. This difference in recruitment pattern aids stabiliza-

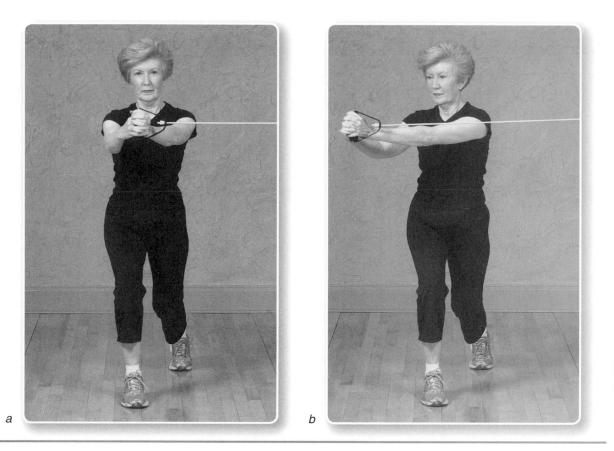

a          b

**Figure 8.5**   Resistance bands can be used in a variety of multiplanar exercises.

tion by enabling the body to respond in many different ways to a given type of resistance.

### Resistance Bands and Cable Equipment

Resistance bands and cable equipment offer similar benefits as free weights and also possess other advantages. Both are very versatile and provide a means for multiplanar movements (figure 8.5, *a & b*). Bands are inexpensive, portable, and nonthreatening, and they offer variable resistance.

### Stability Balls

Stability balls are excellent for core and stability training (such as push-ups, bridges, or hamstring curls; figure 8.6). They can also be used in conjunction with dumbbells, cables, bands, or medicine balls to add variety, complexity, and progression to a program. Performing exercises that require stability and neural control can improve overall performance and reduce risk of

injury. For example, addressing static and dynamic posture on a stability ball helps improve functional and postural strength and control—an important benefit for women who spend several hours a day sitting at work as in figure 8.14 on page 138.

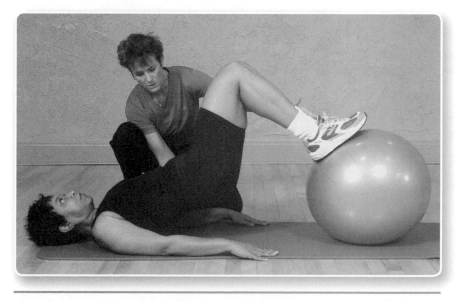

**Figure 8.6**   Supine hamstring curl using the stability ball.

### Advantages of Functional Training Equipment

Functional equipment and functional exercises provide enhanced stability, balance, neural control, and functional strength.

◆ Performing a standing cable chest press (figure 8.7) eliminates the use of a back pad and requires women to stabilize and maintain proper posture in addition to using the pectoral muscles for the chest press exercise.

◆ Performing a bridge on the stability ball (figure 8.8) improves core muscle stability and strength.

◆ Performing a lat pull with resistance bands (figure 8.9) allows for natural shoulder joint movement.

◆ Performing a single-arm cable row (figure 8.10) allows for unilateral movement and strengthening.

◆ Performing exercises with cables, such as woodchops (figure 8.11, *a & b*), provides the opportunity to specifically strengthen and stabilize in many different movement angles.

◆ Performing a lunge with a trunk rotation (figure 8.12) requires the body to move in more than one plane of motion.

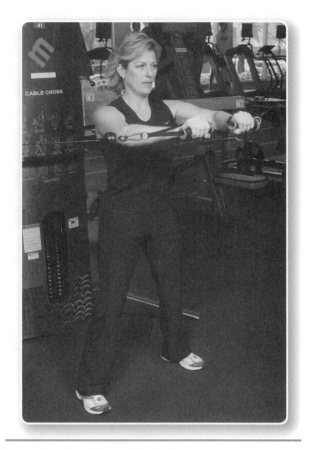

**Figure 8.7** Standing cable chest press.

◆ Performing a squat with a dumbbell overhead press (figure 8.13, *a & b*) requires total body involvement.

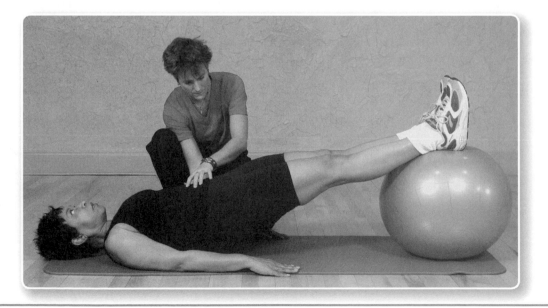

**Figure 8.8** Supine bridge using the stability ball.

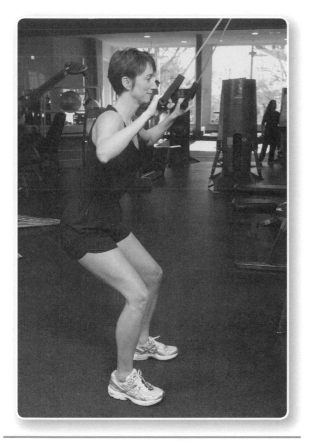

**Figure 8.9** Lat pull exercise using a resistance band.

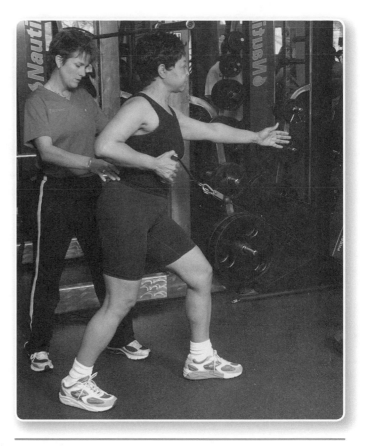

**Figure 8.10** Single-arm cable row.

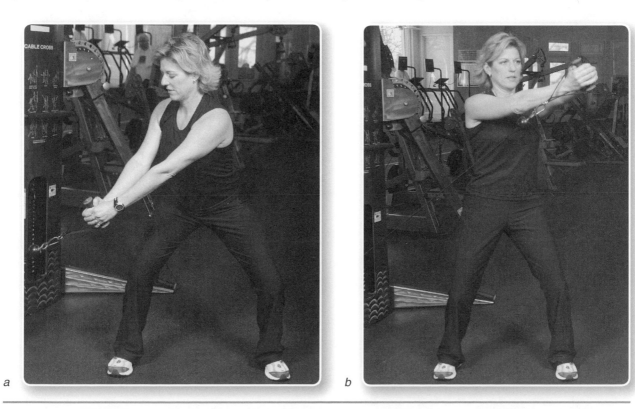

*a*                        *b*

**Figure 8.11** Woodchop movement pattern using the cables.

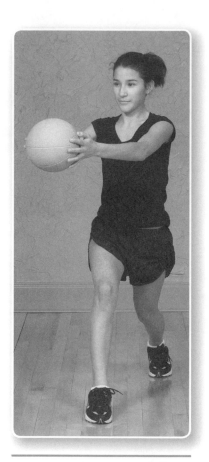

**Figure 8.12** Dynamic lunge with trunk rotation using a medicine ball.

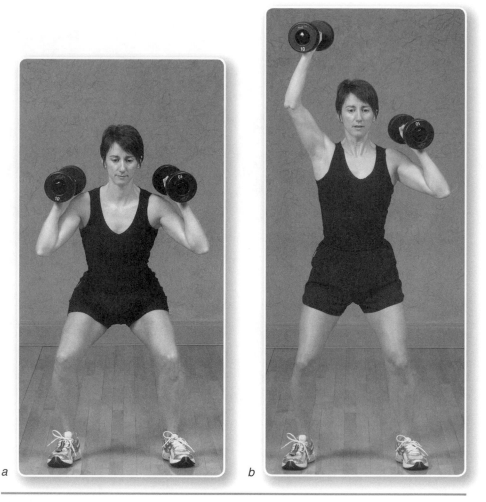

*a*                                                  *b*

**Figure 8.13** Body squat incorporating a dumbbell overhead press.

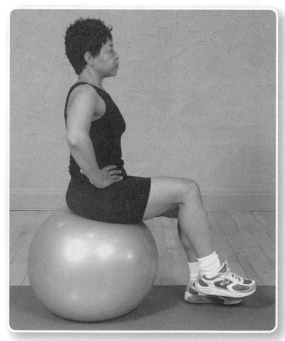

**Figure 8.14** Seated stability ball with a single-foot lift.

◆ Performing seated stability ball exercises (figure 8.14) improves postural stability and strength.

## An Integrated Approach

Traditional strength training exercises are most effective when integrated with functional exercises. It is recommended, however, that during an exercise session, functional-type exercise precede traditional exercise in order to prevent excess fatigue in the muscle and neural system that is needed to perform these types of activities effectively. Functional training leads to increased neural activation of the stabilizing and postural muscles, which can enhance performance during traditional exercises.

Most sports require speed, muscular endurance, power, balance, agility, coordination, and strength. Some athletes believe that too much time spent strength training may hinder their performance in some way. A comprehensive approach that encompasses all aspects of fitness is best. This approach is not only for the performing athlete but also for the recreational exerciser. Improved absolute and functional strength leads to improved performance. Developing basic joint strength and flexibility (muscle balance) provides the base for further strength improvements. For example, if the sport requires power, then maximum power cannot be achieved without maximum strength. Power is the product of strength times acceleration. Optimal strength and power cannot be achieved without the fundamental base of stabilization training.

# Body Mechanics and Spinal Alignment

You should address proper body mechanics and spinal alignment when beginning to train a woman. Explaining basic spinal anatomy and function will help her understand the importance of neutral spinal alignment in preventing injuries. Common injuries that can occur during strength training with improper technique include fractures, sprains, strains, dislocations, and tendinitis.

Proper postural alignment requires the ability to stabilize the spine (back and neck), pelvis, and scapulae. Most people who exercise do not understand that the positioning of their hips (pelvis) and shoulders (scapulae) reflects the positioning of their spine. These three areas, the spine, scapulae, and pelvis, are interconnected and need to work in unison to help maintain proper mechanics. Proper alignment should be maintained in all positions—standing, seated, supine, prone, or lying on the side. A neutral spine should be maintained through the cervical, thoracic, and lumbar curves. This neutral alignment conserves joint, spinal ligament, and intervertebral disc integrity and lessens soft tissue stress and compressive, shear, and rotary torque forces during exercise (figure 8.15). Neutral posture involves avoiding extreme spinal flexion, rotation, and extension. Flexing forward or lifting with improper form places unnecessary strain and pressure on the spine.

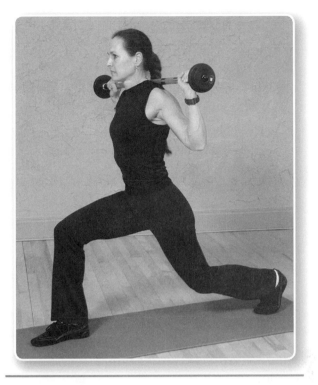

**Figure 8.15** Proper alignment reduces the risk of injury.

## Key Concepts—Postural Alignment and Body Mechanics

- ◆ The position of the pelvis reflects the position of the spine.
- ◆ The spinal (cervical, thoracic, lumbar), scapular, and pelvic areas need to work in proper unison.
- ◆ Proper alignment of the hips, knees, and ankles is necessary.
- ◆ Proper alignment should be maintained in all positions.
- ◆ Avoid extreme spinal flexion, rotation, and extension.
- ◆ Any piece of equipment can be harmful if used improperly.
- ◆ Any exercise or activity that is performed improperly can be harmful.
- ◆ Quality of movement is more important than quantity.
- ◆ Exercises that are too advanced can compromise proper alignment and mechanics, therefore increasing the risk of injury.

# General Strength Training Principles

There are five general strength training principles with which all trainers should be familiar:

- Overload—imposition of demands to elicit specific adaptations
- Variation—changing the training program variables
- Specificity—use of training exercises that are similar to the actual activity
- Individualization—designing a program to address the individual's specific needs
- Progression—adjusting the program to ensure safe and effective progress

In this section we'll discuss the principles as they relate to women's strength training.

**Overload** is a requirement for strength development. The muscles must be exercised at or near maximal strength and endurance for development to occur; the system must experience a load slightly beyond its capacity in order to adapt. Overload provides the pathway for overall progression. The improvements in strength are not governed by the method (type of equipment or resistance), but by the intensity of the overload. A muscle exercised against normally encountered resistances will not improve. Overload occurs through manipulating various training variables (sets, repetitions, frequency, etc.).

Variation refers simply to providing change or modification to variables within the training program. Variation in a training program allows physiological adaptations to occur, reduces the risk of injuries, and prevents overuse. Training variation occurs through specific exercise program planning by manipulation of several program training variables.

**Specificity training** refers to performance of exercises or activities that are specific or similar to the demands of a particular activity. Specificity may involve range of motion, speed, stabilization, planes of motion, or particular resistance demands. The more specifically an exercise matches the actual sport or activity demands, the greater the transfer-of-training effect (Clark 2001). For instance, a golfer could perform trunk rotation stabilization exercises to enhance her golf swing. This is a good example of functional fitness training in which the specific exercise will improve activity (golf) function.

Individualization refers to taking into consideration each individual's personal health, fitness level, and goals. The professional should consider age, injuries, medical history, training goals, exercise background, and the like. The exercise program should be specifically designed for each individual.

Progression is the result of continual adaptation to training stimulus. Progression occurs through overload, variation, specificity, and individualization of training. In order for progression to be continual, the training stimulus must be challenging, be specific to needs and goals, and include systematic manipulation of program variables (periodization). Progression will be safe and effective if the level of difficulty or intensity within each specific training variable is equal to the woman's physical capability level. Progression is the result of a consistent and systematically designed program that includes all the principles just explained.

For proper progression to occur, training variables should be varied or adjusted over time. Altering the training variables in the exercise prescription will advance specific training goals and help avoid overtraining (Kraemer et al. 2004).

## Program training variables

- Volume (sets, reps)
- Intensity
- Speed of movement
- Training frequency
- Training duration
- Rest interval
- Exercise selection
- Exercise order
- Movement patterns
- Plane of motion
- Range of motion
- Progressive difficulty (body position, base of support)

# Periodization

Periodization is a systematically planned exercise regimen lasting for a predetermined period of time, such as a four- to six-week training phase. Length of time depends upon progress and goals. Periodization may entail different training cycles (**microcycles, mesocycles,** and **macrocycles)** or phases, such as a stabilization phase, an endurance phase, a hypertrophy phase, a strength phase, or a power phase. The primary purpose of each training cycle and phase is to focus on one particular training goal more than another. For example, if strength is a long-term goal, then strength will not be maximized without sufficient stabilization. Therefore, a periodized program should be established that focuses on stabilization training before any exclusive strength training phase is begun. Periodization involves the constant manipulation of program training variables throughout each cycle and phase in order to produce a continual adaptation response. If an individual's program consists of the same training variables over a lengthy period of time, then proper progression will not occur.

Furthermore, a periodized training plan should strive to improve specific physical abilities to meet the demands of a sport. A study compared the physiological and performance adaptations between periodized (P) and nonperiodized (NV) resistance training programs in women collegiate tennis athletes (Kraemer et al. 2003). After nine months of training, the periodized group had significantly greater improvements in jump height and ball velocities for the serve, forehand, and backhand tennis strokes. The main finding was that a periodized resistance program produced greater improvements in strength and sport-specific motor performance than traditional resistance training in female tennis players (figure 8.16, *a & b*).

Periodization can also reduce monotony and the risk of injury. Consistently changing a program helps maintain mental interest and reduces boredom. Training stimulus variation also reduces continual repetitive movement patterns in the musculoskeletal system, reducing the risk of an injury. Specifics within a periodized training program are beyond the scope of this chapter; what we have emphasized here is the potential for periodization to produce significant training results.

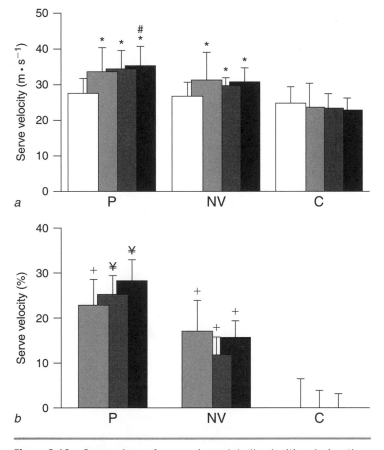

**Figure 8.16** Comparison of women's peak ball velocities during the tennis serve (*a*) and corresponding percent changes (*b*) before □ and after four ▨, six ▨, and nine months ■ of training in P, NV, and C. Values are mean ± SD; P ≤ 0.05 versus corresponding before value; # P ≤ 0.05 versus corresponding 4-month value; + P ≤ 0.05 versus corresponding C value; ¥ P ≤ 0.05 versus corresponding NV and C values. For data in panel A at four, six, and nine months, serve velocity in P > NV (P ≤ 0.05).

Reprinted, by permission, from W.J. Kraemer et al., 2003, "Physiological Changes with Periodized Resistance Training in Women Tennis Players," *Medicine and Science in Sports Exercise* 35(1): 157-168

# Core Training

The core can be defined as the **lumbo-pelvic-hip complex** (Clark 2001). Core training is a way to provide stability, neuromuscular control, and support to the joints and spine. Static and dynamic training of these stabilizing muscles should be the foundation of any exercise program.

## The Core Muscles

The core muscle system has also been categorized and divided into two units: the inner unit or local musculature system and the outer unit or global muscular system (Bergmark 1989). The inner unit consists of muscles that mainly provide joint stabilization. These intrinsic muscles are not responsible for specific movement but provide stability during joint movement (Richardson et al. 1999). The outer unit muscles mainly perform movement of the trunk and limbs and provide support to the spine (Richardson et al. 1999). Both groups should be trained to provide maximum and efficient movement. If the core muscles are functioning optimally, then strength, endurance, power, and neuromuscular control are effectively utilized (Clark 2005). If the extremity muscles are strong and the core is weak, then inefficient movement will occur throughout the kinetic chain (Clark 2001).

It is important to strengthen the inner unit before training the outer unit. If the inner unit is not adequately strengthened, then muscles of the outer unit will compensate and take over as the primary stabilizers. This can result in core dysfunction, which may lead to injury. Exercising with an unstable core, or overtrained superficial muscles and poor posture, creates further muscular imbalance and faulty movement patterns. Inner unit exercises tend to be more isometric such as the draw-in maneuver (figure 8.17) and prone hip extension (figure 8.18). Outer unit exercises are more dynamic such as a ball crunch (figure 8.19).

## Benefits of Core Training

Core muscle system training needs to be incorporated in all methods of strength training—traditional, functional, and sport-specific movements. Core training improves functional performance for women

## The Core Muscle System

**Inner unit (local musculature system)**

- ◆ Multifidus
- ◆ Transverse abdominis
- ◆ Internal oblique
- ◆ Lumbar transversospinalis

**Outer unit (global muscular system)**

- ◆ Rectus abdominis
- ◆ Gluteus maximus
- ◆ Erector spinae
- ◆ Adductors
- ◆ Quadratus lumborum
- ◆ Hamstring
- ◆ External oblique
- ◆ Quadriceps

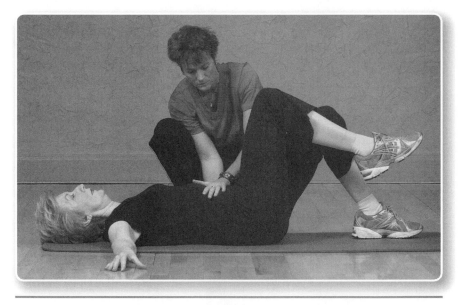

**Figure 8.17**  Inner unit core exercise: draw-in maneuver with single knee to chest.

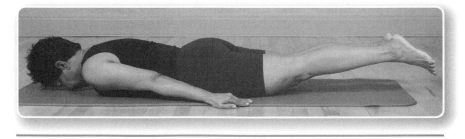

**Figure 8.18**  Inner unit core exercise: prone hip extension.

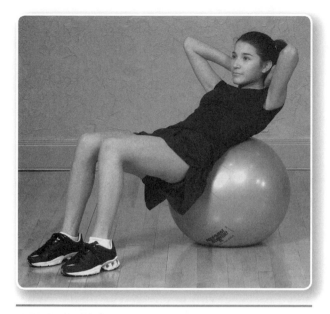

**Figure 8.19** Outer unit core exercise: abdominal crunch using stability ball.

## Core Stabilization Training Benefits

- ◆ Improves static and dynamic postural control
- ◆ Ensures appropriate muscular balance and joint **arthrokinematics**
- ◆ Allows for the safe and maximal expression of functional strength
- ◆ Provides intrinsic stability to the lumbo-pelvic-hip complex, allowing for optimum neuromuscular efficiency of the kinetic chain

Reprinted, by permission, from M.A. Clark, 2001, *Integrated Training for the New Millennium* (Thousand Oaks, CA: National Academy of Sports Medicine).

of all ages and all fitness levels. It improves postural alignment (static and dynamic control), reduces risk of injury, and improves functional strength.

Core strength training produces greater maximal power, which in turn leads to more efficient use of the peripheral muscles (shoulders, arms, legs). This type of training is especially necessary for athletes. Increased core strength improves body control, balance, overall power, and **neuromuscular efficiency,** permitting athletes to safely and effectively execute the necessary movements in their sports. Many sport-related injuries are caused by poor mechanics of movement.

Core training has been effective and useful in the area of rehabilitation (Clark 2005). Core training can be used as a form of injury prevention, including prevention of various lower extremity and lumbo-pelvic-hip complex dysfunctions as outlined in the following (Akuthota and Nadler 2004; Leetun et al. 2004).

For more information on current concepts in human functional anatomy and core stabilization training, contact the National Academy of Sports Medicine (www.nasm.org).

### Specific Benefits of Core Training for Female Athletes

As mentioned in previous chapters, the rate of knee injuries, specifically of the anterior cruciate ligament (ACL), is high in females. The role

of core training in the prevention of this type of injury is significant. Male athletes generally possess greater core stability than female athletes, and this may be one of the reasons men are at lower risk of ACL injury (Leetun et al. 2004). Increasing core strength in women may prevent lower extremity injuries (Ireland and Nattiv 2002; Leetun et al. 2004; Wilson et al. 2004). Increasing core strength will provide the necessary mechanics and stability in the spine, hips, knees, and ankles when multidirectional, pivoting, or jumping activities are required.

Adequate strength in the hip and trunk muscles plays a crucial role in an individual's ability to perform safe and efficient movement in all three planes of motion. The hip abductors and external rotators are important in lower extremity alignment, and weakness in these areas increases risk of injury (Ireland and Nattiv 2002; Leetun et al. 2004).

### Core Training and Prevention of Low Back and Pelvic Pain

A large majority of American women experience low back pain at least once in their lives. Inefficient muscular stabilization of the lumbosacral area is commonly found in women with low back and pelvic pain. Weakness in the transverse abdominis and multifidus muscles is also related to chronic low back pain.

Weakness in the lumbo-pelvic-hip complex may put the sacroiliac (SI) joint at risk. Stability of the SI joint is important because this joint supports a large portion of the body's weight. Shifting weight from one leg to the other involves movement at the SI joint. Sacroiliac joint injuries can be the result of soft tissue failure, direct trauma, or overload. Athletic activities can produce stress or unwanted force on the two SI joints. Muscle imbalances in the kinetic chain or improper sport-specific mechanics can also cause increased stress. Athletes may report a history of foot, ankle, knee, hip, or spine injury before SI joint pain syndrome is exhibited (Chen et al. 2002). Strengthening the hip abductors (gluteus medius) and preventing tightness, or overactivity, in the piriformis, hamstrings, and quadratus lumborum reduce the amount of force on the SI. Also, tightness in the adductors inhibits the gluteus medius. So stretching the adductors may help reduce SI joint injury as well.

The lumbosacral area is stabilized by the transverse abdominis, multifidi, erector spinae, quadratus lumborum, and psoas. The pelvic floor muscles work synergistically with the transverse abdominis (TA), multifidi, and diaphragm (Richardson et al. 1999). The TA, multifidi, and diaphragm assist in trunk stabilization and are active during pelvic muscle contractions (Richardson et al. 1999). All of these muscles, including the pelvic floor muscles, function to support and stabilize the lumbosacral region. Therefore, strength and stability of these muscles are essential to low back and pelvic pain prevention.

# Balance and Neuromuscular Stability Training

Balance and neuromuscular stability training is a must in any functional exercise program. Balance and stability may be simply defined as the body's ability to maintain a desired position (static and dynamic). Training the central nervous system is crucial for balance and stabilization improvements. Kinesthetic and proprioceptive awareness is the ability of the nervous system to know where all body parts are positioned in space at any point in time. Improper kinetic chain function negatively affects balance, stability, kinesthesia, and proprioception. Individuals who may be training specifically for power, speed, agility, or hypertrophy should include balance and stability training in their workouts. Balance and stabili-

zation are required components for all types of movements, both static and dynamic.

## Stability Training Progressions

Balance and stability training should always begin in a stable environment (on the floor) before progressing to unstable environments such as a balance board. Safety should always come first! Whether the environment is stable or unstable, the woman should be able to perform every exercise in a controlled and proficient manner. Being in control means being able to efficiently sustain a static or dynamic position safely and effectively. If an individual cannot be in control during an exercise in a stable environment, then an unstable environment is not appropriate. Stable and unstable environments can be manipulated, adjusted, and modified for proper progression. The following are examples of different types of progressions that can be used in balance and stability training. Progressions vary for both lower- and upper-body exercises. Balance and stability progressions should involve all three planes of motion. Progress from the sagittal, to the frontal, to the transverse, and finally to a combination of all three planes. When appropriate, each balance and stability training progression should include multiplanar movements prior to advancement.

### Lower-Body Balance and Stability Training Progression

Two legs

Two legs in a staggered position

One leg in a stationary position (figure 8.20)

One leg in a squatting position

Two legs in an unstable environment

Two legs staggered in an unstable environment

One leg in an unstable environment (figure 8.21)

### Upper-Body Balance and Stability Training Progression

Two arms

Alternate arms

One arm

One arm with torso rotation

All the preceding on one leg in a stable environment

Two arms in an unstable environment

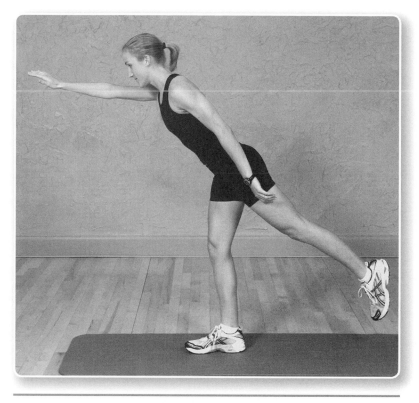

**Figure 8.20** Single-leg balance with opposite arm/leg reach.

Alternate arms in an unstable environment

One arm in an unstable environment

All the preceding on one leg in an unstable environment (figure 8.22)

Lower- and upper-body progressive exercises can be independent. For example, if an individual could effectively perform a single-leg balance, the next step in the progression would be a single-leg squat. The squat position increases the level of strength, balance, and stability required. An example of an upper extremity progression is a standing floor, two-arm (bilateral) overhead press, advancing to alternating arms followed by one-arm (unilateral) movement.

Lower- and upper-body progressions can be combined. For example, an individual can perform

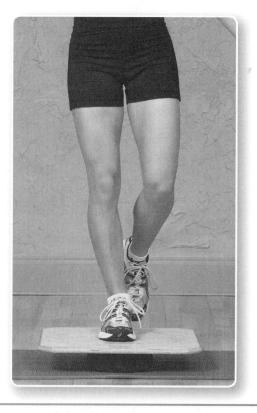

**Figure 8.21** Single-leg balance on an unstable surface (rocker board).

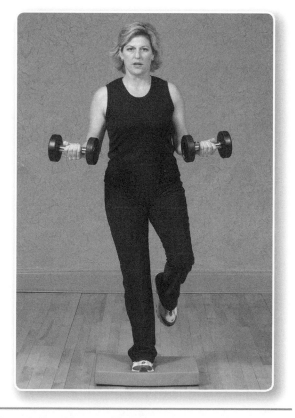

**Figure 8.22** Single-leg bilateral biceps curl in an unstable environment (Airex pad).

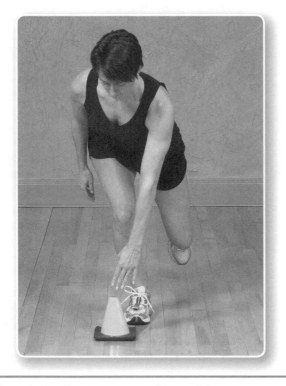

**Figure 8.23** Single-leg squat with multiplanar movement.

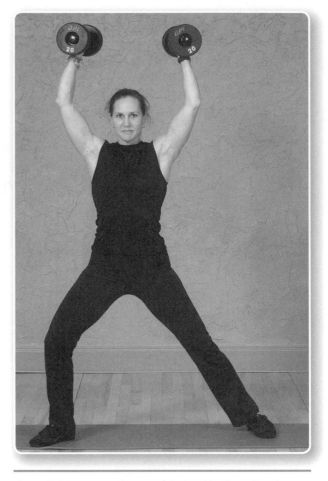

**Figure 8.24** Lateral lunge with dumbbell overhead press.

a bicep curl with two arms while standing on one leg on the floor, then progress to an alternating-arm bicep curl. This individual could eventually progress to standing on the air pad. Progressions vary and are dependent on the individual's ability to perform the easier exercise before moving on to a more difficult exercise. Adequate strength and stability are prerequisites for advancement.

Incorporating different planes of motion is essential in progression. Performing an exercise in the sagittal plane requires less balance and stabilization than in the frontal plane or transverse plane (figure 8.23). Advancing to different planes of motion should be incorporated in lower- and upper-body progressions (figures 8.24 and 8.25). There are multiple ways in which a trainer can use each lower-body, upper-body, and plane-of-motion progression. The most important factor is the individual's ability to perform a specific activity effectively before progressing to the next level.

## Tools for Balance and Stability Training

Different types of balance modalities can be used to create an unstable surface. Following is a common list of tools for stability training organized by levels of difficulty, beginning with the easiest and progressing to the most difficult. These progressions take into account surface size, plane of movement, level of support, and directional instability. Even though each tool has a general level of difficulty, the actual level of difficulty depends upon the specific exercise chosen. Progressions should also move from static to dynamic exercises. For example, an individual needs to effectively balance on a half foam roller before adding any dynamic movement (squat, multiplanar movements, upper extremity exercises, etc.) to the exercise.

While tools can add variety and provide for progression, don't forget the numerous body weight exercises that can be an effective functional training method for providing resistance and challenge. For example, squats, multiplanar lunges, single-leg squats, jumps, and push-ups are advanced exercises for some, even without external resistance or tool use. Always be sure to match the exercise to the woman's physical

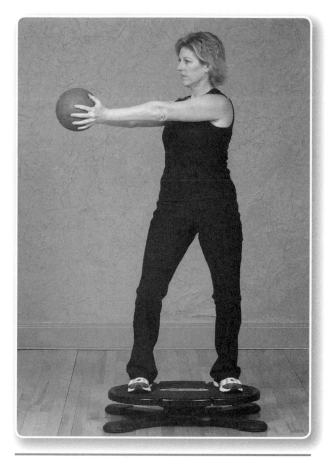

**Figure 8.25** Trunk rotation using medicine ball on a core board.

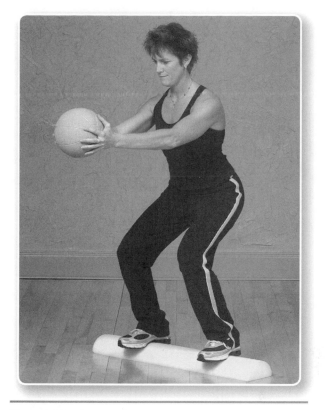

**Figure 8.26** Squat on the half foam roller with a medicine ball.

## Stable to Unstable Progressions (Easiest to Most Difficult)

◆ Floor
◆ Balance beam
◆ Airex pad
◆ Half foam roller (figure 8.26)
◆ Core board (figure 8.27)
◆ Balance (rocker) board
◆ Bosu
◆ Disk pillow (figure 8.28)

abilities. A woman may progress from a stable to an unstable training surface only if she has the required strength, flexibility, and stabilization to do so safely and effectively.

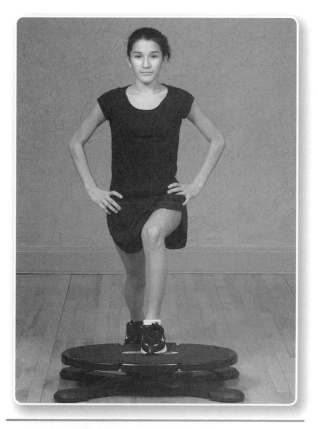

**Figure 8.27** Forward lunge onto a core board.

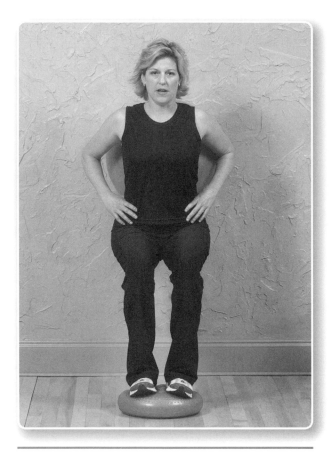

**Figure 8.28** Standing on a disc pillow during a stability ball squat.

# Strength Training Choices

Every trainer will eventually be asked the question, "Can I exercise at home or do I need to join a fitness center?" Strength benefits and progress can be achieved in either environment. The decision about where to exercise depends on the individual woman. What are her personal needs? What environment will be more motivating and provide for long-term consistency? The professional should be prepared to educate women on the advantages and disadvantages of home and fitness club training, as well as to help match their personal needs with the appropriate environment. Whether the woman decides to exercise at home or at a club, she may benefit by hiring a qualified personal trainer to assist with her exercise program. See tables 8.1 and 8.2 for advantages and disadvantages of health or fitness club training and at-home training.

◆ **TABLE 8.1** ◆

## Health and Fitness Clubs

| Advantages | Disadvantages |
| --- | --- |
| Variety (equipment and classes) | Fees |
| Safety (exercise specialist, group leaders) | Travel time |
| Social atmosphere, group support | Distance from home, work |
| Fewer distractions than home exercise | Intimidating environment |
| Expert advice | Limited hours of operation |
| Facility services, amenities (locker rooms, showers, sauna) | |
| Commitment, accountability | |

◆ **TABLE 8.2** ◆

## Home Training

| Advantages | Disadvantages |
| --- | --- |
| No fees | Less equipment/variety |
| Convenient and time efficient | Space requirements |
| Private | Need to purchase some equipment |
| More relaxed environment | No supervision or instruction |
| Not limited to hours of operation | Lack of social support |
| | Distractions from other responsibilities |

◆ Conclusion ◆

In this chapter we have contrasted traditional strength training, which involves single-planar or single-joint exercises, with functional strength training. Functional strength training incorporates stabilizing muscles and natural movement patterns to help women prepare for real-life movements and activities—the activities they perform at home, at work, or in leisure pursuits. In addition to reviewing and applying the principles of traditional strength training, we have introduced the important concepts of body mechanics and spinal alignment, core strength, balance and stability, and neural control. We don't advocate doing away with traditional strength training exercises; rather, we encourage an integrated approach that has the advantages of increasing motivation and activity performance and reducing boredom and risk of injury.

Throughout the chapter we provided numerous examples and illustrations of functional strength training progressions using a variety of tools, including free weights, resistance bands, stability balls, and cable machines. Tips were included for individualizing exercises for women at various skill levels, from beginners to athletes. Because strength training exercises are not limited to the gym, the chapter concludes by outlining the advantages and disadvantages of health or fitness club training and at-home training programs. The benefits of strength training are clearly significant for women of all ages. When the goal is to improve health, function, and quality of life, strength training is closely associated with flexibility training, which is the focus of the next chapter.

# CHAPTER 9

# Flexibility for Women

## Topics in This Chapter

- Benefits of flexibility training
- Types of flexibility training
- Recent flexibility research
- Including flexibility in the workout
- Kinetic chain dysfunction
- Corrective exercise training
- Corrective flexibility training
- Postural alignment
- Factors affecting flexibility

- American College of Sports Medicine flexibility guidelines
- Stretching tools
- Flexibility classes

> I define health simply as successful adaptation to life. To achieve this goal, it is important to maintain a balance of physical and mental fitness.
>
> Pamela Peeke, MD, MPH, author of *Fight Fat After Forty*

Flexibility is one of the key components of fitness, but it could very well be the most misunderstood and poorly addressed aspect of exercise. Fitness professionals usually think of speed, power, force, strength, endurance, or agility when improving performance is the goal. Flexibility is often neglected.

Awareness of the importance of flexibility training has increased. Part of the reason may be an increase in the number of research studies focusing on the validity, significance, and protocols of flexibility training for performance enhancement. This increase in research has encouraged fitness professionals to examine flexibility training more directly. The type of flexibility training in exercise programs today is different from what was included years ago. With further research, flexibility training is likely to continue to change over the coming years as well.

In this chapter we review current research on stretching and suggest ways to fit stretching into an exercise program. It is also important to understand how integral flexibility is in maintaining function of the kinetic chain. Finally, tools for flexibility and flexibility classes are reviewed.

Flexibility appears to improve performance and reduce risk of injury; therefore, flexibility training is key to the success of any woman's fitness program. It should be viewed as a critical component of a balanced fitness program and an integral part of every workout.

## What Is Flexibility?

Simply stated, flexibility is the ability of a joint to move through its complete range of motion (Franklin et al. 2000). We know that flexibility is specific to the type of joint (ball and socket, hinge, etc.) involved and is dependent on the muscles and connective tissue (ligaments, tendons, **fascia**) surrounding that joint. Range of motion is affected by both muscle length and joint integrity.

Joints should move effectively and safely for a specific action. For example, full range of motion of the shoulder is needed to correctly serve a tennis ball (figure 9.1). Of course, it is obvious that muscles must be strong and joints must be stable to perform specific actions. But it is just as important to prepare muscle groups and associated joints for the range of motion required for a particular activity.

The structural and functional benefits of good flexibility are outlined in the following list. For the individual woman, proper flexibility training improves posture and appearance, decreases chance of overuse injuries, prevents joint dysfunction, improves strength and power, improves function for daily activities, and enhances sport performance (figure 9.2).

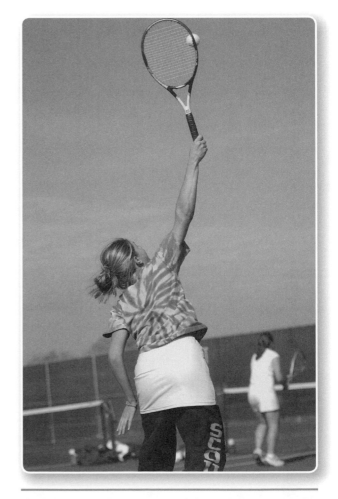

**Figure 9.1**　The tennis serve requires full joint range of motion.

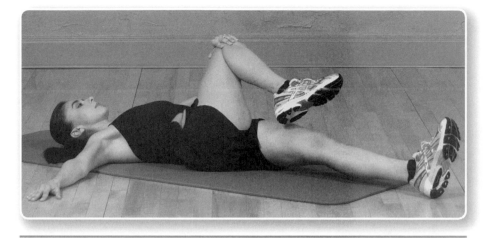

**Figure 9.2** Supine static piriformis stretch: Stretching overly tight muscles can reduce the risk of injury.

## Benefits of Flexibility Training

Proper flexibility training can

- help correct muscle imbalances,
- increase joint range of motion,
- decrease muscle soreness,
- decrease muscle **hypertonicity,**
- relieve joint stress,
- avoid microtrauma to the muscle tissue,
- improve the extensibility of the musculo-tendinous junction, and
- maintain the normal functional length of all muscles.

Reprinted, by permission, from M.A. Clark, 2001, *Integrated Training for the New Millennium* (Thousand Oaks, CA: National Academy of Sports Medicine), 109.

## Types of Flexibility Training

There are two general categories of flexibility training: **static (passive)** and **dynamic (active) stretching.** Static stretching (holding a position) involves passively moving a joint or limb to the point of mild discomfort, then holding it for a fixed period of approximately 15 to 30 seconds. In a static stretch, the shortest muscle involved will receive the tension. An example of a static stretch is the adductor stretch shown in figure 9.3. This type of stretching is easy to measure and is safe and effective. Static type stretching has

been the focus of most of the scientific literature on flexibility.

**Proprioceptive neuromuscular facilitation** (PNF) is a type of static stretching that focuses on the contract–relax and hold–relax mechanisms. A muscle group is passively stretched, contracted against resistance while in the stretched position, then passively stretched again with increased range of motion. This type of stretching, which usually requires a partner, facilitates increased range of motion, increased strength, and movement pattern control.

Dynamic stretching involves actively moving a muscle through the joint's available range of motion. Examples of dynamic stretching are controlled leg swings, lunge or adductor (figure 9.4). This type of stretching involves the

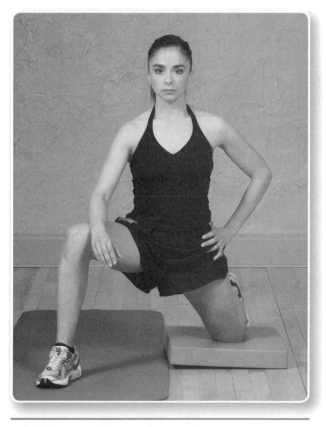

**Figure 9.3** Static lower extremity adductor stretch.

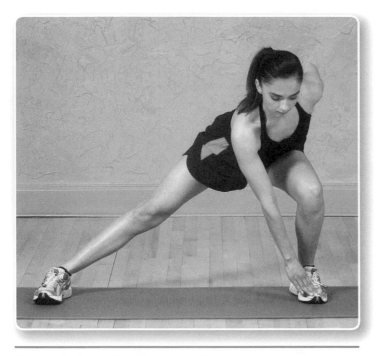

**Figure 9.4** Dynamic adductor stretch.

contraction of the **agonist** muscle while producing a stretch on the **antagonist** muscle.

**Ballistic** stretches, another dynamic stretch, are rapid, jerking, or bouncing motions. With ballistic stretches, traumatic injuries can occur to the muscles, tendons, or ligaments because the joint or muscles (or both) can be taken to a greater length than they are designed for. Ballistic stretches are effective for only certain activities, such as a sport or activity involving explosive movements (sprints, martial arts, ballet). Because ballistic stretches place increased stress on the tissue, they should not be performed by the general public. Only individuals with the acquired knowledge of this type of stretching or those involved in specificity training under supervision should perform ballistic stretches.

Both types of stretching, static and dynamic, are important and effective if performed in the proper manner. No single stretching technique can address every need of a flexibility program.

# Recent Research on Flexibility

For many years, exercise leaders and trainers have encouraged people to warm up prior to exercise by walking or using cardiovascular machines and by performing stretches to reduce the risk of injury. However, despite an increase in the number of studies pertaining to injury prevention and stretching techniques, there remain unanswered questions about the merits of and protocols for a flexibility program. The literature reveals varied opinions, lack of consensus for specific accepted protocols (frequency, duration), and an increased need for evidence in the correct application of stretching techniques for a given individual. Not only is there clinical debate about how to stretch; there is also debate about the relationship between flexibility training and injury prevention. As old theories and practices regarding flexibility and exercise are challenged, flexibility training protocols will need to be modified to achieve optimal and efficient human movement and performance.

## Flexibility and Injury Prevention

A recent systematic review of literature (including studies on men and women) was conducted to investigate the validity of flexibility training as a means to reduce risk of injury (Thacker et al. 2004a). The authors found that there was not sufficient evidence to endorse or discontinue routine pre- or postevent stretching to prevent injury among competitive or recreational athletes. They suggested that better research was needed to determine the proper role of stretching in sports, especially given the increasing numbers of athletes and a growing recognition that all people need to increase their physical activity to improve their health and quality of life.

In support of flexibility training, the researchers pointed out that stretching increases muscle

## Types of Flexibility Training Techniques

- ◆ Static
  - Passive
  - Proprioceptive neuromuscular facilitation
- ◆ Dynamic
  - Active
  - Ballistic

and joint flexibility, which would include the possibility of preventing injuries and improving performance. It is important to note that extremes of hyperflexibility and inflexibility can increase risk of injury. Strong evidence suggested that a program including an adequate warm-up, activity-specific stretching, and other exercise activities (strength and proprioception training, plyometrics) enhances performance and prevents certain kinds of injuries. There was also evidence that strength training, conditioning, and warm-up have an important role in injury prevention. The authors noted that stretching should be performed in the context of adequate conditioning and appropriate warm-up. A follow-up comment by the same authors stated that pre-exercise stretching does not protect athletes from injury. However, maintaining flexibility through a regular stretching program may be important in preventing injuries (Thacker et al. 2004b).

## Pre-Exercise Flexibility: Static Versus Dynamic

Opinions differ on the effectiveness of static versus dynamic stretching. Even though static stretching has been used pre- and postexercise for a number of years, more recent protocols favor combining static and dynamic stretching prior to exercise. Importantly, pre-exercise static stretching performed in a *corrective* manner to reduce muscle imbalances is being highly recommended. Correcting muscle imbalances through flexibility training is addressed in detail later in this chapter.

It is thought that static stretching alone does not adequately prepare the body for the dynamic movements that are performed during exercise and sport activities. Static stretching is usually performed in only one plane of movement. However, most physical activities and exercises occur in all three planes of motion. Therefore, dynamic stretching should follow a light aerobic warm-up and precede the sport or exercise activity. This type of routine is more effective in preparing the muscles and joints for a variety of exercises and functional activities.

Some research has shown that static stretching prior to activity may even have a negative effect on performance. Static stretching in women prior to activity may change the mechanical properties of the muscle, for example altering the **length–tension relationship** or a central

nervous system inhibitory mechanism (Cramer et al. 2004). These are all important points to keep in mind when one is prescribing specific types of stretching exercises for athletes prior to competition or for individuals participating in strenuous activities.

## Flexibility and Training Techniques

Research on the effectiveness of various methods and techniques of flexibility training is inconsistent. Differences in these studies are primarily due to the vast number of variables that are involved, such as type of stretching technique used; stretching with and without prior exercise; the frequency, duration, and number of repetitions and sets; and consistency of the stretching program over time.

While some studies show no difference in the effectiveness of various stretching techniques, such as static (passive) versus PNF, other studies show PNF stretching to be more effective than static (passive) stretching. The duration of the isometric contraction in PNF stretching (at least 5 seconds) has been found to be a factor in stretching effectiveness in some studies as well. There are also differences when one compares flexibility studies as to the amount of warm-up time, such as 10 minutes or greater. Differences in these studies raise questions: Which stretching techniques are best? How frequent and long should a static stretch be held in order to be the most beneficial? How long should a warm-up be to be effective?

Flexibility improvements may also vary with total stretch time (total number of minutes spent stretching over a given period) and length of stretching program (number of weeks). A study pertaining to stretch time in PNF hamstring stretching was performed in women and men (Chan et al. 2001). The two groups in this study had a total stretching time of 3,600 seconds (60 minutes). One group performed the total stretching time over eight weeks and the other over four weeks. Both groups increased hip flexion range of motion, with no significant differences found. The eight-week group had only a slight increase in flexibility over the four-week group (11.2 and 8.9 degrees, respectively). Given the results of these studies, no single stretching protocol is mandated. Rather, a stretching program can be customized for each individual woman's needs.

## Flexibility and Muscle Soreness

One study, including men and women, demonstrated a relationship between muscle stiffness and muscle damage after eccentric exercise (McHugh et al. 1999). This study helps explain the susceptibility to exercise-induced muscle damage and delayed-onset muscle soreness (DOMS). The least flexible subjects in this study felt more muscle pain and tenderness, experienced a loss of isometric strength, and had higher creatine kinase levels (a muscle enzyme) on the days after exercise as compared to their more flexible counterparts. The results indicated that more flexible people are less susceptible to exercise-induced muscle damage. The authors also suggested that more flexible people may be able to exercise at a higher intensity or for a greater duration on the days after a bout of eccentric exercise. It is not known whether stretching to improve flexibility before eccentric exercise will limit subsequent muscle damage. However, there is some evidence indicating that pre-exercise aerobic warm-up may reduce subsequent symptoms of muscle damage. Most importantly, the recurring theme in the literature seems to be that *regular* stretching is what reduces various risks, not pre-exercise stretching.

# Incorporating Stretching Into an Exercise Program

Dynamic stretching, static stretching, and stretching for correction of muscle imbalance are all important parts of an exercise program. In this next section, we'll show you how to incorporate each of these into an individual's program. For daily guidelines, see table 9.1.

## Dynamic Stretching for Warm-Up

There is agreement about the importance of an aerobic warm-up prior to moderate or vigorous activity. A proper warm-up increases heart rate and blood flow, deep muscle and core temperature, and muscle elasticity, and activates the central nervous system. These factors allow for improved performance and a decreased risk for musculotendinous injuries. Many injuries can be prevented with adequate warm-up, especially activities performed in colder climates.

Ideally, a light aerobic warm-up is followed by dynamic stretching. The proposed benefit of dynamic stretching is that it effectively prepares the musculoskeletal and neuromuscular systems for total body movement training or specific sport activity. Dynamic warm-ups are particularly important in preparing athletes for the biomechanical nature of the sport activity. For example, a tennis player could perform controlled lateral shuffles, front-to-back leg lateral crossovers, multiplanar lunges, or lunges with trunk rotation (figure 9.5). Body weight exercises performed for warm-up should be done in controlled motions only. Other examples of these exercises are body squats (figure 9.6), push-ups, stationary skipping (high knees), and walking gluteal kicks. This type of warm-up may prevent needless injuries and improve overall performance.

## Static Stretching for Cool-Down

A cool-down should always end an exercise session. It is important to take time to reduce the intensity of the exercises from vigorous to moderate to mild before performing any prone or supine stretching. The cool-down helps minimize blood pooling and lowers body temperature. Recovery time is dependent on individual fitness levels. Static stretching is appropriate for cooling down

◆ TABLE 9.1 ◆

### Stretching Guidelines for Adults (General Population)

| Type | Exercises for the major muscle and tendon groups using static stretching that focuses on the groups having reduced range of motion; a warm-up should precede stretching |
| --- | --- |
| Frequency | Minimum of 2 days per week; ideally 5-7 days per week |
| Intensity | To the point of end-range motion tightness without inducing discomfort or pain |
| Duration and repetitions | Static: hold 15-30 seconds; two to four times per stretch |

Data from American College of Sports Medicine, 2006, *ACSM guidelines for exercise testing and prescription*, 7th ed. (Lippincott, Wiliams, and Wilkins).

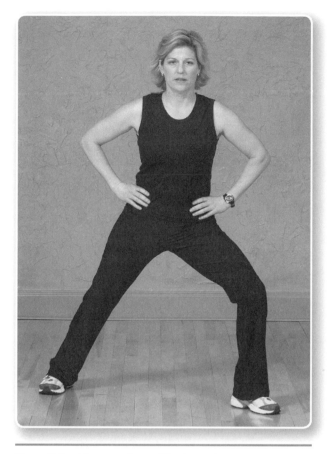

**Figure 9.5**  Movement-specific dynamic warm-ups: dynamic lateral lunges are a good warm-up for tennis or any multi-planar activity.

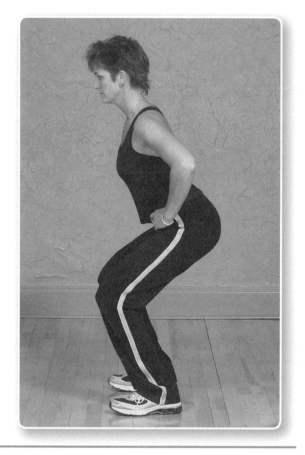

**Figure 9.6**  Body squats can be performed in a dynamic warm-up.

after activity. These stretch-and-hold positions don't tax the muscles in the way that dynamic flexibility movements do prior to exercise.

## Static Stretching to Correct Dysfunctions

Static type stretching is beneficial for maintaining and improving muscle length and range of motion over the long term, as well as for correcting muscle imbalances. Static stretching and **self-myofascial release** (soft tissue release technique) can be used prior to the warm-up to address any musculoskeletal imbalances and dysfunctions in the kinetic chain. Static stretching elongates the musculotendinous unit to create length of a muscle as well as a decrease in passive tension. When this initial soft tissue extensibility is produced in the overly tight muscles, then more appropriate movement patterns during exercise training can occur, thereby improving proper kinetic chain function. These types of stretches should also be used in the cool-down portion of the training program to restore tissue length

and joint range of motion. The health and fitness professional should realize that injury prevention through corrective training is a key factor for achieving effective program results and attaining a woman's fitness, sport, or functional goals.

## Including Flexibility Training in an Exercise Session

The following is an appropriate sequence for incorporating flexibility training into an exercise session:

◆ Corrective stretching, if needed
◆ Light aerobic warm-up
◆ Dynamic warm-up with stretching
◆ Exercise activity or sport
◆ Cool-down with general static and corrective stretching

# Flexibility Training and Kinetic Chain Dysfunction

Patterns of dysfunction can occur in the muscular, neural, and articular systems (kinetic chain) of the body if imbalances are not properly addressed. Inadequate or altered flexibility leads to kinetic chain dysfunction, resulting in muscle imbalances (Clark 2000). Dysfunctions in the kinetic chain can occur over time due to overuse patterns, compensations, and lack of activity. Tissue injury can lead to synergistic muscle compensation (**synergist** muscles are the muscles that assist the prime movers during functional movements) and altered muscle recruitment patterns, causing faulty movement patterns (Edgerton et al. 1996).

Muscle imbalance is a primary cause for kinetic dysfunction. A woman who jogs and consistently avoids stretching specific muscle groups (low back, hamstrings, quadriceps, gluteals, tensor fasciae latae, hip flexors, and calves) could eventually experience muscle imbalance issues. Muscular imbalances affect quality of muscle and joint movement and create incorrect repetitive movement patterns. Prolonged static activity in

## Common Causes of Muscle Imbalance

◆ Postural stress
◆ Lack of core strength
◆ Pattern overload
◆ Lack of neuromuscular control
◆ Repetitive movement
◆ Aging
◆ Cumulative trauma
◆ Immobilization
◆ Poor technical skill (motor patterns)
◆ Decreased recovery and regeneration following activity

Reprinted, by permission, from M.A. Clark, 2001, *Integrated Training for the New Millennium* (Thousand Oaks, CA: National Academy of Sports Medicine), 109.

a constrained, poor posture is a common reason for muscular imbalances. Women whose jobs or personal routines involve sitting most of the day, at a desk, in a car, or on an airplane, are subject to certain postural issues (figure 9.7). Another cause of muscle imbalance is repetition of movement. Any job or activity that requires the same constant joint motion or position (working on a computer, using a telephone without a headset, regular golfing) for prolonged periods can cause tightness in specific muscles. These types of improper postural and repetitive movement activities can be addressed and improved through flexibility training.

## Corrective Exercise Training

Muscle imbalances can be corrected with proper flexibility and strength training, or corrective exercise training. Corrective exercise training to address muscular imbalances involves targeting the specific muscles that have become restricted and weak. An example of corrective exercise training for prolonged sitting with improper posture (flexed spine) is as follows:

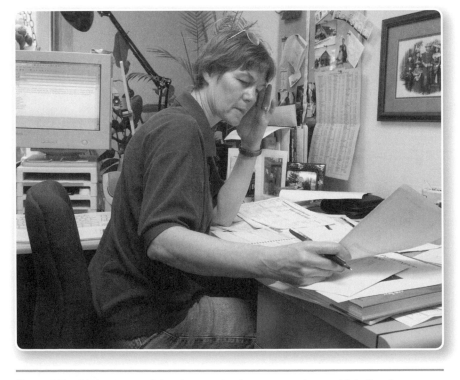

**Figure 9.7** Sitting most of the day can lead to poor posture, which if not addressed can cause muscle imbalances.

◆ Identify the muscles that are possibly shortened from sitting—hip flexors and quadriceps, chest and anterior shoulder, hamstrings, adductors, latissimus dorsi, and calf complex. Stretch these muscles to reestablish musculoskeletal balance.

◆ Identify the muscles that have possibly become overly lengthened and weak from sitting—gluteals, tibialis, posterial deltoid, and core and scapulae stabilizers (upper and mid back). Strengthen these muscles to reestablish musculoskeletal balance.

◆ Note: In this example, any specific cervical muscle imbalances will depend on the positioning of the neck during the prolonged seated position.

This type of training can be used to correct any muscle imbalances, joint or postural dysfunctions, neuromuscular deficiency, and overuse injuries that occur (Clark 2001). More information on corrective exercise training is provided in chapter 10. Because corrective training can improve overall proper kinetic chain function, it is a critical part of the overall exercise program.

## Corrective Flexibility Training

**Corrective flexibility training** is the application of appropriate stretches to improve muscle imbalances, postural distortions, and joint dysfunctions. Specific stretches that address any kinetic chain dysfunction should be done prior to the warm-up. A warm-up (light aerobic activity followed by dynamic stretching) should always precede any strenuous activity. Corrective stretching can be addressed through static and self-myofascial release techniques. Methods for assessing and identifying particular muscle imbalances, as well as ways to correct them, are examined in depth in chapter 10.

Muscle imbalance is the result of certain muscles which have become tight and overused while others have become elongated and weak (Clark 2001). This imbalance can result in improper neuromuscular movement patterns during an activity and incorrect postural alignment (figure 9.8). Neuromuscular and neurodynamic stretching are also appropriate for corrective flexibility training (Clark 2001). More information on neuromuscular and neurodynamic stretching can be

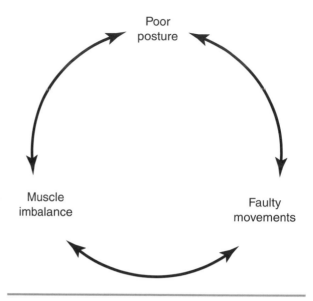

**Figure 9.8** Poor posture, faulty movements, and muscle imbalance are all interrelated.

found through the National Academy of Sports Medicine continuing education and certification programs.

## Postural Alignment

To adequately evaluate an individual's postural imbalances, the fitness professional should focus on posture and alignment issues, as well as observe faulty movement patterns. A postural analysis can be a very effective tool for identifying overly tight and lengthened muscles and prescribing specific flexibility and strengthening exercises. Observing a woman's natural posture during standing (anterior, posterior, and lateral view) provides postural muscle imbalance information necessary for prescribing her specific exercises (figure 9.9, *a & b*). The lateral view is particularly helpful in observing certain imbalances, such as lordosis and kyphosis.

Posture is the specific alignment of the kinetic chain at any given moment. Proper postural alignment can be attained only through kinetic chain balance (figure 9.9*c*). Optimum postural alignment provides optimum structural and functional efficiency to the kinetic chain. For example, if a woman sits or stands in either a lumbar extended or thoracic and cervical flexed spinal posture for extended periods of time, she will most likely develop poor postural alignment because of the altered length of the muscles at the joints.

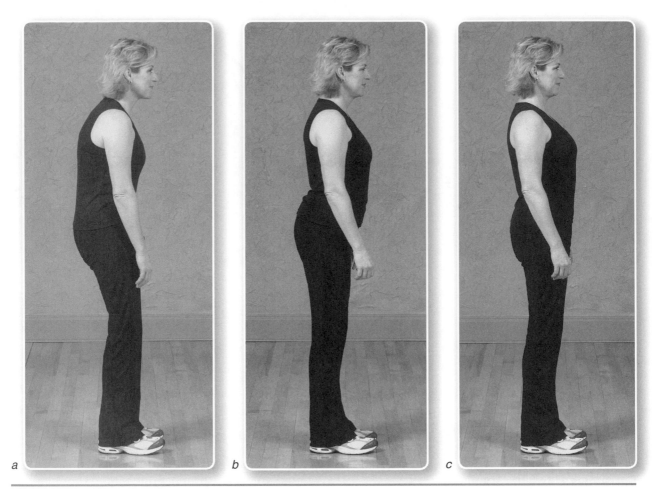

a          b          c

**Figure 9.9** Observing postural imbalance assists in stretching exercise selection. Proper postural alignment enhances kinetic chain function; (*a*) kyphotic posture, *(b)* lordotic posture, *(c)* neutral posture.

There are two forms of postural alignment: static and dynamic. Static posture is the alignment of the muscles and joints in a motionless position (standing or sitting). Dynamic posture is the alignment during moving (walking or housework). Keeping proper body alignment during static and dynamic activity is important for efficient functioning and to reduce unwanted stress.

When the body is in proper alignment (neutral positioning), it is more efficient in performing any static or dynamic activity. Flexibility training can correct postural misalignment. Continual microtrauma due to misalignment can lead to tissue overload and joint stress, causing future injury. In many cases, there are multiple misalignments. Correcting only a single misalignment will not result in optimum postural alignment. Postural alignment is dependent on adequate flexibility, strength,

and stabilization in all the key postural muscle groups.

There are several posture checks and cues that you can use with the women you work with. Good posture habits can be developed through education and training, in and out of the exercise session. To develop postural awareness, advise clients to use mirrors or reflections in windows for frequent posture checks and cues.

◆ Make sure the woman keeps the head aligned over her shoulders with the shoulders slightly pulled back. A forward head position is quite common and can be the result of tight and weak neck muscles, weak upper back muscles, and tight chest and anterior shoulder muscles.

◆ Check the positioning of the low back and pelvis. An excessively arched low back and

## Factors Affecting Flexibility

**Internal influences**

- Type of joint—some joints are genetically limited for stability (sacroiliac joint)
- Bony structures that limit movement (ulnar olecranon)
- Inelastic nature of soft tissue (scar tissue is inelastic)
- Internal resistance (fibrous capsule)
- Elasticity of the skin
- Elastic nature of tendons and ligaments (ligamentous laxity is a precursor to joint hypermobility, which may cause injury)
- Neuromuscular efficiency
- Soft tissue and joint temperature
- Preexisting injuries, muscle imbalances, and tender areas

**External influences**

- Temperature of training conditions (warmer climates are more suitable for increasing flexibility)
- Age (flexibility declines with age)
- Technical skill level (poor motor patterns)
- Time of day (flexibility improves in the afternoon)
- Psychological restraints (lack of personal commitment to improving flexibility)
- Equipment or clothing restrictions

Reprinted, by permission, from M.A. Clark, 2001, *Integrated Training for the New Millennium* (Thousand Oaks, CA: National Academy of Sports Medicine), 109.

protruding abdomen can be the result of weak gluteals and abdominal and core stabilizers, as well as tight hip flexors and tight low back.

- Check for positioning of the feet and knees. Excessive foot pronation, knee flexion and internal rotation during static and dynamic activities are definite patterns that can increase risk of injury. This can be the result of tight calves, hamstrings, adductors, iliopsoas, and iliotibial band, as well as weak tibialis, gluteals, and vastus medialis.

## Stretching Tools

Numerous tools can be used to aid in stretching. Items such as foam rollers, tennis balls, and The Stick can be used for self-myofascial release (figure 9.10). These tools are inexpensive, easy to use, and very effective. The stability ball can be used as a stretching tool as well (figure 9.11) The Bosu and medicine balls are valuable tools that can be used for dynamic-type stretching and warm-ups (figure 9.12). These tools add value to the dynamic warm-up by challenging postural, core, joint, and neuromuscular strength and stabilization.

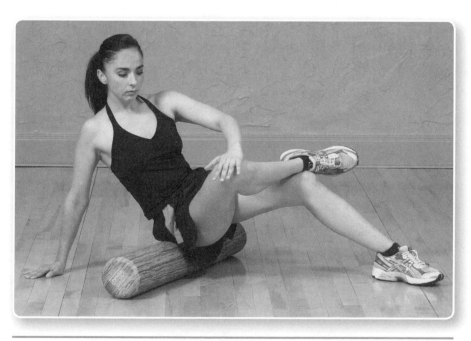

**Figure 9.10**    Self-myofascial release of the piriformis using the foam roller.

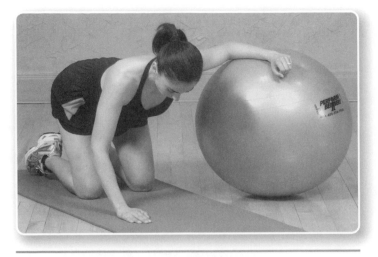

**Figure 9.11**  Chest stretch using the stability ball.

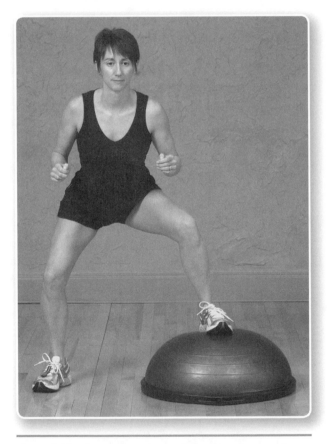

**Figure 9.12**  Dynamic warm-up: lateral squat on a Bosu.

# Flexibility Classes for the Body and Mind

The past few years have seen added interest on the part of women and increased participation in different types of stretching classes. Stretch-ing exercises that connect the body and mind are effective for stress management and are especially popular. Because of the recent growth in the number of independent yoga and Pilates studios, a wide selection of classes is available to active women. Many are conveniently located and may offer a more private setting than the typical fitness center.

## Pilates

Women have been drawn to Pilates because of its nonimpact, nonaerobic, deep muscle condi-tioning benefits (figure 9.13). Pilates, named for founder Joseph Pilates, was once called "control-ogy." It is designed to achieve suppleness, natural grace, and skill in all movements—functional, recreational, and vocational. Whether women are interested in improving overall fitness or recovering from childbirth, an injury, or surgery, Pilates strengthens the body's core—such as the abdominal, gluteal, and back muscles. It improves flexibility, stability, and posture while strength-

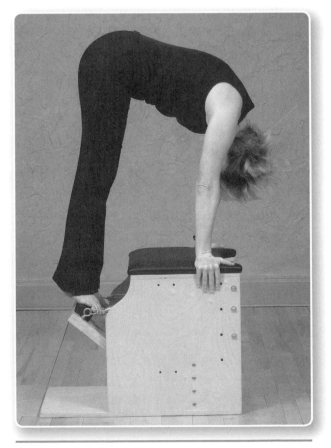

**Figure 9.13**  Pilates can provide the necessary stabiliza-tion, strength, and flexibility for daily function.

ening the muscles deep in the torso (multifidus, transverse abdominis) and around the spine (erector spinae, quadratus lumborum). Pilates can help improve balance, coordination, efficiency of movement, and body awareness and can help to prevent or correct muscle imbalances. Pilates provides total body conditioning without the hypertrophy results of intense weight training. Pilates requires control and concentration to confer the most benefit and can be performed using a mat or Pilates equipment. Exercises can be modified to range from gentle to challenging, depending on fitness level and goals. The Pilates method is useful in correcting postural dysfunctions, as well as managing other conditions such as fibromyalgia, incontinence and pelvic floor dysfunctions, and scoliosis and other back disorders.

The goal of Pilates is improved quality of movement that leads to improved quality of life.

The manner in which the exercises are performed is more important than the number of repetitions. When performing the exercises, one should remember that they are functional movements, not structured exercises. For example, imagine walking up the stairs while feeling the hamstrings firmly in control. Or imagine picking up a baby with the stomach supporting the back. Ideally, these movements take place without one's having to think about the muscles. The principles that are the foundation of the Pilates technique are presented in the sidebar below.

## Yoga

Yoga, often synonymous with stretching, is more than a flexibility program. It includes meditation, relaxation, and body control and results in increased muscular strength and improved flexibility (figure 9.14). The goals of yoga are gener-

## Pilates Principles

◆ Concentration—focusing on muscles as they move. To accomplish even the simplest exercise, the mind needs to focus on small movements (kinesthetic, proprioceptive, and postural awareness with visualization).

◆ Control—essential in preventing injuries. Maintaining control of every movement takes concentration, effort, and awareness of what the rest of the body is doing at a given time. Repetition, dedication, and application improve the degree of control and the perfection of movement. Physical motion must be controlled.

◆ Centering—efforts of movement, force, balance, and strength coming from the center. Abdominal strength provides support, while abdominal control provides fluidity of movement from the center. All movements come from a stable center (core stability).

◆ Flow—fluidity of movement that leads to fluidity of movement in daily living. Continue the movement as if 10 repetitions were one, rather than one repetition repeated 10 times. Stiff movements occur in muscles that are too tight. Fluid movements may initially require some shortening of overextended muscles and lengthening of shortened muscles. Smooth movements are projected outward from a strong center.

◆ Precision—proper and specific movement patterns that maximize the effectiveness and value of the exercise. Working through small steps is required to achieve exactness from simple to complex exercises. When all the movements are put together, the overall exercise becomes graceful and effortless.

◆ Breathing—a vital part of the Pilates work. Expand the rib cage during inhalation to increase flexibility in the intercostal muscles and decrease tightness of the upper thoracic area. Exhale through relaxed jaw to decrease stress and tension in the body. Synchronize breathing patterns during exercise.

◆ Routine—an established routine improves mental and physical conditioning in all individuals. Perseverance, dedication, energy, and regular practice will vastly improve what is achieved physically.

From J. Pilates, W. Miller, and J. Robbins, 1998, *Return to life through contrology* (Incline Village, NV: Bodymind Books), 109.

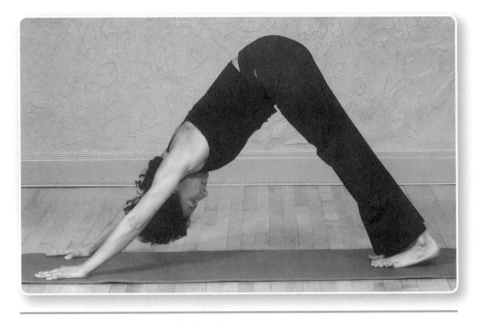

**Figure 9.14** Yoga—downward-facing dog.

ally holistic (true-self or spiritual). The following are four of the more widely practiced forms.

Kundalini yoga is called the noisy yoga. It is an ancient, specific system using physical exercises, yoga postures, sound, chanting, meditation, and breathing techniques. The object is to move energy through the body's energy centers, enhancing creativity, vitality, mental clarity, and personal power. This form of yoga can help improve flexibility and muscle tone, increase mental and physical energy levels, and promote a deep sense of inner calm, strength, and grace.

Vinyasa yoga, or power yoga, builds strength, stamina, and flexibility through a vigorous and physically challenging yoga style. It includes a flowing series of postures linked by the breath. The dynamic flowing stream of *asanas* (poses) cultivates mental and physical balance and tones the whole body while inspiring an overall sense of vitality. Breath work and meditation draw the attention inward, helping to create a calm, peaceful state.

Hatha yoga is the ancient practice of yoga as an experiential path of self-discovery and holistic health. Hatha is not a specific style, but an umbrella for any type of physical yoga. It is a transformational practice that can help improve physical fitness, flexibility, mental clarity, self-understanding, relaxation, stress management, and overall well-being. It is a therapeutic methodology that recognizes the individual's needs and capabilities at different stages of life. This style is grounded in the connection to the earth and a natural release and expansion within the poses facilitated by the wave of the breath.

Bikram yoga is performed in a room heated to a temperature of 105 degrees Fahrenheit. It is the only yoga that is copyrighted, and all 26-pose classes are consistent. Each pose is performed twice, and this class does not include any chanting or meditation.

## Hybrid Classes

The hybrid class has developed as a way to maximize time in a rushed life. One example is the combination of yoga, tai chi, and Pilates into a PiYo class. Classes fuse the basics of the tai chi yang short-form and adapted hatha yoga asanas. Participants benefit from both isometric and isotonic muscular contractions, balance enhancement, and improved relaxation through meditation with visualization. Hybrid classes follow principles of both functional alignment and core stability while incorporating breathing techniques, yoga, tai chi, and Pilates-inspired movements.

## ◆ Conclusion ◆

For women of all ages, good flexibility means improved posture and appearance, decreased chance of overuse injuries, prevention of joint dysfunction, improved strength and power, improved function for daily activities, and enhanced sport performance. However, research on the effectiveness of specific methods and techniques of flexibility training is somewhat inconsistent, as evidenced by studies cited throughout this chapter. With further research, guidelines for flexibility training are likely to continue to evolve over the next few years.

Protocols combine static stretching and dynamic stretching prior to exercise. In this chapter, we promoted both types of stretching for individualized programs: static (passive and proprioceptive neuromuscular facilitation) and dynamic (active and ballistic). Pre-exercise and postexercise stretching to correct muscle imbalances and kinetic chain dysfunctions was also recommended.

We included numerous examples and illustrations of flexibility exercises to prevent muscular imbalances and correct postural misalignment. Because women need to be more aware of their posture, we have suggested posture checks and cues for assessment, education, and training purposes. As with strength training, a variety of static and dynamic stretching tools can be incorporated, including foam rollers, the Bosu, medicine balls, and stability balls. These devices assist in flexibility improvement and help maintain interest in the stretching component. Many women enjoy the mind–body connection experienced in flexibility classes such as Pilates, yoga, and tai chi, as well as various hybrid classes—all excellent options.

Part IV of this book uses the information from all previous chapters to show how to develop an individualized fitness program for a particular woman—one that is enjoyable, effective, and safe.

# Designing Individualized Training Programs

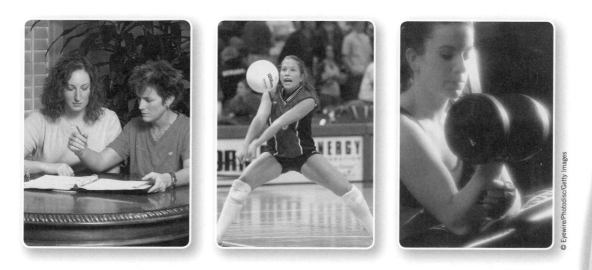

© Eyewire/Photodisc/Getty Images

# CHAPTER 10

# Individualized Training Programs

## Topics in This Chapter

- ◆ Basic concepts of program design
- ◆ Functional assessments for kinetic chain dysfunction
- ◆ Baseline fitness test
- ◆ Consultation and goal setting
- ◆ Advanced concepts of program design
- ◆ Exercise to correct kinetic chain dysfunction
- ◆ Exercise selection for function or sport-specific activity
- ◆ Exercise progression
- ◆ Common exercise tools
- ◆ Case study

As I said before, exercise is individual, as individual as the makeup you choose for yourself. It's got to fit your needs, your desires, what you're best at. . . .

Millie Cooper, author of *Aerobics for Women*

While most of this book has covered information that is of interest to a variety of health professionals (physicians, nurses, health educators, wellness professionals), this chapter will probably be most useful to the fitness professional who designs individualized training programs for particular women in a nonmedical setting.

Fitness trainers generally know what women want to accomplish with a personal training program (table 10.1). Younger women usually express concerns about their appearance. They want to lose weight and get toned to look attractive. As women get older, usually around their 40s and 50s, they can and should expect more than appearance benefits from their fitness programs.

The training goals that individual women set for themselves may differ from the public health goals of fitness programs for women. The fitness trainer has the challenge of meeting the needs of the specific woman and achieving disease prevention and management goals through increased physical activity and fitness.

## Basic Concepts of Program Design

While broad public health goals are appropriate for women in general, to the fitness professional

working with a particular woman, these goals lack specificity for program design. To design an individualized program, several steps are necessary. First, a PAR-Q is completed (see appendix A, page 198). Second, a functional assessment and fitness test must be done. Third, an in-depth consultation with the woman is mandatory.

The PAR-Q provides some quick baseline information that guides functional and fitness testing. By doing a functional assessment, you will identify problem areas that may need corrective action, such as muscle imbalances and compensation patterns, which will be discussed later in further detail. These will take precedence over virtually everything else as you design an initial program in order to restore overall musculoskeletal balance. Fitness testing provides a baseline that is then used to set goals and assess progress. Consultation affords the opportunity to learn each woman's individual goals, which will then be incorporated into the program. Consultation also provides useful information for exercise selection.

Once these steps are completed, certain questions and issues will become obvious to the trainer that may not have been obvious to the woman, such as these:

◆ Can she go through pregnancy and then carry around her infant for the next two years and not experience any significant structural changes?

◆ Can she train for a 5K fun run or a new sport without an injury?

◆ Can she bend over and pick up something without harming her bones, joints, or muscles?

The trainer is then faced with the challenge of merging the data from the functional assess-

◆ **TABLE 10.1** ◆
## Goals of Fitness Programs by Age

| Adolescence (teens) | Childbearing years (20s to 40s) | Menopause and beyond |
|---|---|---|
| Offer programs that appeal to the "whole" girl—that she will enjoy and do<br>Help avoid risky behaviors<br>Help girls grow into healthy women<br>Prevent chronic diseases later in life | Help women:<br>Have a healthy baby<br>Use exercise to deal with the stresses of pregnancy and the postpartum period<br>Recover quickly from delivery<br>Develop lifelong habits of physical activity<br>Assess risks for chronic diseases<br>Encourage their children to be physically active | Help women:<br>Build strength and coordination<br>Maintain function<br>Manage chronic conditions, if necessary<br>Enjoy optimal quality of life<br>Live independently for as long as possible |

ment, fitness testing, and consultation to create a program that achieves both public health and personal fitness goals. To do this, a program must include these three key concepts as part of every workout (Kraemer et al. 2004):

- ◆ Correction of kinetic chain imbalances
- ◆ Attention to functional or sport-related needs
- ◆ Incorporation of individual health and fitness goals

## Functional Testing

The first step in developing an individualized training program is to conduct a functional assessment. To help women attain optimal physical performance and decrease the risk of injury, trainers need to do functional assessments to identify any kinetic chain imbalances. Some examples of a functional assessment are gait analysis, single-leg stance test, goniometric measurements, static postural analysis, overhead squat, and single-leg squat test (Clark 2001; table 10.2). The particular functional assessments in this chapter as well as other types of assessments are taught by the National Academy of Sports Medicine. There are a variety of different assessments that leading fitness experts in the field perform; these assess musculoskeletal function as well. All of these functional assessments provide information about a woman's overall function.

It is very important to be involved in continuing educational seminars, certification classes, and related membership associations to keep constantly updated on the most current approaches in the industry.

One test, the overhead squat test, is especially useful (figure 10.1). It provides a vast amount of information about a woman's functional movement patterns. Ask the woman to perform a squat while holding a light weighted rod or stick raised over her head with elbows fully extended. As the woman continues to repeat the overhead squat movement, look for abnormal movement patterns in the kinetic chain. Table 10.3 shows compensation patterns to note, as well as some related structural involvement (tight or weak muscles) that could be present (Clark 2001). Functional tests for seniors are discussed in chapter 6.

## Fitness Testing

There are five main components of physical fitness testing in nonmedical settings: absolute strength, dynamic strength/endurance, flexibility, cardiorespiratory fitness, and body composition (table 10.4). An example of a personal training assessment sheet, which would include testing results from girth measurement, body composition, and resting metabolic rate, is provided on page 208 in Appendix A. This testing sheet is beneficial to the professional, as well as the

◆ **TABLE 10.2** ◆

## Functional Assessments for Kinetic Chain Imbalances

| | |
|---|---|
| Static postural analysis | Observing static postural alignment in the anterior, posterior, and lateral positions. Designed to assess static postural dysfunctions in the kinetic chain. |
| Gait analysis | Observing gait from anterior, posterior, and lateral views. Designed to assess specific gait deviations. |
| Goniometric test | Goniometer measurements of side-to-side comparison of individual muscle length and joint range of motion. Designed to assess individual muscle tightness and imbalances. |
| Overhead squat | Observing an individual performing a controlled squat with arms raised overhead, with elbows fully extended, holding a stick. Designed to assess bilateral, symmetrical dynamic flexibility; muscle balance; and integrated strength of the ankles, knees, lumbo-pelvic-hip complex, shoulder complex, and cervical-thoracic spine. |
| Single-leg stance test | Observing deficiencies and length of time an individual can balance on one foot. Designed to assess ankle proprioception, core strength, and hip joint stability. This test can be performed with eyes open or eyes closed. |
| Single-leg squat | Observing a single-leg squat. Designed to assess ankle proprioception, core strength, and hip joint stability. To be performed only if individual is sufficient in single-leg balance test. |

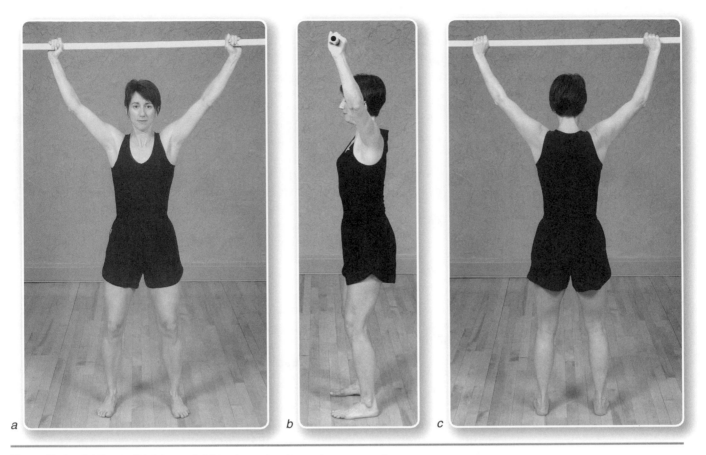

**Figure 10.1** *(a)* Front, *(b)* side, and *(c)* back overhead squat assessments.

client, for baseline measurements and progress checks. Examples of these five physical fitness testing methods are provided on pages 200-207 in appendix A.

Another form of testing that is useful is measuring resting metabolic rate (RMR). Resting metabolic rate is the number of calories a woman burns through the day from normal bodily functions. By knowing this number, as well as an estimate of how many calories a woman burns through general activity during the day and in structured exercise, the professional can make recommendations on general calorie consumption and total calories to burn through exercise to meet weight maintenance or weight loss goals (see the resting metabolic rate section on the personal training assessment sheet on page 208 of appendix A).

The BodyGem by HealtheTech Inc. is a small handheld device that can be used in a nonlaboratory setting for obtaining a valid measure of resting metabolism. This device is precise, easy to use, portable, and relatively inexpensive.

## Consultation

The next step in program design is consulting with the woman. Typically, a consultation, or an interview, is a way to obtain needed information efficiently and effectively. An advantage of an interview is that it provides an opportunity to probe for more details while you are beginning to establish a bond with the woman. Sample consultation forms and health questionnaires are provided on pages 209-214 of appendix A. Generally, this session is similar to taking a medical history. A medical, occupational, and exercise history and some questions about personal fitness goals are appropriate at this session. The following are key consultation topics:

◆ Medical history
◆ Medications
◆ Injury history
◆ Occupational history
◆ Past exercise habits
◆ Current exercise habits
◆ Short-term goals
◆ Long-term goals

◆ TABLE 10.3 ◆

## Compensation Patterns and Related Structural Issues

| Abnormal movement | Tight muscles | Weak muscles |
|---|---|---|
| Feet flatten out (pronate) | Peroneal complex | Posterior tibialis |
| Feet turn out (externally rotate) | Soleus, lateral gastrocnemius | Medial gastrocnemius, posterior tibialis |
| Heel of foot rises | Soleus | Anterior tibialis |
| Hip abducts (externally rotates) | Piriformis, tensor fascia latae, iliopsoas, biceps femoris, sartorius | Adductors, medial hamstrings |
| Hip adducts (internally rotates) | Adductors, medial hamstrings | Gluteus maximus/medius |
| Excessive hip flexion | Calve complex, iliopsoas, tensor fascia latae, rectus femoris | Gluteals, upper hamstring complex, posterior adductor magnus, anterior tibialis |
| Asymmetrical pelvic shifting | Correlate foot, knee, and hip deviations for specifics. Note: Client usually deviates to dominant adductor side (possibly due to opposite ankle restriction) | |
| Increased lumbar extension | Iliopsoas, lumbar erectors, latissimus dorsi, quadratus lumborum | Gluteus maximus, external/internal obliques, rectus abdominis |
| Increased lumbar flexion | External/internal obliques, hamstrings, rectus abdominis, adductor magnus | Iliopsoas, lumbar erectors, latissimus dorsi, quadratus lumborum |
| Protruded abdomen | Iliopsoas, lumbar erectors, quadratus lumborum | Rectus abdominis, obliques, inner unit, gluteus maximus |
| Arm or arms fall forward | Latissimus dorsi, pectoralis major, upper abdominal muscles | Rhomboids, middle trapezius, thoracic erector spinae |
| Elbows flexed | Pectoralis major, latissimus dorsi | Infraspinatus, teres minor, thoracic erector spinae, middle trapezius, rhomboids |
| Abnormal shoulder elevation | Upper trapezius, levator scapulae | Lower trapezius, serratus anterior |
| Shoulder blade winging | Serratus anterior, pectoralis minor | Middle trapezius, rhomboids |
| Protruded head | Cervical spinal extensors | Cervical spinal flexors |

Reprinted, by permission, from M.A. Clark and L. Parracino, 2003, *Advanced integrated flexibility* (Course Manual) (Calabasas, CA: National Academy of Sports Medicine), 96.

◆ TABLE 10.4 ◆

## Five Components of Physical Fitness Testing

| Fitness component | Example of Fitness tests |
|---|---|
| Absolute strength | 1-repetition maximum |
| Dynamic strength and endurance | Abdominal crunches or push-ups |
| Flexibility | Sit and reach |
| Cardiorespiratory fitness | Submaximal bike or run test |
| Body composition | Skinfold caliper measurements |

Data from Physical Fitness Specialist Course and Certification 2005.

### *Medical, Medication, and Injury History*

The medical history includes any conditions, surgeries, or diseases that may exist in the present or past history. Any medical condition that may have an effect on the woman's exercise program must be known prior to program design. For example, a woman with fibromyalgia or rheumatoid arthritis would not be given the same exercise prescription as a healthy woman desiring to gain strength. Any medications being taken are also necessary information. A woman on beta-blockers would not be set up using a target heart zone; rather, her rate of perceived exertion would determine the intensity level (see table 7.1 on page 114 for rate of perceived exertion scale). Previous or present injuries will also be a big factor in program design (exercise selection, workload, etc.). Orthopedic injuries, spinal conditions, or lumbo-pelvic-hip complex issues are common problems the health and fitness professional will face.

### Occupational History

In addition to the medical history questions, the trainer needs information about the woman's environment: her occupation, any repetitive movement patterns, and postural positions that occur throughout the day. For example, if a woman's daily life or occupation involves sitting most of the day, then posture and muscle imbalances may occur. She could be developing tightness in some major muscle groups, such as the chest, shoulder, neck, back, and hips.

Asking questions about the woman's daily activities and occupation is important to determine what stressors her body experiences during the day or week. These findings affect the exercise selection portion of program design. It is especially important to note whether repetitive movements or postures have occurred for a lengthy period of time without exercise correction. Generally, the longer a woman has neglected postural issues, the more essential corrective exercises will be. Some women are completely unaware of postural and overuse issues. The functional assessment brings awareness to the professional about what typical posture, repetitive, and general movement patterns a person might be performing consistently throughout the day or week and therefore determines what corrective measures are needed.

### Exercise Habits

Past exercise habits can give information concerning degree of experience with exercise equipment, activity or sport involvement, or a base knowledge of exercise itself. A woman who has not exercised in the past 10 years will have a very different exercise prescription than a woman who has not exercised in the past two months.

Current exercise habits can determine present level of fitness, related types of future exercise selection, and the recommended cardiovascular and strength training prescription (frequency, intensity, and duration). Both past and present exercise information can also determine the extent of health and fitness education that needs to be involved (biomechanics, benefits of exercise, etc.).

### Reviewing Goals

It is important to know the woman's personal short-term and long-term goals. Short-term goals may cover a period of a few weeks to two to three months. Long-term goals may extend from six months to a year. Most people are not able to focus on goals that are much beyond a year. Listen carefully to what women say they will do in the next month because that is what they are most likely to accomplish.

Answers to these questions help establish goals and make them measurable:

What do you want to achieve?

When do you want to achieve it?

What are you willing to do (or give up) to achieve the goal?

What will enable you to be consistent?

How will you know that you have achieved your goal to your satisfaction?

What's stopping you?

Regardless of the particular time frame, a goal should be realistic. Ask, "Could another woman similar to you be expected to achieve the same goal?" For those involved in athletics or possessing a more competitive nature, the goal should also be challenging, yet realistic. Athletes tend to be very sport specific when establishing goals. For example, a female athlete playing volleyball or basketball has a goal to improve jump height in order to enhance sport performance. A short-term goal to improve vertical height jump 2 inches (5 centimeters) with proper training in 10 to 12 weeks would be realistic; a goal to improve that much by next week's game would be unrealistic. Established long-term goals need to be supported by accomplished short-term goals. Setting and achieving short-term goals will produce greater motivation and desire to achieve long-term goals. A woman has a long-term goal to run a full marathon in eight months. Setting a short-term goal of participating in a 5K run followed by a 10K run would provide motivation and a sense of confidence for achieving the long-term marathon goal.

# Advanced Concepts in Program Design

A general physical activity or exercise program can produce significant health improvements, but not maximal performance improvements. If a woman desires significant performance improvements, a systematically planned program is needed.

Designing exercise programs around isolating the basic eight major muscle groups (chest, shoulder, triceps, back, biceps, quadriceps, hamstring, abdominal) should definitely be a model of the past. Using information about postural dysfunctions and functional assessments provides information about how the human body functions as a whole unit during activities. Don't look at a specific muscle group and its primary movement pattern or action. Rather, look at a muscle group and see how it relates and functions with other muscle groups in the body. This is the premise behind functional training and is why specific muscle isolation training only does not fully prepare our muscle, neural, and articular systems (kinetic chain) for sport-related or daily activity. A woman does not lean over and pick up her child through isolated muscle movement only. Her entire kinetic chain system is interrelated, and no system functions independently. To be even more specific, not only does each system not function independently; each muscle group does not function entirely on its own but relies on other muscle group function and assistance to perform an activity. The philosophy of program design described in this chapter can be used with women of all ages who are involved in any exercise activity and have the goal of enhancing their performance.

## Exercises to Correct Kinetic Chain Dysfunctions

Muscle imbalance is a primary reason for kinetic chain dysfunction. Kinetic chain dysfunction leads to compensation patterns, which in turn can lead to injury. Some causes of kinetic chain dysfunction other than postural stress and repetitive movements are pattern overload, joint dysfunction, and lack of core strength and neuromuscular control (See common causes of muscle imbalances on page 158 in chapter 9). An example is tight chest and weak back muscles contributing to poor posture and shoulder joint instability. As stated in chapters 8 and 9, to achieve maximum muscle performance, it is necessary to build a program around core and neuromuscular training by incorporating multiplanar activities, static and dynamic postural alignment, and proprioceptive awareness.

Developing postural control, core strength, flexibility, joint stabilization, and effective neuromuscular control is critical to a successful program (Clark and Parracino 2003). Fitness professionals need training in assessing and identifying kinetic chain dysfunctions and functional movement patterns and applying corrective exercises. An integrated training approach, which includes kinetic chain function and applying corrective exercises, has been designed by the National Academy of Sports Medicine. More information is available through the educational and certification programs at www.nasm.org.

## Common Postural Dysfunctions

Three common postural dysfunctions that can eventually lead to specific joint and neuromuscular problems and injuries are presented next (Clark 2001). They are lower crossed syndrome (tables 10.5 and 10.6), which is characterized by increased lumbar lordosis (figure 10.2) and anterior pelvic tilt; upper crossed syndrome (tables 10.7 and 10.8), which is characterized by rounded shoulders and a forward head posture (figure 10.3); and pronation-distortion syndrome (tables

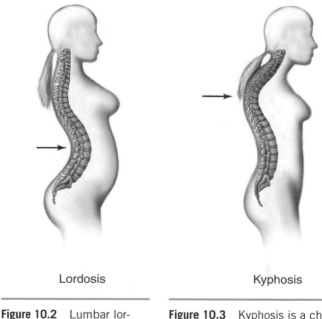

Lordosis                          Kyphosis

**Figure 10.2** Lumbar lordosis is a characteristic of lower crossed syndrome.

**Figure 10.3** Kyphosis is a characteristic of upper crossed syndrome.

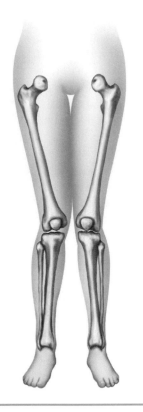

**Figure 10.4** Knock-knees and excessive foot pronation are characteristic of pronation-distortion syndrome.

10.9 and 10.10), which is characterized by excessive foot pronation, knee flexion and internal rotation, and valgus during functional movements (figure 10.4). A postural analysis (anterior, posterior, lateral views) along with other functional testing will identify these imbalance issues. These postural dysfunctions result from tight and weak muscle groups.

Corrective exercises for these syndromes are stretching the tight muscles and strengthening the weak muscles. Every trainer should be familiar with these syndromes and the muscles affected. Knowing the syndromes allows the trainer to target strengthening of weak muscles and stretching of tight muscles.

## Correcting Postural Imbalances in Pregnant Women

A postural analysis of a pregnant woman may identify some of these common postural imbalances (Parracino 2004). Exercise and pregnancy were discussed in chapter 5. The postural changes

◆ TABLE 10.5 ◆
### Lower Crossed Syndrome

| Tight/short muscles | Weak/lengthened muscles |
| --- | --- |
| Iliopsoas | Gluteus maximus |
| Rectus femoris | Hamstrings, gluteus maximus |
| Tensor fasciae latae | Gluteus medius |
| Adductors | Gluteus medius |
| Erector spinae | Transverse abdominis, internal oblique, multifidus |
| Gastrocnemius/soleus | Anterior/posterior tibialis |

Data from M.A. Clark, 2001, *Integrated training for the New Millennium* (Thousand Oaks, CA: National Academy of Sports Medicine).

◆ TABLE 10.6 ◆
### Lower Crossed Syndrome Joint Dysfunctions and Injury Patterns

| Associated joint dysfunctions | Injury patterns |
| --- | --- |
| Sacroiliac | Anterior knee pain |
| Tibiofibular | Hamstring sprains |
| Tibiofemoral | Low back pain |
| Iliofemoral | |
| Subtalar | |
| Iliosacral | |
| Lumbar facet | |

Data from M.A. Clark, 2001, *Integrated training for the New Millennium* (Thousand Oaks, CA: National Academy of Sports Medicine).

◆ TABLE 10.7 ◆
### Upper Crossed Syndrome

| Tight/short muscles | Weak/lengthened muscles |
| --- | --- |
| Pectoralis major | Rhomboids |
| Pectoralis minor, teres major, levator scapulae, upper trapezius | Lower trapezius, serratus anterior |
| Anterior deltoid | Posterior deltoid |
| Subscapularis, teres major, latissimus dorsi | Teres minor, posterior deltoid, infraspinatus |
| Sternocleidomastoid, scalenes, rectus capitus | Longus coli/capitus |

Data from M.A. Clark, 2001, *Integrated training for the New Millennium* (Thousand Oaks, CA: National Academy of Sports Medicine).

◆ TABLE 10.8 ◆
### Upper Crossed Syndrome Joint Dysfunctions and Injury Patterns

| Associated joint dysfunctions | Injury patterns |
| --- | --- |
| Sternoclavicular | Shoulder instability |
| Acromioclavicular | Rotator cuff impingement |
| Thoracic | Biceps tendinitis |
| Cervical facet | Thoracic outlet syndrome |
| | Headaches |

Data from M.A. Clark, 2001, *Integrated training for the New Millennium* (Thousand Oaks, CA: National Academy of Sports Medicine).

◆ TABLE 10.9 ◆

## Pronation-Distortion Syndrome

| Tight/short muscles | Weak/lengthened muscles |
|---|---|
| Peroneals | Posterior tibialis, flexor digitorum/hallucis longus |
| Gastrocnemius | Anterior tibialis |
| Soleus | Posterior tibialis |
| Iliotibial band, hamstrings | Vastus medialis |
| Adductors | Gluteus medius |
| Iliopsoas | Gluteus maximus |

Data from M.A. Clark, 2001, *Integrated training for the New Millennium* (Thousand Oaks, CA: National Academy of Sports Medicine).

◆ TABLE 10.10 ◆

## Pronation-Distortion Syndrome Joint Dysfunctions and Injury Patterns

| Associated joint dysfunctions | Injury patterns |
|---|---|
| Lumbar facet | Plantar fasciitis |
| Sacroiliac | Posterior tibialis tendinitis |
| Subtalar | Anterior knee pain |
| Talocrural | Low back pain |
| Tibiofibular | |
| First metatarsophalangeal (MTP) | |

Data from M.A. Clark, 2001, *Integrated training for the New Millennium* (Thousand Oaks, CA: National Academy of Sports Medicine).

of pregnancy are so common and easy to diagnose and address that they merit being revisited here (see table 10.11).

## Exercise Selection for Function or Sport-Specific Activity

Selecting the appropriate exercises is integral to program design. Understanding the requirements of an activity (what the body needs to do to perform that activity effectively) is the basis of exercise selection. The exercises selected to help enhance performance of a specific activity are dependent on the mechanical and physiological characteristics of the activity. Ask:

What types of biomechanical movements are required?

How often?

For how long?

At what intensity level?

How much trunk or joint stability is needed?

What are the requirements in relation to joint mobility or flexibility?

What planes of motions or movement angles are required?

What is the primary purpose of the skill involved?

What is the risk versus benefit of the exercise?

◆ TABLE 10.11 ◆

## Common Postural Imbalances in Pregnant Women

| Postural imbalance | Probable cause | Stretch exercise |
|---|---|---|
| Excessive lumbar curve with anterior pelvic tilt | Increase in size and weight causes an upward/forward shift in the center of gravity, leading to anterior pelvic tilt. | Hip flexors, adductors, iliotibial band (IT band) and tensor fasciae latae (TFL), posterior pelvic tilts |
| Increased thoracic curvature | This center of gravity shift causes increased lordosis; enlarged breasts also contribute. | Pectoral stretch, chin tuck stretch |
| Excessive scapula abduction | Weight gain in breasts pulls shoulders forward while possibly increasing thoracic curvature. | Pectoral stretch |
| Excessive forward head posture | Increased thoracic curvature and breast enlargement force head forward/upward, increasing curvature of cervical spine. | Cervical spinal extensors (e.g., chin tuck) |
| Overpronated feet | Weight gain, pelvic misalignments, and changes in hormones may contribute to joint laxity; hypermobility may lead to fallen arches. | Calf stretch |

Reprinted, by permission, from L. Parracino, 2004, *Pregnancy trimesters and exercise. Personal training on the net*.

## Case Study

Goal: A 56-year-old woman wants to start playing golf for the first time and needs an updated exercise program to fit the activity. Her usual fitness program included walking on the treadmill and using only standard machines for resistance training.

What should be the approach to exercise selection for this woman? First, identify the functional abilities that are required in swinging a golf club, such as static and dynamic postural stability, multiplanar movement, adequate flexibility, and core and joint stability and strength. After evaluating the specific movement patterns and needed abilities, assess overall muscle balance, flexibility, static and dynamic postural stability, strength, and power. Any dysfunctions found in the functional assessment should be addressed accordingly. For example, if thoracic spinal flexion (kyphosis) is observed in the functional assessment, then adequate torso rotation is restricted due to a disruption in spinal mechanics. See upper crossed syndrome on page 176, tables 10.7 and 10.8.

Initially, this woman's program should focus on any muscular imbalances, inadequate flexibility, and static and dynamic postural stability. After these three areas are adequate, then her program can move into the strength and power phases (Chek 2001). It is important to adequately stabilize the entire kinetic chain in all three planes of motion before more aggressive exercises are performed. Change her previous exercise program by gradually introducing more functional and sport-specific activities. Examples are utilizing free weights, resistance bands, and stability balls, as well as incorporating static and dynamic flexibility, single-leg balancing, alternating upper extremity movements, and especially multiplanar motions for dynamic stability. Training core, postural, and joint stability will enhance performance in any sport or activity. The job of the golf pro is to help the woman with the mechanics of the golf swing. However, the fitness professional's job is to identify the physical ability requirements as they relate to a golf swing and set up an exercise program accordingly. For more information on golf training, education, and certification programs for the fitness or golf professional, go to www.chekinstitute.com.

Also, evaluate the woman's present cardiovascular program and make any changes that are needed. This may not substantially improve her golf game score; however, a variety of cardiovascular activities can reduce repetitive joint movement and promote diverse muscular endurance development. If she walks 18 holes instead of using a golf cart, then adequate endurance is needed to prevent any fatigue, which could affect sport performance.

Educate her about how the specific exercise choices and the functional activity approach are helping her accomplish her sport-specific goal—learning to play golf efficiently. The successful outcome of this training program is a better golfer who has the stamina and functional abilities to progress in her sport.

## Exercise Progression

Progression is a major component of program design. It's key to improving performance and reducing the risk of injury. The more progress a woman experiences, the more motivated she becomes. Motivation contributes to consistency of workouts, which in turn produces further progression and improved performance. Figure 10.5 is an example of lunge pose progressions for women of different abilities, experiences, and circumstances.

These are some important tips for successful progression:

- ◆ Repeat assessments periodically to decipher what types of changes should occur within the program. Ask: Has an area that was previously weak become stronger? Are there new areas that need attention? Have the program goals changed?

- ◆ Always point out specific signs of progress, no matter how small they may be.

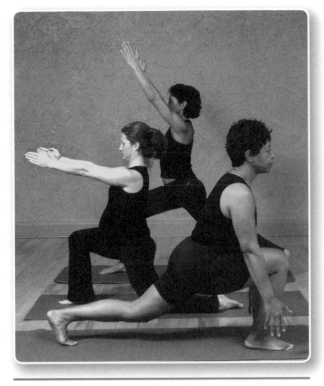

**Figure 10.5** Lunge pose progressions. The lunge pose may be modified for different levels of fitness and conditions such as pregnancy.

- ◆ Encourage gradual and continual progress.
- ◆ Select new exercises that are challenging. Don't prescribe activities that someone can't perform effectively and successfully.
- ◆ Be sure the woman has the proper strength, flexibility, balance, coordination, and neuromuscular efficiency needed to perform the activity.
- ◆ When appropriate use different exercise tools to provide variety and make exercise choices and progressions almost endless (see "Common Exercise Tools and Their Uses" on page 181).
- ◆ Educate the woman about how the principles of exercise progression relate to her life outside the gym. Ask her to choose a functional activity that is currently difficult for her to perform (e.g., climbing stairs, sitting up straight while working on the computer, getting through the second half of the tennis match without fatigue, carrying luggage). Set a short-term functional activity goal to help her identify progress beyond her structured exercise program. Appendix A provides an

example of a weekly exercise plan that is useful to the professional as well as for keeping the individual on track (page 215-216).

See table 10.12 for principles of exercise progression as they relate to functional movement patterns. Figures 10.6 and 10.7 present an example of a stable-to-unstable progression. Figures 10.8 and 10.9 are examples of a progression from static activity to dynamic activity.

◆ **TABLE 10.12** ◆

## Principles of Exercise Progression

| Initial activity | Exercise progression |
|---|---|
| Limited range of motion | Full range of motion |
| Slow movements | Fast movements |
| Single plane | Multiplane |
| Stable surface | Unstable surface |
| Simple movement patterns | Complex movement patterns |
| Lighter weights | Heavier weights |
| Static activity | Dynamic activity |

Data from M.A. Clark, 2001, *Integrated training for the New Millennium* (Thousand Oaks, CA: National Academy of Sports Medicine).

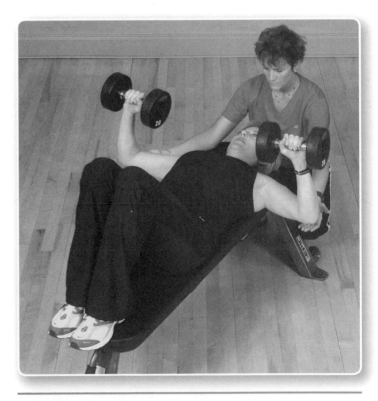

**Figure 10.6** Dumbbell chest press on flat bench is a more stable surface exercise.

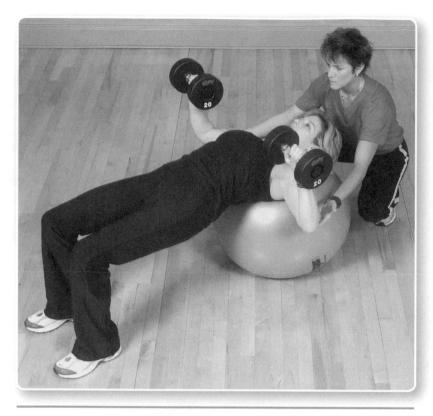

**Figure 10.7** Dumbbell chest press on a stability ball is an unstable surface exercise, and therefore more challenging.

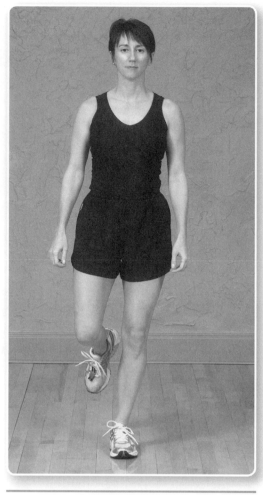

**Figure 10.8** Static single-leg balance.

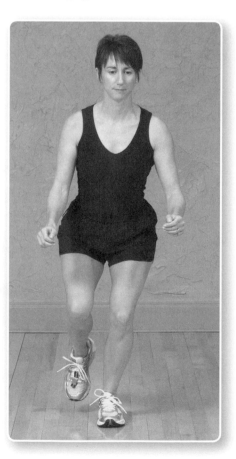

**Figure 10.9** Dynamic single-leg squat.

The National Academy of Sports Medicine also provides the following progressive training principles (Clark 2001):

◆ Develop proper muscle balance.

◆ Correct all kinetic chain imbalances.

◆ Develop proper structural integrity of the kinetic chain before activity-specific training.

◆ Establish optimum multiplanar postural control.

◆ Develop optimum levels of stabilization strength, core strength, and neuromuscular efficiency prior to extremity strength, prime mover strength, or explosive strength.

◆ Establish optimum levels of activity-specific functional strength, neuromuscular efficiency, reactive neuromuscular control, and power.

## Case Study

Here is an example of exercise progression—from a simple movement pattern to a more complex movement pattern. Suppose a woman has the ability to perform a proper lunge. Rather than handing her a barbell or dumbbells and asking her to perform the same activity, challenge her outside of the sagittal plane by giving her a very light weighted object and asking her to perform a lunge while incorporating a controlled trunk rotation (figure 10.10). Remember, the body is made and required to move in all three planes of motion. Train her in the sagittal, transverse, and frontal planes before adding any external resistance. This could also be an example of progressing from a single-planar motion to a multiplanar motion. A sagittal plane lunge incorporated with a dumbbell arm curl or overhead press would also be an example of a simple to more complex movement. Each principle of progression is dependent on the woman's physical capabilities. A woman should never perform exercises out of the scope of her physical capabilities.

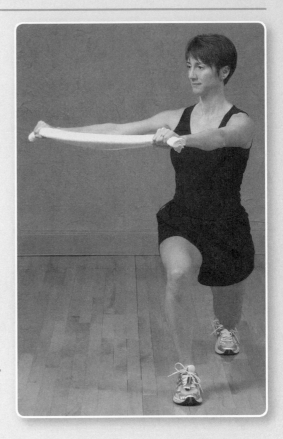

**Figure 10.10** Walking lunge incorporating trunk rotation using a towel. This is a multiplanar and more complex movement pattern.

## Common Exercise Tools and Their Uses

There are many tools that can be used to enhance functional ability and performance. The use of each tool, as well as the level of difficulty of the exercise chosen, depends upon the physical abilities of an individual. Over recent years there has been a vast increase in the number and variety of tools used in facilities and current exercise programs. This increase does not necessarily mandate the use of this equipment. Each tool should be used only in appropriate situations. It is the health and fitness professional's job to ensure that the specific exercise meets the functional ability of an individual. Proper progression through exercise selection is a key factor for ensuring safety and improving functional fitness. Exercise tools may be used to enhance balance, stability, core strength, neural function, multiplanar function, overall strength, or power. The following are types of exercise tools and some valuable uses.

Balance boards, core boards, Bosu, pads, discs—balance, stabilization, strength, and power

Stability balls—balance, and core and joint stabilization training

Foam rollers—self-myofascial release, balance, body alignment, and stabilization

Tubing—variable, multiplanar resistance used for functional and core stabilization and strength

Medicine balls—improving core strength, stabilization, and overall strength and power

For more information on training tools and performance enhancement and rehabilitation, visit www.performbetter.com.

The following case study involves an example of a disease (fibromyalgia) that is more specific to women than to men. It includes the relevant information and results obtained from a consultation and assessment. Also included are tips for training a woman with fibromyalgia, recommendations, program design summary, progressions involved, and goals that were achieved.

# Fibromyalgia Case Study

Age: 74

### Initial Assessment

Medical history—diagnosed with fibromyalgia at age 61, high blood pressure

Injury history—intermittent left shoulder joint pain (no diagnosis)

Medications—Advil when needed, Lopressor 100 milligrams two times a day

Exercise history—active jogger and consistent weightlifter until age 54; since then, irregular walking and no resistance training due to muscle pain and fatigue

Short-term goal—walk up stairs at home without stopping to rest; increase overall strength and endurance

Long-term goal—decrease frequency of muscle aches, pain, and fatigue due to fibromyalgia; decrease percent body fat

### Physical Profile

Body fat—33%

RMR—1,150 kcal

Resting blood pressure—118/74

Resting heart rate—76 beats per minute

### Functional Profile Results

Muscle length: decreased range of motion—pectoralis, infraspinatus/teres minor, latissimus dorsi, gastrocnemius, soleus, adductors, hamstrings, tensor fasciae latae (iliotibial band), and psoas

Static postural and overhead squat assessment: shoulders protracted, arms moved forward, head protracted, scapulae winged, feet flatten out and externally rotate, knees internally rotate, hip adduction, excessive hip flexion, increased lumbar flexion

Single leg balance: poor

## Adjustments Due to Fibromyalgia

If the individual is experiencing increased pain, fatigue, or stiffness on a particular day, the exercise training variables should be changed. Reduce the exercise intensity or even recommend other management tools (massage, warm water) to help avoid additional increase in symptoms. Do not encourage overtraining or risk muscle fatigue and delayed-onset muscle soreness. Light to moderate intensities of resistance training that enhance functional strength should be the primary focus. Encourage stretching on a daily basis but never to the point of pain or tenderness. Aerobic training should be performed at low-intensity levels, and total exercise time may be divided into several 10-minute bouts throughout the day. Educate the woman on the benefits of regular exercise in the management of fibromyalgia, as shown in the sidebar "Symptoms of Fibromyalgia and Benefits of Regular Exercise" on page 184.

## Beginning Training Program

The training program begins with low-intensity levels for cardiovascular and resistance exercises to allow the musculoskeletal system to adapt to additional physical stressors. The main focus is the corrective strategies developed from the kinetic assessment to address postural alignment, muscle imbalances, abnormal movement patterns, and joint dysfunction (specifically the shoulder) to decrease the risk of injury and improve overall performance. The program should not include methods to develop absolute strength or power, but rather ways to develop function to improve movement (neuromuscular) utilizing all three planes of motion.

◆ Corrective flexibility exercises (static, self-myofascial release, neurodynamic, neuromuscular): cervical spine extensors, pectoralis major/minor, serratus anterior, shoulder external rotators, latissimus dorsi, rectus abdominis, upper abdominal muscles, external/internal obliques, adductors, hamstrings, calf complex (peroneals), quadriceps, tensor fasciae latae, hip flexors.

◆ Corrective strengthening exercises: cervical spine flexors, rhomboids, trapezius, rotator cuff, erector spinae, latissimus dorsi, quadratus lumborum, iliopsoas, gluteals, adductor magnus, upper hamstrings, tibialis, medial gastrocnemius

### Recommended Cardiovascular Training

Modes—treadmill walking, outdoor walking (soft surface), stationary bike (recumbent), aquatic walking (heated)

Frequency—three times per week

Intensity—low level to begin

Duration—10 to 20 minutes as tolerated (can use as a warm-up following corrective stretching)

### Recommended Strength and Stability Training

Frequency—two times per week (total body)

Intensity—light weights; 12 to 18 reps; one to two sets; rest as needed

Flexibility program—begin with the corrective stretches listed prior to any dynamic activity; also recommend stretching at regular intervals throughout the day to reduce pain and stiffness

## Progressions in Program Design

Increase cardiovascular frequency to four to five times per week, increase intensity to low-moderate, and increase duration to 20-30 minutes. Resistance exercises should be maintained at light to moderate training loads with adequate rest period, slowly increasing number of sets to a maximum of three, or increasing frequency to three days per week.

Note: All increases are subject to individual and daily symptoms and progress. Corrective strengthening and flexibility exercises should be continued until muscle imbalances, joint dysfunctions, and postural distortions are not evident in kinetic chain assessment. Subsequently, active stretching should take place after the cardiovascular warm-up, while static stretching should end the exercise session.

## Progress After One Year

This woman was very consistent throughout the 12 months of her training program. After approximately 6 months, her body fat had been reduced to 31 percent. At the end of 12 months, her body fat was 29 percent. Also, her RMR was reevaluated at 12 months and was essentially unchanged at 1,167 calories per day.

Her cardiovascular program averaged four days per week with variety. She participated in water aerobics once a week and exercised on an elliptical cardiovascular machine once a week. She continued to walk on the treadmill, slowly improving her speed up to 3.5 miles (6 kilometers) per hour, with some days at a 3 to 5 percent incline. The stationary bike was a challenge to her lower extremity muscular system, but as she improved her strength and endurance, she was able to sustain a light to moderate intensity for 30 minutes.

The resistance training program was her biggest challenge, and in her mind the biggest accomplishment. She performed light weight resistance exercises and stability training three days per week. Her program incorporated both variable resistance and free joint motion machines. Neuromuscular stability, core stabilization, and multiplanar functional strength training was incorporated into her program. Improving neuromuscular stabilization (balance) should be a primary focus when training an older woman.

Her short-term goals, improving strength and endurance and walking upstairs with more ease, were achieved in the desired time frame. This specific improvement motivated and dramatically improved her confidence related to mobility in her daily life.

Regarding the intermittent left shoulder joint pain, improvement occurred over the course of her program. She performed no upper-body exercises that caused any pain or discomfort symptoms. She had minimal complaints of any pain episodes after starting the corrective strengthening and flexibility exercises. The decreased shoulder pain could have been due to the increased joint stability and strength as well as improved joint function that resulted from correcting postural dysfunctions. These results show how integrated training can improve overall function.

The woman also noticed postural changes in a matter of a few weeks. Educating the client on postural positioning and awareness was as important as performance of the corrective exercises. She was diligent in stretching five to six days per week. The muscle length, postural, and overhead squat assessment was performed regularly to evaluate progress in the kinetic chain. With consistency, she improved her range of motion and functional flexibility.

Self-reported fibromyalgia symptoms were reduced in frequency and severity throughout the 12-month period. There were, however, days of intensified musculoskeletal pain, stiffness, and fatigue. On these days, she either reduced the intensity or duration of exercise (or both), compromised with water activity, performed stretching only, or stayed home and took a warm bath. Her progress and success were due to her commitment and consistency over time.

## Symptoms of Fibromyalgia and Benefits of Regular Exercise

**Most Common Symptoms**
- Musculoskeletal pain
- Extreme fatigue
- Generalized stiffness
- Multiple tender points

**Other Symptoms**
- Sleep problems
- Anxiety and depression
- Headaches
- Cognitive impairment
- Gastrointestinal problems
- Temporomandibular joint pain
- Myofascial pain
- Bladder problems

**Benefits of Regular Exercise**
- Improved cardiovascular health and fitness
- Weight management
- Improved muscular work capacity
- Improved sleep patterns
- Improved functional abilities
- Improved pain management
- Increased energy and decreased fatigue
- Increased self-worth and self-esteem
- Increased sense of control
- Less stress, anxiety, and depression

Reprinted, by permission, from M.A. Clark, 2001, *Integrated Training for the New Millennium* (Thousand Oaks, CA: National Academy of Sports Medicine), 225.

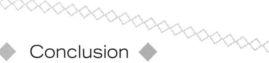

## ◆ Conclusion ◆

Information in the preceding chapters laid the foundation for designing individualized fitness programs for women. While a general physical activity or exercise program can produce important health improvements, the woman who desires significant performance improvements needs a special, systematically planned program. The philosophy of program design described in this chapter can be used with women of all ages whose goals are to enhance their performance. Properly assessing the individual woman and identifying her special needs, goals, and problem areas are important first steps. The fitness assessment also provides the baseline from which to measure progress and make program adjustments. We provided sample tools for conducting and recording information from screenings, functional and fitness tests, and consultations. We summarized program design principles at the end of the chapter by reviewing a detailed case study. Program design is a constantly evolving challenge that yields tremendous reward to the participant as well as to the professional.

# CHAPTER 11

# Female Injury and Safety Issues

## Topics in This Chapter

Please know I am quite aware of the hazards. I want to do it because I want to do it. Women must try like men have tried. When they fail, failure must be but a challenge to others.

Amelia Earhart

**D**espite our best efforts to design safe and effective training programs, some women will sustain injuries, especially lower extremity injuries. In this chapter we discuss common injuries that affect women and strategies to prevent them. In chapter 1, we discussed the anatomical and physiological issues that make women more prone to anterior cruciate ligament (ACL) injuries and patellofemoral stress syndrome. Other lower extremity injuries that aren't as gender specific merit mention here, too, because they affect so many women. These issues include plantar fasciitis, Achilles tendinitis, iliotibial band syndrome, and stress fractures. The factors that may play a role in female lower extremity injury risk are the following:

Decreased lower-extremity muscle mass

Upright landing posture

Increased knee valgus

Larger Q angle

Smaller bones

Smaller ACL ligament*

Smaller width and different shape of intercondylar ACL notch*

Increased ligament laxity*

*Data on these risk factors are inconclusive or insufficient.

## Anterior Cruciate Ligament

Knee pain is an all too common complaint. More than nine million people visited an orthopedic surgeon in 2001 because of some type of knee problem (American Academy of Orthopaedic Surgeons 2000a). Women have experienced increased rates of knee injury due to increasing participation in various sports. But, even

given increased rates of participation, women experience a disproportionately higher risk of knee injury than men (American Academy of Orthopaedic Surgeons 2002a). Musculoskeletal injuries are generally sport specific rather than gender specific, but females participating in certain sports are three to four times more likely to injure their ACL than males (American Academy of Orthopaedic Surgeons 2002b). A majority of these injuries occur between the ages 15 and 25.

Three high-risk sports for ACL injury in females are basketball, soccer, and volleyball (American Academy of Orthopaedic Surgeons 2000b). However, since women participate in a wide variety of sports today, any activity that involves jumping, rapidly changing direction, deceleration of running, or contact should be considered high risk for ACL injury.

According to the American Academy of Orthopaedic Surgeons (2002a), 60 percent of female ACL injuries in basketball players occur during landing from a jump. As discussed in chapter 1, women should be instructed on how to land properly to avoid knee injury (figure 11.1). Women need to flex more at the knees and hips when landing or changing direction. Engaging the hamstring more fully decreases stress on the ACL and reduces the risk of injury.

The authors of one study evaluated the benefit of plyometric training in decreasing the risk of ACL injuries. Female basketball and soccer players participated in a six-week plyometric training program during the off-season (Wilkerson et al. 2004). The control group participated in a basic conditioning program. After six weeks, quadriceps and hamstring peak torque values were tested along with vertical ground force generated from stepping off a platform. The results from the plyometric training group indicated an increase in peak torque generated by the hamstrings. There was a significant increase in the hamstring-to-quadriceps strength ratio, which the authors suggested would play a significant role in decreasing the risk for an ACL injury. See figures 11.2 and 11.3 for examples of plyometric exercises.

The American College of Sports Medicine in a 2004 study proposed that decreased core stability contributed to the onset of lower leg injuries, particularly in females (Leetun et al. 2004). The study compared measures between genders and

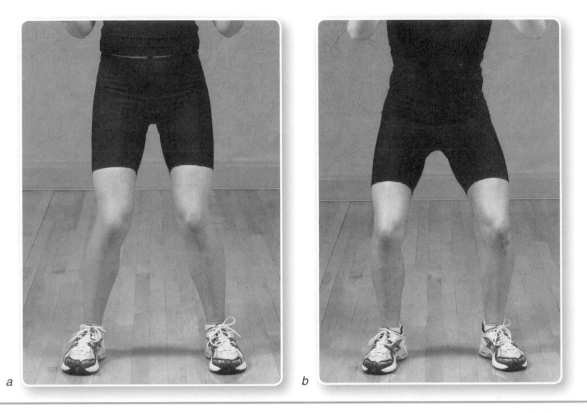

**Figure 11.1** Landing properly from a jump will reduce the risk of injury. Components of a high-risk landing *(a)* include minimal flexion at the hip and knee, excessive valgus knee angulation, and resulting forward shift of body weight. A proper, or low-risk, landing *(b)* emphasizes flexion at the hip and knee with less knee valgus angulation, shifting body weight backward and increasing stability.

also between injured and noninjured athletes during basketball and track season. Prior to their season, 140 intercollegiate basketball and track athletes (80 females, 60 males) were tested for hip external rotation strength and other measures of strength and endurance. Females and injured athletes were statistically significantly weaker in hip external rotation strength than males and noninjured athletes. For this reason, core strengthening, including hip external rotation strengthening, is recommended for lower extremity injury prevention.

Another study determined whether the hormone relaxin was associated with female athlete pain and injury incidence during menses (Ingraham et al. 2003). Relaxin is normally associated with pregnancy. It is known to alter collagen synthesis, reducing the intrinsic strength of connective tissue. Twenty-eight collegiate and postcollegiate female track and field athletes recorded their menstrual cycles, injuries, and pain throughout a season. Analysis revealed a significant increased risk for new injury and pain

during the relaxin phase of the menstrual cycle. It is difficult to translate these findings into practical advice for female athletes. Peak hormone levels vary from cycle to cycle for many women, and certainly vary considerably between women. We don't recommend any specific changes in female exercise training during any phase of the menstrual cycle.

## Anterior Knee Pain

Anterior knee pain is a common complaint for women and has many causes, mainly mechanical. Mechanical sources of anterior knee pain include subluxation, dislocation, patellofemoral stress syndrome (PFSS), and symptomatic medial plica (intra-articular synovial fold) (Ireland and Ott 2001). Inflammatory causes, such as bursitis, tendinitis, and arthritis, are also in the differential diagnosis. Of the many mechanical issues, PFSS is of particular concern due to its frequent occurrence. Patellofemoral stress syndrome is

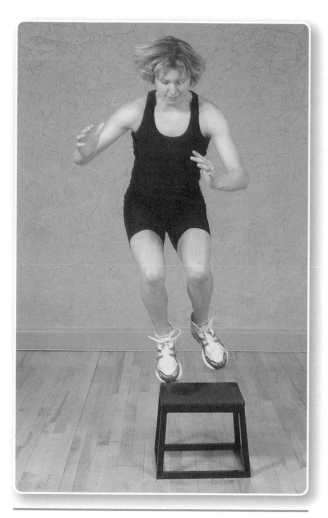

**Figure 11.2** Plyometric lateral box jumps.

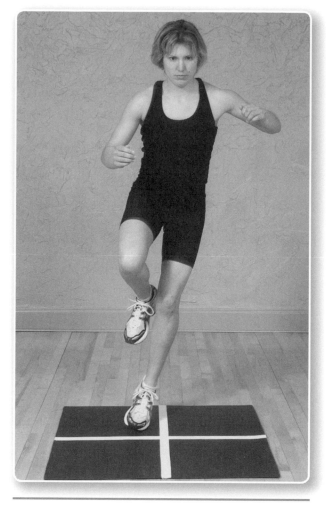

**Figure 11.3** Plyometric four-quadrant hops.

## Tips for Preventing ACL Injuries

◆ Teach women proper landing positions. Women need to flex more at the knees and hips when landing or changing direction.

◆ Strengthen and stretch the quadriceps and hamstrings.

◆ Plyometric training is recommended to prepare the knee for the various forces it is exposed to during certain high-risk activities.

◆ Core strengthening, including hip external rotation strengthening, is recommended for lower-extremity injury prevention.

◆ No specific changes in exercise training are recommended during any phase of the menstrual cycle for injury prevention.

the result of abnormal patellar tracking. The underlying cause of PFSS may be structural or functional. Structural or anatomic issues, such as excessive Q angle and genu valgum, contribute to risk for PFSS and are more difficult to address than functional issues such as quadriceps imbalance or overtraining. Even in women without structural or functional issues, proper patellar tracking may be disrupted by incorrect loading via inappropriate biomechanics during use of machines or performance of other activities or sports.

Patellofemoral stress syndrome may be exacerbated by repetitive knee flexion, as in squatting, stair climbing, hiking, jumping, kneeling, deep knee bends, running, or prolonged sitting. Over time, these stresses can lead to erosion and softening of the cartilage on the undersurface of the patella, a condition known as chondromalacia.

Prevention of PFSS is essential for those who are at risk. Maintain muscle balance through strengthening the quadriceps, especially the vastus medialis obliquus (VMO) (short-arc quad sets, isometric quad sets, straight leg raise with leg externally rotated). Tight hamstrings can disrupt quadriceps function and increase patellofemoral joint load. A tight iliotibial (IT) band and vastus lateralis (lateral quadriceps muscle) can affect lateral tracking of the knee. Correcting these biomechanical imbalances is a recurrent theme for preventing injuries. Also, avoid sudden changes in the frequency, intensity, or duration in exercise activity. Progression should be gradual to avoid these types of injuries.

Treatment can be simple and noninvasive. Proper shoes are necessary for shock absorption, and orthotics are often helpful for overpronators. Orthopedic massage therapy can be very useful as well. Rest, ice, and anti-inflammatory drugs to reduce swelling and inflammation are recommended for those experiencing discomfort and pain. Also, recommend a temporary change in exercise to include non-weight-bearing activities (swimming) in order to prevent further pain and inflammation. Of interest, a symptomatic plica is treated in the same conservative manner. If there is no improvement in symptoms, refer to a physician for further assessment. As a very last resort, arthroscopic or realignment kneecap surgery may be performed.

# Plantar Fasciitis

Plantar fasciitis is one of the most common causes of heel pain in runners. Women are affected by plantar fasciitis twice as often as men (Foye and Stitik 2004).

The plantar fascia is a fibrous band that runs from the forefoot to the middle arch and inserts into the calcaneus bone (figure 11.4). It provides support for the arch of the foot and also shock absorption during foot strike. The inflammation of the fascia occurs at the calcaneus (heel) insertion due to chronic traction on the fascia. Bone spurs may develop on the calcaneus, but it is the inflammation of the fascia that causes the painful symptoms.

Gradual onset of pain can be due to excessive foot pronation, tight or weak calf muscles, weak intrinsic foot muscles, or any other underlying

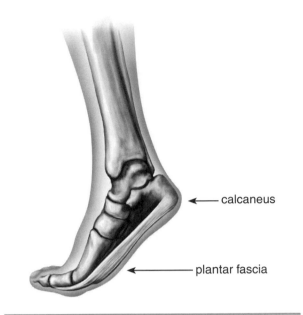

**Figure 11.4** Anatomy of the plantar fascia.

imbalance that changes gait pattern during running. Individuals with high-arched or low-arched feet are at risk for this injury. Reduced heel fat pad is another factor, and this is more common as women age. Overweight women experience added stress and pressure to the plantar fascia (Hills et al. 2001; Milne et al. 2003).

Prevention and treatment programs for plantar fasciitis must include stretching. Reducing calf muscle tightness is essential (figure 11.5). Improved flexibility can aid in overcoming weakness in intrinsic muscles of the foot. Calf complex stretching with rocker boards is recommended (figure 11.6). Proper shoe fit is also necessary, especially to improve

## Causes of Plantar Fasciitis

- ◆ Excessive foot pronation
- ◆ Tight or weak calf muscles
- ◆ Weak intrinsic foot muscles
- ◆ Underlying imbalances that change gait patterns
- ◆ High-arched or low-arched feet
- ◆ Reduced heel fat pad
- ◆ Being overweight

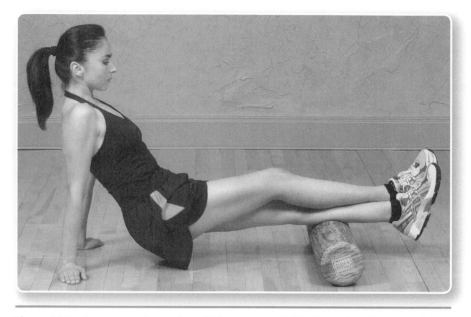

**Figure 11.5** Improve calf muscle soft tissue extensibility through self-myofascial release using the foam roller.

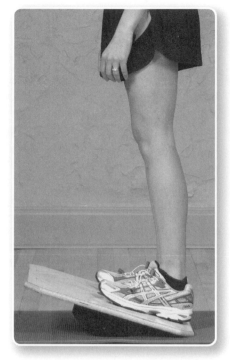

**Figure 11.6** Calf stretch using the rocker board.

midfoot support and reduce impact. Women who don't respond to conservative measures may benefit from referral to an orthopedist for night splints, steroid injections, or other therapies.

# Achilles Tendinitis

The classic presentation of Achilles tendinitis is pain about 2 to 4 inches (5 to 10 centimeters) above the tendon attachment to the heel. The blood supply to this part of the tendon is limited, perhaps contributing to injury susceptibility. Intense, repeated, and/or sustained exercise without proper conditioning, gradual progression, and preparation are risk factors for tendinitis. Tendinitis actually begins as peritendinitis (localized swelling around the tendon), which may progress to tendon degeneration and scar tissue formation. The Achilles is the largest and strongest tendon in the body (figure 11.7). Tight calf muscles, tight hamstrings, tightness in the tendon itself, and foot pronation can cause stress and inflammation of the Achilles tendon. Increasing age and heel deformities may also contribute to risk.

To prevent an Achilles injury, be sure women stretch the calves, hamstrings, and Achilles tendons. Advise women to correct pronation if necessary with proper shoes or orthotics. It is also important to avoid overtraining to reduce the amount of stress placed on the tissue. Repetitive

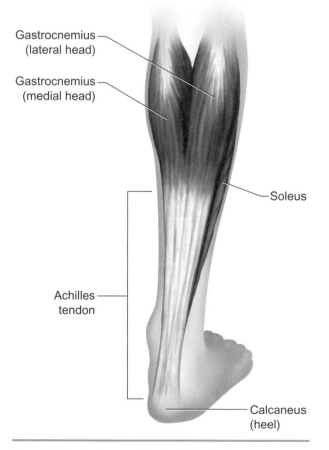

**Figure 11.7** Anatomy of the Achilles tendon.

activities, such as running, hiking, sports that involve frequent jumping, and stair climbing, can produce greater tension on the tendon. Without proper strengthening and stretching, the risk of injury over time is increased. As discussed in previous chapters, muscle balance is a key factor in the prevention of injuries. If, despite a careful exercise program, an Achilles injury occurs, treatment is straightforward. Reduce stressors and institute a stretching program as already noted. Shoe inserts, ice, and anti-inflammatories are all helpful.

## Iliotibial Band Syndrome

Iliotibial band syndrome (ITBS) is one of the most common causes of lateral knee pain in athletes and runners. The syndrome usually occurs to athletes in sports or activities with repetitive knee flexion and extension movements. Marathoners, long-distance cyclists, skiers, and tennis or volleyball players are most at risk for this condition.

The IT band originates at the iliac crest; it is a tendinous extension of the fascia covering the gluteus maximus and tensor fascia latae muscles. Distally, the IT band inserts on the lateral aspect of the proximal tibia (figure 11.8). It aids in knee stabilization. The band performs hip abduction, contributes to internal rotation of the hip, and assists with knee flexion and extension. Proximally, the band is not attached to any bone, so it is allowed to freely move anterior and posterior with continuous knee flexion and extension.

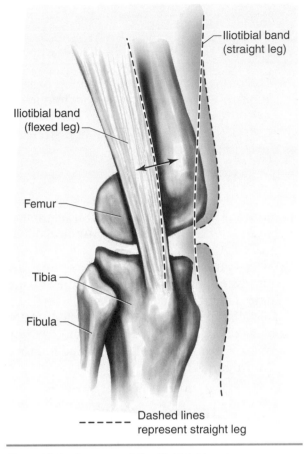

Figure 11.8 Anatomy of the iliotibial band.

Repetitive flexion and extension movements can cause friction and irritation to the band by rubbing it over the lateral femoral epicondyle. Walking or running on a banked surface or frequently running downhill, or misalignment issues that excessively stretch the band, can cause

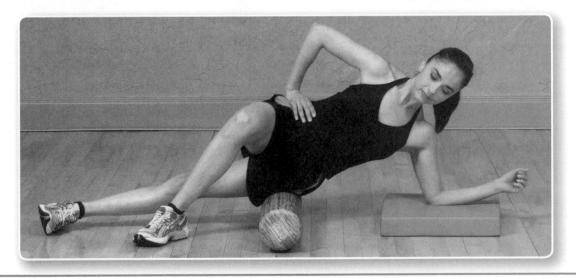

**Figure 11.9** Iliotibial band self-myofascial release using the foam roller.

## Tips for Preventing ITBS

- ◆ Discourage women from walking or running on a banked surface or from frequently running downhill.
- ◆ Emphasize proper warm-up and stretches to maintain flexibility.

microtrauma and inflammation. Misalignment issues can also result from the anatomical differences of the Q angle.

The IT band may also become irritated due to tightness of the band itself. Since the IT band originates lateral to the tensor fascia latae (TFL), the TFL helps to maintain IT band tension. Maintaining flexibility in both the IT band and TFL will reduce the risk of increased tension and improve function (figure 11.9).

## Stress Fractures and Overuse Injuries

Stress fractures appear to result from inadequate or insufficient remodeling of strained bone (Ireland and Nattiv 2002). Stress fractures can be debilitating to the elite as well as the recreational athlete, and females are more susceptible than males (Protzman and Griffis 1997). For women with menstrual irregularities, stress fractures are a particular risk, likely due to decreased bone mineral density. Stress fractures often occur in the bones of the feet but are also reported in the tibia, femur, pelvis, and sacrum.

Prevention of stress fractures should focus on maintaining adequate nutrition for females, including a diet with sufficient calcium. The importance of minimizing menstrual irregularities (whether related to overtraining or disordered eating) cannot be overemphasized. Once again, appropriate progression of exercise in regard to intensity, frequency, and duration is a must. Females should wear appropriate footwear and should exercise on surfaces that minimize bone and joint stress. Treatment of stress fractures varies by site and severity and should be initiated by a physician.

Females are subject to more and certain types of overuse injuries given the same activities as men. A study documenting overuse injuries in

male and female West Point cadets perfectly illustrates this point. From 1989 through 1993, 269 cadets were followed during fitness training in order to track injuries. The male (136) and female (133) cadets participated in the same activities during the summer; but during the academic year, the women were not included in typically male-dominated sports such as boxing, football, wrestling, rugby, and hockey. Despite participating in fewer sports, the women sustained far more overuse injuries (167 vs. 62) than the men (Ireland and Nattiv 2002). In table 11.1, note the high number of lower-extremity overuse injuries that occurred in the women. Of interest, men experienced more traumatic injuries, most likely due to participating in more contact sports.

◆ **TABLE 11.1** ◆

### Overuse Injuries by Gender

|  | Men | Women |
|---|---|---|
| Shoulder | 2 | 2 |
| Arm | 0 | 1 |
| Elbow, forearm | 1 | 3 |
| Wrist | 0 | 2 |
| Hand | 0 | 3 |
| Pelvis/hip | 1 | 9 |
| Thigh | 2 | 2 |
| Knee | 11 | 41 |
| Leg | 13 | 29 |
| Ankle | 2 | 13 |
| Foot | 29 | 56 |
| Back | 1 | 0 |

Reprinted from *The Female Athlete*, M.L. Ireland, pg. 18, Copyright 2003, with permission from Elsevier.

## Safety

Women should carefully observe safety guidelines for aerobic exercise. Most guidelines are common sense, such as wearing helmets for outdoor cycling. Encourage women to follow basic safety guidelines. Then, reinforce these less commonly cited concerns for personal safety while exercising:

- ◆ Avoid wearing headphones when exercising outdoors. Use of headphones limits aware-

## Tips for General Injury Prevention and Treating Injuries

Share with women the following tips for injury prevention and treatment.

**Prevention**

◆ Assess and correct any musculoskeletal imbalances.

◆ Recommend extra time before and after workouts to warm up and cool down the muscular system.

◆ Discourage running or other high-impact activities on concrete surfaces.

◆ Encourage purchasing new exercise shoes when needed.

◆ Refer women for orthotics to correct biomechanical problems.

◆ Discourage very high heels and pointed-toe shoes for daily wear.

◆ Reinforce cross training to avoid repetitive-use injuries.

◆ Make exercise progression gradual.

**Treatment**

◆ Pay attention to pain. Exercising through pain causes secondary problems.

◆ Modify exercise program by modality, frequency, intensity, duration.

◆ Advise medical treatment for acute injuries quickly.

◆ Following recovery, gradually increase the frequency, duration, and intensity of exercise as long as symptoms are not present.

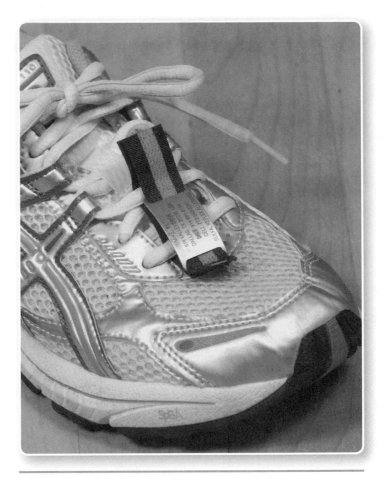

**Figure 11.10**   Wear an ID tag in case of emergency.

ness, making women vulnerable to assault and injury.

◆ Carry identification. Several companies make tiny tags that attach to shoes and include name, address, and emergency phone contact (figure 11.10).

◆ Be aware. Pay attention to slowly moving cars, suspicious people, or isolated areas. Get away from anyone or anything that doesn't seem right.

◆ Carry protection. Pepper spray and an implement called "the Persuader" (a small rod for self-defense) can help women escape attack. Check to be sure pepper spray is legal in your area. Training is needed to use the Persuader.

## Heat, Cold, and Altitude Stress

Avoiding stress from temperature extremes has become easier over the years because of advances in sport apparel. Moisture-wicking fabrics keep exercisers cool and dry in summer, and lightweight layers keep them warm in winter.

In hot and humid environments, it takes 10 to 14 days to acclimate. Advise women to avoid the hottest times of day and limit exercise to 30 minutes or less until acclimated. General recommendations on the amount of fluid to consume aren't that helpful, because sweating varies between individuals and because women generally sweat less than men (see the handout "Hydration Hints" in appendix B). The first sign of dehydration is darker urine, and thirst is one of the last indicators of dehydration. Women should stop exercising immediately with signs of heat stress, such as dizziness, cramps, nausea, and headache. Overheating can lead to heatstroke, which can be fatal.

When it's cool, advise women to wear a hat and mittens, dress in layers, drink plenty of fluids, and shed wet clothing. Women shouldn't hesitate to take a day off or to exercise indoors when the temperature drops below zero.

Acclimating to altitude takes time, usually 5 to 10 days. Even after acclimatization, performance at altitude won't match performance at sea level. Women should be encouraged to ascend gradually, avoid vigorous exercise until acclimated, drink plenty of fluids, and avoid alcohol. For any significant symptoms of altitude sickness, descent is the treatment of choice.

## ◆ Conclusion ◆

In this chapter we discussed common injuries that affect women and strategies to prevent them. Related to each injury, we discussed sports or activities that put the athlete at risk. We provided an anatomical illustration, listed symptoms and possible causes, and suggested specific corrective exercises and noninvasive treatments. Correcting muscle imbalances is a recurring theme for prevention of injuries. Common treatments include proper shoe fit (possibly including orthotics), orthopedic massage, rest, ice, anti-inflammatory drugs, and temporary change to non-weight-bearing exercises. If there is no improvement, the woman should be referred to a physician for further assessment.

The chapter concluded with a discussion of stress fractures and general overuse injuries. Prevention of stress fractures should focus on ensuring proper nutrition (especially adequate calcium), following appropriate exercise progression, selecting appropriate footwear, exercising on surfaces that minimize bone and joint stress, and minimizing menstrual irregularities. Treatment of stress fractures varies by site and severity and should be initiated by a physician. In addition to previously mentioned tips, taking extra time for warm-up and cool-down and cross training may help avoid or prevent repetitive-use injuries. Finally, we gave specific personal safety recommendations for women. Ways to avoid stress from temperature extremes and altitude were also provided.

# Conclusion

**H**ealth professionals who work with women must understand the key anatomic and physiologic differences between men and women, especially regarding the lower extremity. Women are at higher risk for lower-extremity injury than men, due to anterior pelvic tilt, larger Q angle, and increased valgus angulation. Health professionals who understand these differences can design safe and effective exercise programs that address them. By integrating muscle strengthening and flexibility exercises as well as appropriate plyometric training into a woman's program, health professionals encourage safer movement patterns, including more stable landing postures, to minimize lower-extremity injury risk. Achieving proper muscle balance is essential in preventing most other commonly occurring injuries in women.

Women can drastically reduce their risk of premature death and disability by minimizing sedentary behaviors and becoming more physically active. Health professionals must encourage women to be fit to prevent cardiovascular disease and stroke, cancer, diabetes, hypertension, dyslipidemia, dementia, osteoporosis, and obesity. Even women who have already been diagnosed with diseases can benefit by regular exercise. Maintaining or improving fitness reduces complications of disease. It is never too late to start an exercise program. Health professionals must understand that exercise benefits women with a wide variety of illnesses and disabilities.

Health professionals have many opportunities during a woman's lifetime to encourage physical activity. They play a pivotal role in exposing adolescents to a variety of exercise options to promote a healthy lifestyle. Health professionals must understand the important role of exercise in the development of peak bone mass, which is critical at this time of life. In addition to offering their technical expertise, health and fitness professionals can serve as mentors and appropriate role models.

Pregnancy provides an excellent opportunity for health and fitness professionals to reinforce information about the benefits of physical activity. The goals of having a healthy baby, staying fit during pregnancy, and resuming exercise postpartum can be addressed by appropriate prenatal and postpartum exercise programs. Exercise during pregnancy and postpartum does require some modifications, but most women will be able to exercise moderately and safely quite easily during this time. Of critical importance is the role that prenatal exercise plays in reducing risk of preeclampsia and gestational diabetes.

Menopause is another critical juncture in women's lives that can be favorably influenced by physical activity. Exercise reduces some of the symptoms of menopause; this is important for health professionals to understand and use as a motivational tool. Through the menopausal years and beyond, the strength and stability as well as flexibility components of fitness programming deserve added emphasis, especially in forestalling frailty and preventing falls. The ultimate goal of fitness programming for senior women is to be able to perform functions of daily living and remain independent for as long as possible.

Women can achieve aerobic fitness in many ways. Some women attain fitness through regular activities of daily life. Others need structured exercise to achieve fitness. Professionals can assist women in assessing their level of fitness and prescribing an appropriate aerobic exercise program. Even light exercise offers benefits for those who have been sedentary, but moderate-intensity exercise on most days of the week is recommended. Professionals should be aware of the benefits of cross and interval training to assist women in reaching their goals.

Women must be trained in a manner that will prepare them for daily life and activity. This should include functional exercise training that focuses on stabilization, neuromuscular control (balance), strength, endurance, flexibility, speed, and power. Strength training programs for women should address and promote proper mechanics and spinal alignment, core strength, and appropriate exercise progression.

Flexibility training is an integral component of a fitness program for women. Flexibility and strength training help to restore proper kinetic chain function through muscle balance, therefore improving performance and reducing risk of injury. Flexibility training should include both static and dynamic stretching exercises. Further research is needed to determine optimal protocols, methods, and techniques for any individual woman.

The health professional can integrate knowledge from this book into a protocol for exercise program design for women. Program design begins with data collection from a personal consultation, fitness testing, and functional testing. Cardiovascular endurance, strength and stability, and flexibility exercises should be selected with the corrective musculoskeletal needs of the individual in mind. Program design should focus on the needs, interests, and goals of the individual in order to provide optimal performance in and outside of the gym.

The science of understanding sex differences and their relationship to fitness is growing, but incomplete. Ongoing research will continue to address these differences and their impact on exercise prescription, injury prevention, and performance. As women expand the number of activities in which they participate, it becomes increasingly critical to understand and anticipate the sex/gender influences on cardiovascular fitness, muscle strength and endurance, and flexibility.

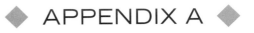
# Tools

The tools in this appendix should be very useful to you in your work. Photocopy them as needed. The tools are the following:

- ◆ Par-Q & You Questionnaire
- ◆ Physical fitness assessment tools
  - – Cardiorespiratory fitness tests for ages 20 to 79
  - – Flexibility—sit and reach
  - – Dynamic strength—1-minute sit-up
  - – Dynamic strength—modified push-up
  - – Dynamic strength—full-body push-up
  - – Absolute strength—1-repetition maximum bench press
- ◆ Personal training assessment sheet
- ◆ Fitness and functional consultation, with example
- ◆ Weekly plan, with example

# PAR-Q & YOU

## (A Questionnaire for People Aged 15 to 69)

Regular physical activity is fun and healthy, and increasingly more people are starting to become more active every day. Being more active is very safe for most people. However, some people should check with their doctor before they start becoming much more physically active.

If you are planning to become much more physically active than you are now, start by answering the seven questions in the box below. If you are between the ages of 15 and 69, the PAR-Q will tell you if you should check with your doctor before you start. If you are over 69 years of age, and you are not used to being very active, check with your doctor.

Common sense is your best guide when you answer these questions. Please read the questions carefully and answer each one honestly: check YES or NO.

| YES | NO | | |
|-----|----|----|---|
| ☐ | ☐ | 1. | Has your doctor ever said that you have a heart condition <u>and</u> that you should only do physical activity recommended by a doctor? |
| ☐ | ☐ | 2. | Do you feel pain in your chest when you do physical activity? |
| ☐ | ☐ | 3. | In the past month, have you had chest pain when you were not doing physical activity? |
| ☐ | ☐ | 4. | Do you lose your balance because of dizziness or do you ever lose consciousness? |
| ☐ | ☐ | 5. | Do you have a bone or joint problem (for example, back, knee or hip) that could be made worse by a change in your physical activity? |
| ☐ | ☐ | 6. | Is your doctor currently prescribing drugs (for example, water pills) for your blood pressure or heart condition? |
| ☐ | ☐ | 7. | Do you know of <u>any other reason</u> why you should not do physical activity? |

**If you answered**

## YES to one or more questions

Talk with your doctor by phone or in person BEFORE you start becoming much more physically active or BEFORE you have a fitness appraisal. Tell your doctor about the PAR-Q and which questions you answered YES.

- You may be able to do any activity you want — as long as you start slowly and build up gradually. Or, you may need to restrict your activities to those which are safe for you. Talk with your doctor about the kinds of activities you wish to participate in and follow his/her advice.
- Find out which community programs are safe and helpful for you.

## NO to all questions

If you answered NO honestly to <u>all</u> PAR-Q questions, you can be reasonably sure that you can:
- start becoming much more physically active — begin slowly and build up gradually. This is the safest and easiest way to go.
- take part in a fitness appraisal — this is an excellent way to determine your basic fitness so that you can plan the best way for you to live actively. It is also highly recommended that you have your blood pressure evaluated. If your reading is over 144/94, talk with your doctor before you start becoming much more physically active.

**DELAY BECOMING MUCH MORE ACTIVE:**
- if you are not feeling well because of a temporary illness such as a cold or a fever — wait until you feel better; or
- if you are or may be pregnant — talk to your doctor before you start becoming more active.

**PLEASE NOTE:** If your health changes so that you then answer YES to any of the above questions, tell your fitness or health professional. Ask whether you should change your physical activity plan.

<u>Informed Use of the PAR-Q</u>: The Canadian Society for Exercise Physiology, Health Canada, and their agents assume no liability for persons who undertake physical activity, and if in doubt after completing this questionnaire, consult your doctor prior to physical activity.

**No changes permitted. You are encouraged to photocopy the PAR-Q but only if you use the entire form.**

NOTE: If the PAR-Q is being given to a person before he or she participates in a physical activity program or a fitness appraisal, this section may be used for legal or administrative purposes.

"I have read, understood and completed this questionnaire. Any questions I had were answered to my full satisfaction."

NAME _____

SIGNATURE _____  DATE _____

SIGNATURE OF PARENT _____  WITNESS _____
or GUARDIAN (for participants under the age of majority)

> **Note: This physical activity clearance is valid for a maximum of 12 months from the date it is completed and becomes invalid if your condition changes so that you would answer YES to any of the seven questions.**

continued on other side...

# PAR-Q & YOU

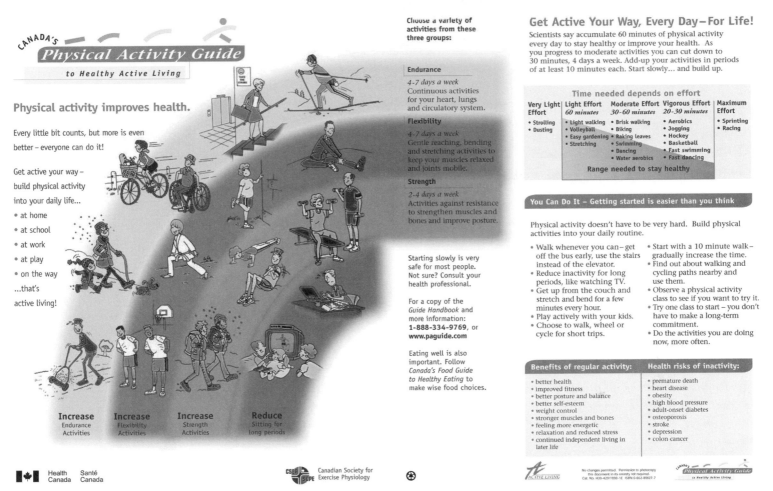

## Canada's *Physical Activity Guide* to Healthy Active Living

**Physical activity improves health.**

Every little bit counts, but more is even better – everyone can do it!

Get active your way – build physical activity into your daily life...

* at home
* at school
* at work
* at play
* on the way

...that's active living!

**Increase** Endurance Activities

**Increase** Flexibility Activities

**Increase** Strength Activities

**Reduce** Sitting for long periods

Health Canada    Santé Canada

CSEP SCPE  Canadian Society for Exercise Physiology

**Choose a variety of activities from these three groups:**

**Endurance**
*4-7 days a week*
Continuous activities for your heart, lungs and circulatory system.

**Flexibility**
*4-7 days a week*
Gentle reaching, bending and stretching activities to keep your muscles relaxed and joints mobile.

**Strength**
*2-4 days a week*
Activities against resistance to strengthen muscles and bones and improve posture.

Starting slowly is very safe for most people. Not sure? Consult your health professional.

For a copy of the *Guide Handbook* and more information:
**1-888-334-9769**, or **www.paguide.com**

Eating well is also important. Follow *Canada's Food Guide to Healthy Eating* to make wise food choices.

## Get Active Your Way, Every Day – For Life!

Scientists say accumulate 60 minutes of physical activity every day to stay healthy or improve your health. As you progress to moderate activities you can cut down to 30 minutes, 4 days a week. Add-up your activities in periods of at least 10 minutes each. Start slowly... and build up.

### Time needed depends on effort

| Very Light Effort | Light Effort *60 minutes* | Moderate Effort *30-60 minutes* | Vigorous Effort *20-30 minutes* | Maximum Effort |
|---|---|---|---|---|
| • Strolling<br>• Dusting | • Light walking<br>• Volleyball<br>• Easy gardening<br>• Stretching | • Brisk walking<br>• Biking<br>• Raking leaves<br>• Swimming<br>• Dancing<br>• Water aerobics | • Aerobics<br>• Jogging<br>• Hockey<br>• Basketball<br>• Fast swimming<br>• Fast dancing | • Sprinting<br>• Racing |
| | | **Range needed to stay healthy** | | |

### You Can Do It – Getting started is easier than you think

Physical activity doesn't have to be very hard. Build physical activities into your daily routine.

* Walk whenever you can – get off the bus early, use the stairs instead of the elevator.
* Reduce inactivity for long periods, like watching TV.
* Get up from the couch and stretch and bend for a few minutes every hour.
* Play actively with your kids.
* Choose to walk, wheel or cycle for short trips.

* Start with a 10 minute walk – gradually increase the time.
* Find out about walking and cycling paths nearby and use them.
* Observe a physical activity class to see if you want to try it.
* Try one class to start – you don't have to make a long-term commitment.
* Do the activities you are doing now, more often.

| Benefits of regular activity: | Health risks of inactivity: |
|---|---|
| • better health<br>• improved fitness<br>• better posture and balance<br>• better self-esteem<br>• weight control<br>• stronger muscles and bones<br>• feeling more energetic<br>• relaxation and reduced stress<br>• continued independent living in later life | • premature death<br>• heart disease<br>• obesity<br>• high blood pressure<br>• adult-onset diabetes<br>• osteoporosis<br>• stroke<br>• depression<br>• colon cancer |

ACTIVE LIVING  No changes permitted. Permission to photocopy this document in its entirety not required. Cat. H39-429/1998-1E  ISBN 0-662-86627-7

Canada's *Physical Activity Guide* to Healthy Active Living

---

**FITNESS AND HEALTH PROFESSIONALS MAY BE INTERESTED IN THE INFORMATION BELOW:**

The following companion forms are available for doctors' use by contacting the Canadian Society for Exercise Physiology (address below):

The **Physical Activity Readiness Medical Examination (PARmed-X)** – to be used by doctors with people who answer YES to one or more questions on the PAR-Q.

The **Physical Activity Readiness Medical Examination for Pregnancy (PARmed-X for Pregnancy)** – to be used by doctors with pregnant patients who wish to become more active.

References:
Arraix, G.A., Wigle, D.T., Mao, Y. (1992). Risk Assessment of Physical Activity and Physical Fitness in the Canada Health Survey Follow-Up Study. **J. Clin. Epidemiol.** 45:4 419-428.
Mottola, M., Wolfe, L.A. (1994). Active Living and Pregnancy, In: A. Quinney, L. Gauvin, T. Wall (eds.), **Toward Active Living: Proceedings of the International Conference on Physical Activity, Fitness and Health**. Champaign, IL: Human Kinetics.
PAR-Q Validation Report, British Columbia Ministry of Health, 1978.
Thomas, S., Reading, J., Shephard, R.J. (1992). Revision of the Physical Activity Readiness Questionnaire (PAR-Q). **Can. J. Spt. Sci.** 17:4 338-345.

---

To order multiple printed copies of the PAR-Q, please contact the:

Canadian Society for Exercise Physiology
202-185 Somerset Street West
Ottawa, ON  K2P 0J2
Tel. 1-877-651-3755 • FAX (613) 234-3565
Online: www.csep.ca

The original PAR-Q was developed by the British Columbia Ministry of Health. It has been revised by an Expert Advisory Committee of the Canadian Society for Exercise Physiology chaired by Dr. N. Gledhill (2002).

Disponible en français sous le titre «Questionnaire sur l'aptitude à l'activité physique - Q-AAP (revisé 2002)».

CSEP SCPE  © Canadian Society for Exercise Physiology

Supported by:  Health Canada    Santé Canada

# Cardiorespiratory Fitness Tests

## Females

| Percentile | Age 20-29 | | | | Age 30-39 | | | | |
|---|---|---|---|---|---|---|---|---|---|
| | Balke Treadmill (time) | Max V̇O$_2$ (ml/kg/min) | 12 min run distance (miles) | 1.5 mile run (time) | Balke Treadmill (time) | Max V̇O$_2$ (ml/kg/min) | 12 min run distance (miles) | 1.5 mile run (time) | |
| 99 | 27:43 | 55.0 | 1.84 | 9:23 | 26:00 | 52.5 | 1.77 | 9:52 | Superior |
| 95 | 24:24 | 50.2 | 1.71 | 10:20 | 22:06 | 46.9 | 1.62 | 11:08 | |
| 90 | 22:30 | 47.5 | 1.63 | 10:59 | 20:34 | 44.7 | 1.56 | 11:43 | Excellent |
| 85 | 21:00 | 45.3 | 1.57 | 11:34 | 19:03 | 42.5 | 1.50 | 12:23 | |
| 80 | 20:04 | 44.0 | 1.54 | 11:56 | 18:00 | 41.0 | 1.45 | 12:53 | |
| 75 | 19:42 | 43.4 | 1.52 | 12:07 | 17:30 | 40.3 | 1.43 | 13:08 | Good |
| 70 | 18:06 | 41.1 | 1.46 | 12:51 | 16:30 | 38.8 | 1.39 | 13:41 | |
| 65 | 17:45 | 40.6 | 1.44 | 13:01 | 16:00 | 38.1 | 1.37 | 13:58 | |
| 60 | 17:00 | 39.5 | 1.41 | 13:25 | 15:02 | 36.7 | 1.33 | 14:33 | |
| 55 | 16:00 | 38.1 | 1.37 | 13:58 | 15:00 | 36.7 | 1.33 | 14:33 | Fair |
| 50 | 15:30 | 37.4 | 1.35 | 14:15 | 14:00 | 35.2 | 1.29 | 15:14 | |
| 45 | 15:00 | 36.7 | 1.33 | 14:33 | 13:30 | 34.5 | 1.27 | 15:35 | |
| 40 | 14:11 | 35.5 | 1.30 | 15:05 | 13:00 | 33.8 | 1.25 | 15:56 | |
| 35 | 13:36 | 34.6 | 1.27 | 15:32 | 12:03 | 32.4 | 1.21 | 16:43 | Poor |
| 30 | 13:00 | 33.8 | 1.25 | 15:56 | 12:00 | 32.3 | 1.21 | 16:46 | |
| 25 | 12:04 | 32.4 | 1.22 | 16:43 | 11:00 | 30.9 | 1.17 | 17:38 | |
| 20 | 11:30 | 31.6 | 1.19 | 17:11 | 10:20 | 29.9 | 1.15 | 18:18 | |
| 15 | 10:42 | 30.5 | 1.16 | 17:53 | 9:39 | 28.9 | 1.12 | 19:01 | Very poor |
| 10 | 10:00 | 29.4 | 1.13 | 18:39 | 8:36 | 27.4 | 1.08 | 20:13 | |
| 5 | 7:54 | 26.4 | 1:05 | 21:05 | 7:16 | 25.5 | 1.02 | 21:57 | |
| 1 | 5:14 | 22.6 | 0.94 | 25:17 | 5:20 | 22.7 | 0.94 | 25:10 | |

n = 1,350                    n = 4,394

Total n = 5,744

Reprinted, by permission, from The Cooper Institute, 2005, *Physical fitness specialist course and certification* (Dallas, TX: The Cooper Institute), 30.

# Cardiorespiratory Fitness Tests

## Females

| | Age 40-49 | | | | Age 50-59 | | | | |
|---|---|---|---|---|---|---|---|---|---|
| Percentile | Balke Treadmill (time) | Max $\dot{V}O_2$ (ml/kg/min) | 12 min run distance (miles) | 1.5 mile run (time) | Balke Treadmill (time) | Max $\dot{V}O_2$ (ml/kg/min) | 12 min run distance (miles) | 1.5 mile run (time) | |
| 99 | 25:00 | 51.1 | 1.74 | 10:09 | 21:00 | 45.3 | 1.57 | 11:34 | Superior |
| 95 | 20:56 | 45.2 | 1.57 | 11:35 | 17:16 | 39.9 | 1.42 | 13:16 | |
| 90 | 19:00 | 42.2 | 1.49 | 12:25 | 16:00 | 38.1 | 1.37 | 13:58 | Excellent |
| 85 | 17:20 | 40.0 | 1.43 | 13:14 | 15:00 | 36.7 | 1.33 | 14:33 | |
| 80 | 16:34 | 38.9 | 1.40 | 13:38 | 14:00 | 35.2 | 1.29 | 15:14 | |
| 75 | 16:00 | 38.1 | 1.37 | 13:58 | 13:15 | 34.1 | 1.26 | 15:47 | Good |
| 70 | 15:00 | 36.7 | 1.33 | 14:33 | 12:23 | 32.9 | 1.23 | 16:26 | |
| 65 | 14:14 | 35.6 | 1.30 | 15:03 | 12:00 | 32.3 | 1.21 | 16:46 | |
| 60 | 13:56 | 35.1 | 1.29 | 15:17 | 11:23 | 31.4 | 1.19 | 17:19 | |
| 55 | 13:02 | 33.8 | 1.25 | 15:56 | 11:00 | 30.9 | 1.17 | 17:38 | Fair |
| 50 | 12:39 | 33.3 | 1.24 | 16:13 | 10:30 | 30.2 | 1.15 | 18:05 | |
| 45 | 12:00 | 32.3 | 1.21 | 16:46 | 10:00 | 29.4 | 1.13 | 18:39 | |
| 40 | 11:30 | 31.6 | 1.19 | 17:11 | 9:30 | 28.7 | 1.11 | 19:10 | |
| 35 | 11:00 | 30.9 | 1.17 | 17:38 | 9:00 | 28.0 | 1.09 | 19:43 | Poor |
| 30 | 10:10 | 29.7 | 1.14 | 18:26 | 8:30 | 27.3 | 1.07 | 20:17 | |
| 25 | 10:00 | 29.4 | 1.13 | 18:39 | 8:00 | 26.6 | 1.05 | 20:55 | |
| 20 | 9:00 | 28.0 | 1.09 | 19:43 | 7:15 | 25.5 | 1.02 | 21:57 | |
| 15 | 8:07 | 26.7 | 1.06 | 20:49 | 6:40 | 24.6 | 1.00 | 22:53 | Very poor |
| 10 | 7:21 | 25.6 | 1.03 | 21:52 | 6:00 | 23.7 | 0.97 | 23:55 | |
| 5 | 6:17 | 24.1 | 0:98 | 23:27 | 4:48 | 21.9 | 0.92 | 26:15 | |
| 1 | 4:00 | 20.8 | 0.89 | 27:55 | 3:00 | 19.3 | 0.85 | 30:34 | |

*n* = 4,834

*n* = 3,103

Total *n* = 7,937

Reprinted, by permission, from The Cooper Institute, 2005, *Physical fitness specialist course and certification* (Dallas, TX: The Cooper Institute), 30.

# Cardiorespiratory Fitness Tests

## Females

| Percentile | Age 60-69 | | | | Age 70-79 | | | | |
|---|---|---|---|---|---|---|---|---|---|
| | Balke Treadmill (time) | Max $\dot{V}O_2$ (ml/kg/min) | 12 min run distance (miles) | 1.5 mile run (time) | Balke Treadmill (time) | Max $\dot{V}O_2$ (ml/kg/min) | 12 min run distance (miles) | 1.5 mile run (time) | |
| 99 | 19:00 | 42.4 | 1.49 | 12:25 | 19:00 | 42.4 | 1.49 | 12:25 | Superior |
| 95 | 15:09 | 36.9 | 1.34 | 14:28 | 15:00 | 36.7 | 1.33 | 14:33 | |
| 90 | 13:33 | 34.6 | 1.27 | 15:32 | 12:50 | 33.5 | 1.25 | 16:06 | Excellent |
| 85 | 12:28 | 33.0 | 1.23 | 16:22 | 11:46 | 32.0 | 1.20 | 16:57 | |
| 80 | 12:00 | 32.3 | 1.21 | 16:46 | 10:30 | 30.2 | 1.15 | 18:05 | |
| 75 | 11:04 | 31.0 | 1.18 | 17:34 | 10:00 | 29.4 | 1.13 | 18:39 | Good |
| 70 | 10:30 | 30.2 | 1.15 | 18:05 | 9:15 | 28.4 | 1.10 | 19:24 | |
| 65 | 10:00 | 29.4 | 1.13 | 18:39 | 8:43 | 27.6 | 1.08 | 20:02 | |
| 60 | 9:44 | 29.1 | 1.12 | 18:52 | 8:00 | 26.6 | 1.05 | 20:54 | |
| 55 | 9:11 | 28.3 | 1.10 | 19:29 | 7:37 | 26.0 | 1.04 | 21:45 | Fair |
| 50 | 8:40 | 27.5 | 1.08 | 20:08 | 7:00 | 25.1 | 1.01 | 22:22 | |
| 45 | 8:15 | 26.9 | 1.06 | 20:38 | 6:39 | 24.6 | 1.00 | 22:54 | |
| 40 | 8:00 | 26.6 | 1.05 | 20:55 | 6:05 | 23.8 | 0.98 | 23:47 | |
| 35 | 7:14 | 25.4 | 1.02 | 22:03 | 5:28 | 22.9 | 0.95 | 24:54 | Poor |
| 30 | 6:52 | 24.9 | 1.01 | 22:34 | 5:00 | 22.2 | 0.93 | 25:49 | |
| 25 | 6:21 | 24.2 | 0.99 | 23:20 | 4:45 | 21.9 | 0.92 | 26:15 | |
| 20 | 6:00 | 23.7 | 0.97 | 23:55 | 4:16 | 21.2 | 0.90 | 27:17 | |
| 15 | 5:25 | 22.8 | 0.95 | 25:02 | 4:00 | 20.8 | 0.89 | 27:55 | Very poor |
| 10 | 4:40 | 21.7 | 0.92 | 26:32 | 3:00 | 19.3 | 0.85 | 30:34 | |
| 5 | 3:30 | 20.1 | 0.87 | 29.06 | 2:00 | 17.9 | 0.81 | 33:32 | |
| 1 | 2:10 | 18.1 | 0.82 | 33:05 | 1:00 | 16.4 | 0.77 | 37:26 | |

n = 1,088

n = 209

Total n = 1,297

Reprinted, by permission, from The Cooper Institute, 2005, *Physical fitness specialist course and certification* (Dallas, TX: The Cooper Institute), 30.

# Flexibility—Sit and Reach

## Females

### Age

| Percentile | <20 | 20-29 | 30-39 | 40-49 | 50-59 | 60+ | |
|:---:|:---:|:---:|:---:|:---:|:---:|:---:|:---|
| 99 | >24.3 | >24.5 | >24.0 | >22.8 | >23.0 | >23.0 | Superior |
| 95 | 24.3 | 24.5 | 24.0 | 22.8 | 23.0 | 23.0 | |
| 90 | 24.3 | 23.8 | 22.5 | 21.5 | 21.5 | 21.8 | Excellent |
| 85 | 22.5 | 23.0 | 22.0 | 21.3 | 21.0 | 19.5 | |
| 80 | 22.5 | 22.5 | 21.5 | 20.5 | 20.3 | 19.0 | |
| 75 | 22.3 | 22.0 | 21.0 | 20.0 | 20.0 | 18.0 | Good |
| 70 | 22.0 | 21.5 | 20.5 | 19.8 | 19.3 | 17.5 | |
| 65 | 21.8 | 21.0 | 20.3 | 19.1 | 19.0 | 17.5 | |
| 60 | 21.5 | 20.5 | 20.0 | 19.0 | 18.5 | 17.0 | |
| 55 | 21.3 | 20.3 | 19.5 | 18.5 | 18.0 | 17.0 | Fair |
| 50 | 21.0 | 20.0 | 19.0 | 18.0 | 17.9 | 16.4 | |
| 45 | 20.5 | 19.5 | 18.5 | 18.0 | 17.0 | 16.1 | |
| 40 | 20.5 | 19.3 | 18.3 | 17.3 | 16.8 | 15.5 | |
| 35 | 20.0 | 19.0 | 17.8 | 17.0 | 16.0 | 15.2 | Poor |
| 30 | 19.5 | 18.3 | 17.3 | 16.5 | 15.5 | 14.4 | |
| 25 | 19.0 | 17.8 | 16.8 | 16.0 | 15.3 | 13.6 | |
| 20 | 18.5 | 17.0 | 16.5 | 15.0 | 14.8 | 13.0 | |
| 15 | 17.8 | 16.4 | 15.5 | 14.0 | 14.0 | 11.5 | Very poor |
| 10 | 14.5 | 15.4 | 14.4 | 13.0 | 13.0 | 11.5 | |
| 5 | 14.5 | 14.1 | 12.0 | 10.5 | 12.3 | 9.2 | |
| 1 | <14.5 | <14.1 | <12.0 | <10.5 | <12.3 | <9.2 | |
| *n* | 19 | 183 | 376 | 332 | 192 | 44 | |

Total *n* = 1,146

Reprinted, by permission, from The Cooper Institute, 2005, *Physical fitness specialist course and certification* (Dallas, TX: The Cooper Institute), 30.

# Dynamic Strength
## 1-Minute Sit-Up

### Females

### Age

| Percentile | <20 | 20-29 | 30-39 | 40-49 | 50-59 | 60+ | |
|---|---|---|---|---|---|---|---|
| 99 | >55.0 | >51.0 | >42.0 | >38.0 | >30.0 | >28.0 | Superior |
| 95 | 55.0 | 51.0 | 42.0 | 38.0 | 30.0 | 28.0 | Superior |
| 90 | 54.0 | 49.0 | 40.0 | 34.0 | 29.0 | 26.0 | Excellent |
| 85 | 49.0 | 45.0 | 38.0 | 32.0 | 25.0 | 20.0 | Excellent |
| 80 | 46.0 | 44.0 | 35.0 | 29.0 | 24.0 | 17.0 | Excellent |
| 75 | 40.0 | 42.0 | 3.0 | 28.0 | 22.0 | 15.0 | Good |
| 70 | 38.0 | 41.0 | 32.0 | 27.0 | 22.0 | 12.0 | Good |
| 65 | 37.0 | 39.0 | 30.0 | 25.0 | 21.0 | 12.0 | Good |
| 60 | 36.0 | 38.0 | 29.0 | 24.0 | 20.0 | 11.0 | Good |
| 55 | 35.0 | 37.0 | 28.0 | 23.0 | 19.0 | 10.0 | Fair |
| 50 | 34.0 | 35.0 | 27.0 | 22.0 | 17.0 | 8.0 | Fair |
| 45 | 34.0 | 34.0 | 26.0 | 21.0 | 16.0 | 8.0 | Fair |
| 40 | 32.0 | 32.0 | 25.0 | 20.0 | 14.0 | 6.0 | Fair |
| 35 | 30.0 | 31.0 | 24.0 | 19.0 | 12.0 | 5.0 | Poor |
| 30 | 29.0 | 30.0 | 22.0 | 17.0 | 12.0 | 4.0 | Poor |
| 25 | 29.0 | 28.0 | 21.0 | 16.0 | 11.0 | 4.0 | Poor |
| 20 | 28.0 | 24.0 | 20.0 | 14.0 | 10.0 | 3.0 | Poor |
| 15 | 27.0 | 23.0 | 18.0 | 13.0 | 7.0 | 2.0 | Very poor |
| 10 | 25.0 | 21.0 | 15.0 | 10.0 | 6.0 | 1.0 | Very poor |
| 5 | 25.0 | 18.0 | 11.0 | 7.0 | 5.0 | 0.0 | Very poor |
| 1 | <25.0 | <18.0 | <11.0 | <7.0 | <5.0 | 0.0 | Very poor |
| n | 15 | 144 | 289 | 249 | 137 | 26 | |

Total n = 860

Reprinted, by permission, from The Cooper Institute, 2005, *Physical fitness specialist course and certification* (Dallas, TX: The Cooper Institute), 30.

# Dynamic Strength
## Modified Push-Up

### Females

#### Age

| Percentile | 20-29 | 30-39 | 40-49 | 50-59 | 60+ | |
|:---:|:---:|:---:|:---:|:---:|:---:|:---:|
| 99 | 70 | 56 | 60 | 31 | 20 | Superior |
| 95 | 45 | 39 | 33 | 28 | 20 | Superior |
| 90 | 42 | 36 | 28 | 25 | 17 | Excellent |
| 85 | 39 | 33 | 26 | 23 | 15 | Excellent |
| 80 | 36 | 31 | 24 | 21 | 15 | Excellent |
| 75 | 34 | 29 | 21 | 20 | 15 | Good |
| 70 | 32 | 28 | 20 | 19 | 14 | Good |
| 65 | 31 | 26 | 19 | 18 | 13 | Good |
| 60 | 30 | 24 | 18 | 17 | 12 | Good |
| 55 | 29 | 23 | 17 | 15 | 12 | Fair |
| 50 | 26 | 21 | 15 | 13 | 8 | Fair |
| 45 | 25 | 20 | 14 | 13 | 6 | Fair |
| 40 | 23 | 19 | 13 | 12 | 5 | Fair |
| 35 | 22 | 17 | 11 | 10 | 4 | Poor |
| 30 | 20 | 15 | 10 | 9 | 3 | Poor |
| 25 | 19 | 14 | 9 | 8 | 2 | Poor |
| 20 | 17 | 11 | 6 | 6 | 2 | Poor |
| 15 | 15 | 9 | 4 | 4 | 1 | Very poor |
| 10 | 12 | 8 | 2 | 1 | 0 | Very poor |
| 5 | 9 | 4 | 1 | 0 | 0 | Very poor |
| *n* | 579 | 411 | 246 | 105 | 12 | |

Total *n* = 1,353

Reprinted, by permission, from The Cooper Institute, 2005, *Physical fitness specialist course and certification* (Dallas, TX: The Cooper Institute), 30.

# Dynamic Strength
## Full-Body Push-Up*

### Females

#### Age

| Percentile | 20-29 | 30-39 | 40-49 | |
|---|---|---|---|---|
| 99 | 53.0 | 48.0 | 23.0 | Superior |
| 95 | 42.0 | 39.5 | 20.0 | Superior |
| 90 | 37.0 | 33.0 | 18.0 | Excellent |
| 85 | 33.0 | 26.0 | 17.0 | Excellent |
| 80 | 28.0 | 23.0 | 15.0 | Excellent |
| 75 | 27.0 | 19.0 | 15.0 | Good |
| 70 | 24.0 | 18.0 | 14.0 | Good |
| 65 | 23.0 | 16.0 | 13.0 | Good |
| 60 | 21.0 | 15.0 | 13.0 | Good |
| 55 | 19.0 | 14.0 | 11.0 | Fair |
| 50 | 18.0 | 14.0 | 11.0 | Fair |
| 45 | 17.0 | 13.0 | 10.0 | Fair |
| 40 | 15.0 | 11.0 | 9.0 | Fair |
| 35 | 14.0 | 10.0 | 8.0 | Poor |
| 30 | 13.0 | 9.0 | 7.0 | Poor |
| 25 | 11.0 | 9.0 | 7.0 | Poor |
| 20 | 10.0 | 8.0 | 6.0 | Poor |
| 15 | 9.0 | 6.5 | 5.0 | Very poor |
| 10 | 8.0 | 6.0 | 4.0 | Very poor |
| 5 | 6.0 | 4.0 | 1.0 | Very poor |
| 1 | 3.0 | 1.0 | 0.0 | |

*Full-body push-ups are generally used by law enforcement and public safety organizations. These norms are baed on >1,000 female U.S. Army soldiers who were tested in the 1990s by the U.S. Army.

Reprinted, by permission, from The Cooper Institute, 2005, *Physical fitness specialist course and certification* (Dallas, TX: The Cooper Institute), 30.

# Absolute Strength
## 1-Repetition Maximum Bench Press

Bench press weight ratio = $\dfrac{\text{weight pushed in pounds}}{\text{body weight in pounds}}$

### Females

| | | | Age | | | | |
|---|---|---|---|---|---|---|---|
| Percentile | <20 | 20-29 | 30-39 | 40-49 | 50-59 | 60+ | |
| 99 | >.88 | >1.01 | >.82 | >.77 | >.68 | >.72 | Superior |
| 95 | .88 | 1.01 | .82 | .77 | .68 | .72 | |
| 90 | .83 | .90 | .76 | .71 | .61 | .64 | Excellent |
| 85 | .81 | .83 | .72 | .66 | .57 | .59 | |
| 80 | .77 | .80 | .70 | .62 | .55 | .54 | |
| 75 | .76 | .77 | .65 | .60 | .53 | .53 | Good |
| 70 | .74 | .74 | .63 | .57 | .52 | .51 | |
| 65 | .70 | .72 | .62 | .55 | .50 | .48 | |
| 60 | .65 | .70 | .60 | .54 | .48 | .47 | |
| 55 | .64 | .68 | .58 | .53 | .47 | .46 | Fair |
| 50 | .63 | .65 | .57 | .52 | .46 | .45 | |
| 45 | .60 | .63 | .55 | .51 | .45 | .44 | |
| 40 | .58 | .59 | .53 | .50 | .44 | .43 | |
| 35 | .57 | .58 | .52 | .48 | .43 | .41 | Poor |
| 30 | .56 | .56 | .51 | .47 | .42 | .40 | |
| 25 | .55 | .53 | .49 | .45 | .41 | .39 | |
| 20 | .53 | .51 | .47 | .43 | .39 | .38 | |
| 15 | .52 | .50 | .45 | .42 | .38 | .36 | Very poor |
| 10 | .50 | .48 | .42 | .38 | .37 | .33 | |
| 5 | .41 | .44 | .39 | .35 | .31 | .26 | |
| 1 | <.41 | <.44 | <.39 | <.35 | <.31 | <.26 | |
| n | 20 | 191 | 379 | 333 | 189 | 42 | |

Total n = 1,154

Reprinted, by permission, from The Cooper Institute, 2005, *Physical fitness specialist course and certification* (Dallas, TX: The Cooper Institute), 30.

# Personal Training Assessment Sheet

Name: _____     Age: _____

## Girth measurements: tape measure

| *Date:* | _____ | _____ | _____ | _____ | _____ |
|---|---|---|---|---|---|
| Chest | _____ | _____ | _____ | _____ | _____ |
| Waist | _____ | _____ | _____ | _____ | _____ |
| Hips | _____ | _____ | _____ | _____ | _____ |
| Thighs | _____ | _____ | _____ | _____ | _____ |
| Calves | _____ | _____ | _____ | _____ | _____ |
| Arms | _____ | _____ | _____ | _____ | _____ |

## Body composition: skin calipers

| *Date:* | _____ | _____ | _____ | _____ | _____ |
|---|---|---|---|---|---|
| Weight | _____ | _____ | _____ | _____ | _____ |
| Height | _____ | _____ | _____ | _____ | _____ |
| Chest | _____ | _____ | _____ | _____ | _____ |
| Triceps | _____ | _____ | _____ | _____ | _____ |
| Midaxillary | _____ | _____ | _____ | _____ | _____ |
| Subscapular | _____ | _____ | _____ | _____ | _____ |
| Suprailiac | _____ | _____ | _____ | _____ | _____ |
| Abdomen | _____ | _____ | _____ | _____ | _____ |
| Thigh | _____ | _____ | _____ | _____ | _____ |
| **Total** | _____ | _____ | _____ | _____ | _____ |
| Body fat % | _____ | _____ | _____ | _____ | _____ |
| Lean % | _____ | _____ | _____ | _____ | _____ |
| Fat wt. (lb) | _____ | _____ | _____ | _____ | _____ |
| Lean wt. (lb) | _____ | _____ | _____ | _____ | _____ |

## Resting metabolic rate: RMR device

| *Date:* | _____ | _____ | _____ | _____ | _____ |
|---|---|---|---|---|---|
| RMR reading | _____ | _____ | _____ | _____ | _____ |

## Daily calorie expenditures:

| Activities of daily living | _____ | _____ | _____ | _____ | _____ |
|---|---|---|---|---|---|
| Strength training | _____ | _____ | _____ | _____ | _____ |
| Cardiovascular | _____ | _____ | _____ | _____ | _____ |
| Exercise classes | _____ | _____ | _____ | _____ | _____ |
| Total energy used daily | _____ | _____ | _____ | _____ | _____ |
| Daily calories consumed | _____ | _____ | _____ | _____ | _____ |
| Weight gain/loss | _____ | _____ | _____ | _____ | _____ |

From *Women's Health and Fitness Guide* by Michele Kettles, Colette Cole, and Brenda Wright, 2006, Champaign, IL: Human Kinetics.

# Fitness and Functional Consultation

Name: _____   Date: _____   Age: _____

Resting Blood Pressure _____                    Resting Heart Rate _____

Medical/Injury history: _____

_____

_____

_____

_____

Medications: _____

_____

_____

Occupation: _____

Exercise history (past/present):_____

_____

_____

_____

_____

## Health/Fitness goals:

Short-term:_____

_____

_____

Long-term: _____

_____

_____

## Fitness assessment category results:

Absolute strength:_____

_____

_____

*(continued)*

From *Women's Health and Fitness Guide* by Michele Kettles, Colette Cole, and Brenda Wright, 2006, Champaign, IL: Human Kinetics.

## Fitness and Functional Consultation *(continued)*

Dynamic strength:_____

_____

_____

Flexibility: _____

_____

_____

Body composition: _____

_____

_____

Cardiorespiratory: _____

_____

_____

## Functional assessment results relevant to program design:

_____

_____

_____

Corrective strengthening muscles: _____

_____

_____

_____

Corrective flexibility muscles: _____

_____

_____

_____

Recommended cardiovascular training:_____

_____

_____

_____

Frequency: _____ Intensity: _____ Duration: _____

From *Women's Health and Fitness Guide* by Michele Kettles, Colette Cole, and Brenda Wright, 2006, Champaign, IL: Human Kinetics.

## Appropriate modes of exercise:

| | | |
|---|---|---|
| _____Walking | _____Upright bike | _____Jogging |
| _____Stair stepping | _____Swimming | _____Rowing |
| _____Elliptical | _____Spin class | _____Mind/body |
| _____Water class | _____Group classes | _____Other indoor activities |
| _____Other outdoor activities | _____Recumbent bike | |

Specific notes:_____

_____

_____

_____

_____

Recommended resistance training: _____

_____

_____

_____

_____

Warm-up: _____    Cool-down: _____

Type (total/split): _____    Frequency: _____

Volume (reps): _____    Sets: _____

Rest period: _____    Exercise phase: _____

Specific notes:_____

_____

_____

_____

From *Women's Health and Fitness Guide* by Michele Kettles, Colette Cole, and Brenda Wright, 2006, Champaign, IL: Human Kinetics.

# Fitness and Functional Consultation (Example)

Name: _Faye Fitness_     Date: _4/01/05_     Age: _40_

Resting Blood Pressure _102/64_     Resting Heart Rate _72_

Medical/Injury history: _Frequent foot pain (plantar fasciitis) and back pain_

_____

_____

_____

_____

Medications: _Ibuprofen when needed_

_____

_____

Occupation: _Part-time legal assistant_

Exercise history (past/present): _Ran marathon 4 months ago, active with sporadic tennis,_
_outdoor biking, swimming, and snow skiing._
_Currently jogging around neighborhood 2-3 × a week for 30-45 minutes when pain free_

_____

_____

## Health/Fitness goals:

Short-term: _Short-term: Improve muscle tone, improve flexibility, and prevent foot and_
_back pain_

_____

Long-term: _Maintain cardiovascular fitness and health, maintain bone density, maintain_
_% body fat, play tennis regularly_

_____

## Fitness assessment category results:

Absolute strength: _Fair_

_____

_____

Dynamic strength: *Good*

Flexibility: *Poor*

Body composition: *21.9%—good*

Cardiorespiratory: *Excellent*

## Functional assessment results relevant to program design:

*Tight muscles—chest, latissimus dorsi, anterior deltoid, cervical spinal extensors, hamstrings, hip flexors, calf, hip adductors*

*Posture—rounded shoulders, forward head, slight foot pronation*

Corrective strengthening muscles: *Rhomboids, trapezius, posterior deltoid, teres minor, infraspinatus, cervical spinal flexors, gluteals, tibialis, vastus medialis. Core, neuromuscular, postural, and joint stabilization.*

Corrective flexibility muscles: *Chest, latissimus dorsi, anterior deltoid, cervical extensors, teres major, hamstrings, calf complex, iliotibial band, hip flexors, hip adductors.*

Recommended cardiovascular training: *Temporarily reduce jogging frequency. Add variety to cardio program—bike, swim, elliptical, etc.*

Frequency: *3 × wk*     Intensity: *Mod-high*     Duration: *30-45 min*

*(continued)*

From *Women's Health and Fitness Guide* by Michele Kettles, Colette Cole, and Brenda Wright, 2006, Champaign, IL: Human Kinetics.

## Fitness and Functional Consultation *(continued)*

### Appropriate modes of exercise:

| | | |
|---|---|---|
| _____ Walking | _X_ Upright bike | _____ Jogging |
| _____ Stair stepping | _X_ Swimming | _____ Rowing |
| _____ Elliptical | _X_ Spin class | _X_ Mind/body |
| _X_ Water class | _____ Group classes | _____ Other indoor activities |
| _X_ Other outdoor activities | _____ Recumbent bike | |

Specific notes: *Outdoor biking with family on the weekends*

_____

_____

_____

_____

Recommended resistance training: *Core, postural, balance training. Specifically scapular retraction, scapular depression, and cervical retraction. Incorporate stability ball, unilateral and alternating upper extremity with cables, and single-leg exercises.*

_____

_____

Warm-up: *Corrective flex/cardio—5 min*     Cool-down: *Static stretch/Self-MFR*

Type (total/split): *Total body*     Frequency: *3 × wk*

Volume (reps): *15-25*     Sets: *1-3*

Rest period: *45-90 sec*     Exercise phase: *Corrective*

Specific notes: *Corrective strengthening and stretching for upper crossed and pronation-distortion syndrome. Use foam roller for self-myofascial release. Reevaluate in 4 weeks.*

_____

_____

_____

# Weekly Exercise Plan

Name: _____ Date: _____

New program date: _____ Weeks/phase: _____ Training phase: _____

| | Flexibility Training | Cardiovascular Training | Resistance/Stability/ Balance Training | Mind/Body Training |
|---|---|---|---|---|
| Monday | | | | |
| Tuesday | | | | |
| Wednesday | | | | |
| Thursday | | | | |
| Friday | | | | |
| Saturday | | | | |
| Sunday | | | | |

Short-term goals:_____

_____

_____

_____

Specific areas of focus: _____

_____

_____

_____

Health/injury concerns: _____

_____

_____

_____

From *Women's Health and Fitness Guide* by Michele Kettles, Colette Cole, and Brenda Wright, 2006, Champaign, IL: Human Kinetics.

# Weekly Exercise Plan—Example

Name: _Faye Fitness_                    Date: _4/1/05_

New program date: _5/1-5/15_     Weeks/phase: _4-6_     Training phase: _Stabilization_

| | Flexibility Training | Cardiovascular Training | Resistance/Stability/ Balance Training | Mind/Body Training |
|---|---|---|---|---|
| Monday | Dynamic 5-10 min, static 5 min | | Total body, 40-45 min | |
| Tuesday | Static 5-10 min | Spin class, 30-45 min | | |
| Wednesday | Dynamic 5-10 min, static 5 min | | Total body, 40-45 min | |
| Thursday | Static 5-10 min | Elliptical, 30-45 min | | Pilates class |
| Friday | Dynamic 5-10 min, static 5 min | | Total body, 40-45 min | |
| Saturday | | Swim or outdoor bicycle, 30-45 min | | |
| Sunday | | | | |

Short-term goals: _Cardiovascular and weight training consistency_
_Improve body positioning awareness during workouts and daily living_
_Improve core and postural stabilization_

Specific areas of focus: _Balance, lumbo-pelvic-hip stabilization, scapular and cervical_
_retraction, and scapular depression. Flexibility and strength exercises to improve muscular_
_imbalances._

Health/injury concerns: _Intermittent back pain and plantar fasciitis_

From *Women's Health and Fitness Guide* by Michele Kettles, Colette Cole, and Brenda Wright, 2006, Champaign, IL: Human Kinetics.

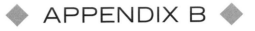

# ◆ APPENDIX B ◆

# Handouts

We have provided the handouts in this appendix for your use. Photocopy them and hand them out to clients as appropriate. These are the handouts:

- Building a Better Body Image*
- Healthy Eating Practices for Weight Management*
- Hydration Hints*
- Recommendation for Developing Maximum Bone Mass (Ages 14 to 35)
- Taking a Calcium Supplement*
- General Exercise Safety Guidelines During Pregnancy
- Recommendations for Pregnant Swimmers
- Recommendations for Pregnant Joggers and Runners
- Tips for Dealing with Common Discomforts of Pregnancy
- Tips for Physically Active Nursing Mothers
- Living with Osteoarthritis
- Urinary Incontinence
- Reduce Risks for Falls and Fractures

*Appropriate for various ages.

# Building a Better Body Image

- You cannot change your body type. You inherited it from your parents, just as you inherited your eye and hair color. Your body type does not guarantee success in a specific sport or profession or happiness in life.

- Try to adopt a positive and realistic attitude about your body. The standards that you set for yourself related to your appearance (your body image) are your personal choice.

- Stop comparing yourself to others or to the ideal that is portrayed in the media. You can be healthy, happy, and fit regardless of your body type.

- Respect your body and celebrate what your body can do when it is fit and healthy.

- Remember that every body type has its advantages. Focus on yours.

- Identify your best physical features and plan ways to emphasize them.

- Focus on your positive individual qualities and talents.

- Wear clothes that fit comfortably—not too tight, not too baggy.

- Listen for and accept compliments.

- Practice positive self-talk. You will believe the inner dialogues that you have with yourself.

- Be physically active. It's a great way to improve your body image and boost your confidence in other areas as well.

- Start a diary or journal. Write about things you do well, physically and mentally, and work on those. Express your feelings. Identify problems and look for options. Look back at your progress after six months.

- Find other women with whom you can share your feelings and concerns about your body image. Nurture and support each other.

- Seek professional help if necessary. You may need to consult with a psychologist, medical doctor, nutritionist, or registered dietitian.

From *Women's Health and Fitness Guide* by Michele Kettles, Colette Cole, and Brenda Wright, 2006, Champaign, IL: Human Kinetics.

# Healthy Eating Practices for Weight Management

♦ Keep a food diary to be more aware of what, how much, and why you eat. Do you eat when you are not hungry? Do you eat when feeling happy, sad, angry, or stressed?

♦ Eat a healthy breakfast every day. Eat four to six small meals instead of three larger ones.

♦ Try to eat at the same time of day every day.

♦ Try to eat at home or prepare or take your food with you so you will have more control over what you eat.

♦ Have nutritious snacks (fruit, raw veggies, nuts, fat-free yogurt or cheese, whole-grain breads and cereals) available so you don't go hungry.

♦ Avoid choosing empty-calorie fast foods (beverages sweetened with sugar, candies, cookies, pastries, salty snacks such as high-fat chips and crackers).

♦ Avoid foods high in simple sugar (sweets, jams and jellies, sweetened beverages) and saturated fats or trans fats (high-fat meats, butter, cream, stick margarine, hydrogenated peanut butter, commercially prepared baked goods).

♦ Drink plenty of fluids, especially water, daily. Low-calorie hot beverages, such as herbal teas or bouillon, are filling and count as fluids.

♦ Take a drink of water between bites of food.

♦ Try to chew your food thoroughly.

♦ Eat slowly.

♦ Eat only while seated at the table (not while watching TV, reading, talking on the phone, or at the computer).

♦ Control your portion sizes. When eating at home, use smaller plates, bowls, and glasses.

♦ When eating in a restaurant, order an appetizer as an entrée or plan in advance to take some food home.

♦ Eat with someone who will help support your healthy eating practices.

From *Women's Health and Fitness Guide* by Michele Kettles, Colette Cole, and Brenda Wright, 2006, Champaign, IL: Human Kinetics.

# Hydration Hints

Take your body weight and divide it in half. The resulting number is the total ounces of fluid you should consume each day. For example, a woman weighing 140 pounds (63.5 kilograms) should drink about 70 ounces of fluids per day (about 9 cups or 2+ liters). All fluids count, even those containing caffeine. When you urinate, your urine should be pale yellow, not dark. If the urine is dark, more fluids are needed to maintain adequate hydration. Remember, thirst is a very late and unreliable signal of hydration.

When exercising, depending on intensity and heat exposure, consume more fluids (about 8 to 10 ounces [236 to 296 milliliters] for 30 to 60 minutes of exercise). For women who perform endurance exercise or who sweat heavily during exercise, a more precise measure of fluid loss during activity can be made. The woman should weigh herself before and after an hour of exercise. For every pound of weight lost in an hour, she should consume 13 to 16 ounces (394 to 473 milliliters) of fluid. Ideally, these fluids are consumed during exercise and spread throughout the workout.

It is possible to overhydrate and cause hyponatremia (low sodium in the blood), which can be life threatening. This is generally more of an issue in endurance events lasting more than 4 hours. For this reason, endurance athletes need to calculate their "sweat rate" per hour, as noted earlier. Keep in mind that sport drinks do *not* protect against hyponatremia.

From *Women's Health and Fitness Guide* by Michele Kettles, Colette Cole, and Brenda Wright, 2006, Champaign, IL: Human Kinetics.

# Recommendations for Developing Maximum Bone Mass (Ages 14 to 35)

◆ Participate in regular weight-bearing exercise to gain peak bone mass, particularly during puberty when growing taller. High-impact activities such as jogging, jumping rope, gymnastics, and aerobic dance are best.

◆ Add strength training to build muscle mass and make bones stronger.

◆ Eat a balanced and varied diet.

◆ Get adequate amounts of calcium (1,200 to 1,500 milligrams a day).

◆ Seek professional help immediately if you think you may have an eating disorder.

◆ Don't smoke or abuse alcohol.

◆ Have regular menstrual periods. See a doctor if menstrual cycles stop for more than three months.

◆ If you develop amenorrhea, you need 1,500 milligrams of calcium a day. Young women with amenorrhea and low estrogen levels lose as much as 1 to 5 percent of their total bone mass each year that they lack estrogen. This rate of bone loss is similar to what is experienced by women after menopause. Poor nutrition increases the risk of losing even more bone.

◆ Remember that pregnancy and breast-feeding require more calcium. If you are pregnant, consume 1,500 milligrams of calcium per day, whether through food or a supplement.

From *Women's Health and Fitness Guide* by Michele Kettles, Colette Cole, and Brenda Wright, 2006, Champaign, IL: Human Kinetics.

# Taking a Calcium Supplement

- Calcium supplements are available over the counter. Calcium must be combined with other elements to get it into a tablet form. You will find it available as calcium carbonate, calcium citrate, calcium gluconate, calcium phosphate, and in other forms.

- Select a calcium supplement that contains a high amount of calcium in each pill, such as 400 to 600 milligrams. Calcium carbonate (such as Tums) and calcium citrate are good choices.

- Be aware that calcium derived from bone meal (from animals, dolomite, and oyster shells) has been found to contain substances that can be harmful, such as arsenic, lead, or mercury. These types of calcium are not recommended.

- If you have difficulty swallowing large tablets, choose a flavored, chewable calcium supplement.

- Know that low-cost generic or pharmacy-brand calcium carbonate or calcium citrate tablets are as good as name-brand products.

- To avoid side effects, begin by taking half a tablet and gradually build up to the amount you need. Side effects include gas, bloating, nausea, diarrhea, and constipation.

- Take calcium carbonate supplements after a meal when there is plenty of acid in your stomach to help dissolve the tablet. If the tablet doesn't dissolve, it can't be absorbed and used by the body. Calcium citrate supplements are readily absorbed on an empty stomach.

- Don't take more than 1,000 to 1,500 milligrams of calcium a day, and don't take more than 600 milligrams at one time. The body can't absorb more than 600 milligrams at one time. Excess calcium is filtered out by the kidneys and can cause kidney stones in women who have had prior kidney stones. Staying well hydrated helps prevent kidney stones.

- Be sure to get adequate vitamin D to help your body absorb calcium. Vitamin D is found in fortified milk or soy milk and also in multivitamin supplements. Look for supplements containing 400 to 800 IU (international units) of vitamin D. Exposing your skin to sunlight for 15 to 20 minutes a day without sunscreen will also allow your body to make the vitamin D it needs.

From *Women's Health and Fitness Guide* by Michele Kettles, Colette Cole, and Brenda Wright, 2006, Champaign, IL: Human Kinetics.

# General Exercise Safety Guidelines During Pregnancy

- Don't work out so hard that you are out of breath or very hot.
- Don't exercise if you have a fever.
- Avoid performing exercises while lying on your back after the third or fourth month.
- Avoid standing still on your feet for more than 20 to 30 minutes at a time.
- Do not suddenly change your position.
- Don't exercise when feeling overly fatigued.
- Avoid overtraining and binge exercise.
- Avoid motions that produce discomfort or pain.
- Eat often and in small amounts (have a small carbohydrate snack and water or juice available).
- Include adequate protein (eggs, milk, nuts, seeds, fish, chicken, meat, soy, and dried beans) to maintain energy over the long term.

- Drink water and avoid hot, humid environments.
- Wear good shoes, dress in layers, and make sure any equipment you use is in good condition.
- Breathe slowly and deeply during all phases of exercise.
- Include a thorough cool-down to prevent pooling of blood in the extremities.
- Take a rest on your side during the day in the second and third trimesters.
- If you experience any of these signs or symptoms, see your health care provider:
  - Bleeding or a large amount of discharge
  - Frequent light-headedness, seeing stars, or having an ongoing headache
  - Swelling in your face or hands
  - Regular contractions or cramps that continue when you stop exercising
  - Discomfort in the low back

Adapted from Cowlin AF. *Women's Fitness Program Development*

From *Women's Health and Fitness Guide* by Michele Kettles, Colette Cole, and Brenda Wright, 2006, Champaign, IL: Human Kinetics.

# Recommendations for Pregnant Swimmers

- Wear a comfortable swimsuit. Some maternity suits become too heavy when wet, making swimming difficult. Experiment with different fabrics, styles, and sizes until you find something that gives you support where you need it and still lets you swim comfortably.

- Don't swim alone. However, avoid crowded pools to minimize the risk of being kicked.

- Be sure the water and air temperatures are comfortable. Leave the water if you feel uncomfortably chilled or overheated.

- Take time to warm up. Try doing some stretching on land or in the water. Start off swimming slowly until you loosen up.

- Swim according to your abilities. Use moderation and be sure to breathe properly. Avoid diving or jumping into the water feet first.

- Remember to drink water both before and after exercise.

- If you experience contractions, leg cramps, or joint pain, be ready to stop swimming or change your swimming style. You may need to try different strokes, kicks, or turns. Modify or stop your exercise program if you develop medical problems such as early dilation.

Adapted from Lutter and Jaffee (1996)

From *Women's Health and Fitness Guide* by Michele Kettles, Colette Cole, and Brenda Wright, 2006, Champaign, IL: Human Kinetics.

# Recommendations for Pregnant Joggers and Runners

- Jog or run in the coolest part of the day and in appropriate clothing. Be sure to drink plenty of fluids before exercising, even if you may have to stop for bathroom breaks more often.

- Exercise with others, if possible. Always let people know when and where you are jogging or running. Carry a cell phone in case you need to call for help.

- Take the time for adequate warm-up and cool-down before and after exercise.

- Be willing to modify your run's intensity, frequency, and speed. Increasing weight and fatigue may dictate shorter, slower runs, eliminating hills and speed work. Stop and walk if necessary. You may feel a need to slow down because of heat, ligament or joint pain, or Braxton-Hicks contractions (painless uterine tightenings).

- Wear comfortable clothing. Well-cushioned, stable running shoes, a good bra, and comfortable shorts are important. Some women find that a lightweight maternity girdle offers support for the back and ligaments.

- Be kind to your back. Pay attention to your posture and balance. You may want to experiment with posture changes that make you more stable while running.

- Modify or stop your exercise program if medical problems such as unusual discomfort, early dilation, or bleeding develop.

Adapted from Lutter and Jaffee (1996)

From *Women's Health and Fitness Guide* by Michele Kettles, Colette Cole, and Brenda Wright, 2006, Champaign, IL: Human Kinetics.

# Tips for Dealing with Common Discomforts of Pregnancy

## Nausea and Vomiting

- Eat often and in small amounts to prevent extremes in blood glucose levels.
- Eat something first thing in the morning and at bedtime.
- Eat adequate amounts of protein (70 to 90 grams per day or an additional 30 grams per baby per day above nonpregnancy needs).
- Avoid foods that seem noxious.
- Try drinking a sport drink, ginger ale, or ginger tea.
- Try a wristband for seasickness.
- Take a prenatal vitamin (with food) as prescribed by the health care provider to ensure adequate micronutrients. Cut the vitamin into smaller pieces and take them several times during the day.

## Fatigue

- Rest on the side to maximize blood flow.
- Eat small meals over the course of the day to regulate blood glucose levels.
- Stay well hydrated.
- Get plenty of sleep, especially during the first trimester.
- Get checked for anemia.

## Tender Breasts

Wear a new, larger, supportive bra.

## Constipation, Gas, Hemorrhoids

- Get adequate fluids and fiber to prevent constipation.
- Assume the deeply folded position to open the bowels and relieve gas.
- Do Kegel exercises to relieve hemorrhoids.

## Backache

- Rest on the side with a pillow between the legs, under the abdomen, between the arms, and under the head to stabilize the spine.
- Get up or change position slowly.

## Anxiety and Insomnia

- Practice stress management and relaxation techniques (deep breathing, stretching).
- Drink chamomile tea before bed to help with sleep.

## Leg Cramps

- Get off your feet and lie on your side.
- Allow for adequate cool-down after aerobic activity.
- For leg cramps at night—flex ankles or apply ice on the calves for 10 minutes before going to bed.

## Varicosities

- Use support stockings or a prenatal support girdle.
- Use ice to relieve discomfort.

Adapted from Cowlin (2002)

From *Women's Health and Fitness Guide* by Michele Kettles, Colette Cole, and Brenda Wright, 2006, Champaign, IL: Human Kinetics.

# Tips for Physically Active Nursing Mothers

- If you drink an extra 6 to 8 ounces (177 to 236 milliliters) of water before working out, the volume of milk you produce will not be compromised.

- If your infant won't accept your postexercise milk, you should express milk prior to exercise to give to your infant afterward. You can express and discard postexercise breast milk.

- Nurse first and then exercise to avoid the discomfort of overly full breasts.

- As support for the breasts during exercise, you should wear a sports bra or stretch top over a nursing bra. Remove any binding immediately following your exercise.

- Use a lubricant or pad to protect your nipples from abrasion during exercise.

- Perform strengthening and stretching exercises for muscles of the upper back, shoulders, and chest to help relieve the discomforts associated with nursing.

From *Women's Health and Fitness Guide* by Michele Kettles, Colette Cole, and Brenda Wright, 2006, Champaign, IL: Human Kinetics.

# Living with Osteoarthritis

The key to living with osteoarthritis is getting proper medical help early and faithfully staying with the treatment program even during periods of remission. Tips for managing your osteoarthritis are discussed below.

## Medications

- Take your medications exactly as your doctor instructs.

- Do not skip a dose unless your doctor recommends it. This can increase your pain to a large degree.

- Don't take an over-the-counter medication in addition to a prescribed medicine unless your doctor recommends it.

- Keep in mind that it takes some medications longer to work than others.

## A Balanced Exercise Program

- Participate in a regular, balanced exercise program that includes aerobic, strength-building, flexibility, and balance exercises. A modified exercise program can be developed if you need to use a wheelchair.

- Exercise in water so there is less stress on the hips, knees, and spine. Exercising in warm water is especially good for stiff, sore joints. The water temperature should be between 83 and 90 degrees. Stationary cycling is also a good way to improve fitness without putting too much stress on the hips, knees, and feet. Start slowly and use limited or no resistance. Walking is an appropriate exercise for osteoarthritis. However, walking for exercise may not be recommended for people with severe hip, knee, ankle, or foot problems.

- Exercise at the time of day when you are feeling less pain and stiffness.

- Massage the stiff or sore areas or apply heat treatments to the area before beginning to exercise.

- If you have a flare-up, do only gentle flexibility exercises.

- If you develop muscle pain or a cramp, gently rub and stretch the muscle. You may need to change the position or the way you are doing the exercise.

- Listen to your body. Learn the difference between normal discomfort and the pain associated with too much exercise.

## Heat and Cold Treatments and Topical Pain Relievers

- Take a hot bath or shower first thing in the morning to help relax muscles and relieve morning stiffness. Heat may also be applied with hot packs, heat lamps, electric pads, and electric mitts. People with diabetes must use heat cautiously, since their sensation may be impaired.

- Use cold compresses to reduce swelling and to numb the area so less pain is felt. They are especially good for severe joint pain caused by a flare-up of arthritis.

- Don't use cold or heat if the skin has cuts or sores. Also, use extra padding to protect the skin over any bone that is close to the surface of the skin.

- Consider using topical pain relievers, such as creams, rubs, or sprays, to temporarily relieve the pain of osteoarthritis. They work by decreasing the ability of the nerve endings in the skin to sense pain or by distracting from the actual pain. Topical pain relievers can also increase the blood flow and produce a feeling of warmth to the affected area.

## Joint Protection and Good Posture

- Learn to perform daily activities in ways that will be less stressful to joints. Using a cane, walker, or crutches may help take some of the weight off the hips, knees, feet, or spine. Splints can also be used to rest and protect painful joints. Splints should be fitted by health professionals because they can do more harm than good if they are used improperly.

- Keep your back comfortably straight when lying down, sitting, standing, walking, or lifting. Hold your stomach in.

- Use a firm mattress or bed board while you sleep or rest in bed.

- When possible, sit in straight-backed chairs with armrests, and try not to slump while sitting.

- Avoid sitting for long periods of time. Get up and walk around every 30 to 60 minutes, if possible.

From *Women's Health and Fitness Guide* by Michele Kettles, Colette Cole, and Brenda Wright, 2006, Champaign, IL: Human Kinetics.

## Living with Osteoarthritis *(continued)*

### Weight Control

Maintain a healthy weight or lose weight if overweight to help prevent osteoarthritis of the knees. For people who already have osteoarthritis, losing weight can lessen pain by reducing stress on the hips, knees, back, and feet.

### Coping Skills

- Learn coping skills to relieve stress or depression, help you feel more in control, and improve your outlook on life.

- Learn as much as possible about osteoarthritis.
- Be flexible by planning alternative activities for the good and bad days that come with arthritis.
- Focus on what you *can* do and discover new activities that give you pleasure and a sense of purpose.
- Talk over your feelings and problems with family and friends.
- Think positively.

From *Women's Health and Fitness Guide* by Michele Kettles, Colette Cole, and Brenda Wright, 2006, Champaign, IL: Human Kinetics.

# Urinary Incontinence

Urinary incontinence is the loss of bladder control or the leakage of urine. It can happen to anyone, but it is common among women after menopause. Approximately one-third of women over age 60 experience some degree of urinary incontinence. But urinary incontinence is not a natural part of aging. Incontinence in the majority of women can be treated, controlled, and even cured. Unfortunately, most women affected by urinary incontinence do not consult their health care provider about the condition.

## How Your Body Makes, Stores, and Releases Urine

When you eat and drink, your body absorbs the liquid. The kidneys filter out waste products from the body fluids and make urine that is stored in a muscular sac, the bladder. When you need to empty your bladder, your brain tells your system to relax. Urine travels out of your bladder through a tube called the urethra. You release urine by relaxing the urethral sphincter and contracting the bladder muscles.

There are several types of urinary incontinence. It is possible to have more than one type.

- Stress incontinence occurs when urine is leaked following coughing, laughing, straining, sneezing, or other conditions that cause abrupt increases in abdominal pressure. Stress incontinence is very common in older women, probably due to weakened pelvic muscles after childbirth. This type of incontinence can almost always be cured.

- Urge incontinence happens when someone can't hold urine long enough to reach a toilet. Someone with urge incontinence may go to the bathroom very often—every 2 or 3 hours during the day and night—or even wet the bed. Although healthy women can have urge incontinence, it is often found in people who have diabetes, stroke, dementia, Parkinson's disease, or multiple sclerosis. It can also be an early sign of bladder cancer.

- Overflow incontinence occurs when the bladder cannot empty properly and the bladder always remains full. People with overflow incontinence have the feeling that their bladder has not emptied completely, experience difficulty starting to void, and note that their urinary stream is weak and dribbly. Overflow incontinence can result from poor bladder contractions due to severe diabetes, from diseases of the spinal cord, or when the flow of urine from the bladder is blocked by a kidney stone or tumor.

- Functional incontinence occurs in people who have a normal urinary system but who cannot reach the toilet in time because of poor fitness, arthritis, or other crippling disorders.

## Diagnosis and Treatment

If you are experiencing urinary incontinence, the first and most important step is to see your health care provider. Your medical history will be reviewed and you will be given a physical exam. You may be asked to keep a record of your bladder activity. A urine sample may be taken to determine if an infection is present. Your treatment will be designed to meet your specific needs. Many options are available, and the least dangerous procedures should be tried first.

You may want to avoid high-impact, weight-bearing exercises (jogging, jumping movements) if you experience stress incontinence. Also, be sure to empty your bladder before exercising.

- Stay strong and fit so you can get to the bathroom when you need to go.

- Pelvic muscle exercise can help control urination and delay voiding until you can reach a toilet. There are no risks for this type of treatment. See the following description of how to do Kegel exercises.

- Medicines can be prescribed to treat incontinence. However, these drugs may cause side effects such as dry mouth, eye problems, and urine buildup.

- Surgery may improve or cure incontinence if it is caused by a structural problem such as an abnormally positioned bladder. With any surgery there is a possibility of a risk or complication.

## Kegel Exercises

Identify the correct muscles to exercise by stopping and starting the urinary stream while sitting on the toilet. Once the correct muscles are identified, Kegel exercises can be done daily, anytime, anywhere. Two to three sets of 10 to 15 contractions are recommended. Hold each contraction for 3 seconds and release for 3 seconds.

From *Women's Health and Fitness Guide* by Michele Kettles, Colette Cole, and Brenda Wright, 2006, Champaign, IL: Human Kinetics.

# Reduce Risks for Falls and Fractures

These conditions could increase the risk of falling:

- Cataracts or vision problems
- Arthritis
- Stroke
- Parkinson's disease
- Poor hearing
- Low back problems
- Low blood pressure
- Balance and gait disorders
- Dizziness caused by medications

## Preventing Falls

Approximately 30 percent of people over 65 who live independently fall each year. Of these, one-half fall repeatedly. Falls can cause painful bruises and fractures and limit your ability to function. Once you have fallen, it is common to fear falling again.

Over 75 percent of falls occur at home. You may be surprised to know that most falls are not associated with climbing on a ladder or standing on a chair. The most common cause of falls is tripping over an object or on stairs or steps. Falls are most likely to occur when you are walking or changing from one position to another.

Be careful when changing positions. Don't get in too much of a hurry or move too quickly. Your coordination may not be what it used to be. Because of changes in blood circulation, you could become dizzy. Think before you move. Plan your move when

- bending over to pick up something;
- reaching for something overhead;
- getting out of bed;
- getting out of the tub or shower;
- going up and down stairs or steps, especially when carrying objects; or
- getting up from a sofa or low chair.

Many hip fractures happen when older adults with bone or joint problems get up from a sofa or low chair. To reduce your risk of falls and hip fractures, avoid sitting in sofas and chairs that put your hips lower than your knees. Get up from a sofa or chair in the following way:

- If you are getting up from a sofa, sit next to the armrest. If the chair has arms, use them for support.

- Before standing up, put your feet parallel, with your toes pointing straight ahead.
- Stand slowly, using the armrest to help you. If the chair doesn't have armrests, use the edge of the chair.
- Hold on to the chair or sofa until you have your balance.

## Home Safety

Check the safety of your home. The following list identifies what you can do to make your home safer and to decrease your chances of falling. If there are improvements you could make, it's a good idea to plan ahead and make changes before you need to.

### Lights

- Keep hallways, stairs, and rooms well lit.
- Install night-lights in hallways, bathrooms, and bedrooms.
- Keep a flashlight beside your bed and use it if you get up during the night.

### Floors

- Clean up spills or water on the floor immediately.
- Keep traffic paths clear of furniture and obstacles.
- Avoid throw rugs. If you must use them, make sure they have nonslip backing.
- Replace deep-pile carpet with shallow-pile carpet. Tack carpet edges securely.
- Use nonskid wax on floors or don't wax floors.
- Keep electrical cords away from high-traffic areas.

### Stairs

- Install light switches at the top and bottom of stairways.
- Cover stairs with a nonslip surface.
- Keep clutter off stairways.
- Install sturdy handrails on both sides of stairways.
- Use handrails when walking up and down stairs.

*(continued)*

From *Women's Health and Fitness Guide* by Michele Kettles, Colette Cole, and Brenda Wright, 2006, Champaign, IL: Human Kinetics.

### Bathroom

- Install grab bars for the tub or shower and toilet.
- Use a rubber mat or rubberized decals in the bathtub.
- Keep soap in an easy-to-reach holder.
- Add a shower chair with a handheld shower.
- Use nonslip rugs.
- Raise the toilet seat.

### Kitchen

- Make sure that commonly used items are within easy reach.
- Avoid climbing and reaching high shelves, but if you must, use a stable stepstool with handrails to reach items on top shelves.

### Outside

- Make sure exterior doors and pathways are well lighted.
- Keep walkways cleared of ice and wet leaves.

## Safety Tips

- Wear shoes with firm nonskid, nonfriction soles, low heels, and a snug fit. Proper footwear can help prevent falls.

- If you need a walking aid, don't be embarrassed to use one.
- Avoid drinking alcoholic beverages. Alcohol impairs your balance and slows your reflexes.
- Have your vision and hearing checked regularly. You don't want to trip over something you could have seen. Keen hearing (horns, bells, sirens, voices) can warn you of potential dangers.
- Exercise regularly to increase your endurance and strength and improve your flexibility and balance.
- Be sure you understand exactly how your medications should be taken. Certain medications can also affect balance and coordination and put you at risk for falls.

## If You Fall

- Don't panic. If you fall and are not seriously injured, here's how to get up from the floor safely.
  - Roll to your hands and knees and crawl to a piece of furniture that will support your weight, such as a sofa or armchair.
  - Use the furniture to pull yourself up gently.
  - Sit for a few minutes before trying to stand up.
- If you can't get up, call for help. If you are alone, crawl slowly to the phone and call 911.

From *Women's Health and Fitness Guide* by Michele Kettles, Colette Cole, and Brenda Wright, 2006, Champaign, IL: Human Kinetics.

# Glossary

**abduction**—Movement away from the midline of the body.

**active stretch**—Controlled movement of an agonist muscle using individual's own muscle action to dynamically move the joint(s) through the desired range of motion.

**adduction**—Movement toward the midline of the body.

**agonist**—The muscle primarily responsible for the movement involved; prime mover.

**angiotensin converting enzyme (ACE) inhibitor**—A class of medications used to treat high blood pressure (and other conditions). Their mechanism of action is to inhibit angiotensin converting enzyme.

**angiotensin receptor blocker (ARB)**—A class of medications used to treat high blood pressure (and other conditions). Their mechanism of action is to block the angiotensin receptor.

**antagonist**—The muscle opposing the prime mover (agonist).

**anterior**—Referring to a position toward or on the front of the body.

**arthrokinematic**—Referring to normal joint motion of two joint surfaces on one another during movement.

**autonomic dysreflexia (also known as hyperreflexia)**—A condition in which the blood pressure in a person with a spinal cord injury (SCI) above T5-6 becomes excessively high due to the overactivity of the autonomic nervous system. Autonomic dysreflexia is usually caused when a painful stimulus occurs below the level of spinal cord injury.

**ballistic**—Referring to dynamic-type movements that include fast, jerky, or bouncing motions.

**beta-blockers**—A class of medications used to treat high blood pressure (and other conditions). Their mechanism of action is to slow the heart rate.

**calcium channel blocker**—A class of medications used to treat high blood pressure (and other vascular problems). Their mechanism of action is to block calcium channels.

**claudication**—Pain in the calf or thigh muscle that occurs with walking. Claudication occurs because not enough blood is flowing to a muscle.

**corrective flexibility training**—Specific and appropriate flexibility exercises incorporating a variety of stretching techniques designed to correct muscle imbalances, postural distortions, or joint dysfunctions.

**diuretic**—A class of medications used to treat high blood pressure (and fluid overload). Their mechanism of action is to promote the excretion of urine.

**dynamic stretching**—Stretching that involves the movement of a muscle through the joint's available range of motion; dynamic stretching is used to improve functional flexibility.

**dyslipidemia**—Abnormal cholesterol.

**dysmenorrhea**—Difficult and painful menstruation.

**fascia**—Connective tissue that surrounds muscles and various organs of the body.

**functional strength**—Ability of the neuromuscular system to perform dynamic, isometric, and isotonic muscle contractions efficiently when executing multiplanar functional movements.

**hypertonicity**—Abnormally high tension or tone of the muscles.

**hypoxia**—Lack of oxygen in tissues.

**iliotibial band**—A tendinous extension of the fascia covering the gluteus maximus and tensor fasciae latae muscles proximally. It descends distally to attach to the lateral condyle of the tibia. It also sends fibers to the lateral aspect of the patella (kneecap). Essentially, the ITB is the linkage between the pelvis, upper leg, and lower leg.

**inhibit**—To hold back or keep from some action.

**ischemic stroke**—Stroke caused by lack of blood flow to a part of the brain; as opposed to hemorrhagic stroke, which is caused by bleeding in the brain.

**ketoacidosis**—Condition occurring when the body has high blood sugar and a buildup of acids called ketones. If it isn't treated, it can lead to coma and even death. It mainly affects people who have type 1 diabetes. However, it can also happen with other types of diabetes, including type 2 diabetes and diabetes during pregnancy.

**ketosis**—A process in which the body converts fats into energy. The result of ketosis is to obtain energy from the body's stored fats.

**kinetic chain**—The interrelation of the muscular, articular, and neural systems.

**kinetic chain dysfunction**—A condition that occurs when any or all of the muscular, articular, or neural systems are not functioning properly.

**lateral**—Referring to a position farther away from the midline or toward outside of the body.

**length–tension relationship**—Relation between length of the muscle and the amount of force or tension produced by that muscle.

**libido**—Sexual drive or desire.

**lordosis**—An abnormal extension deformity, anteroposterior curvature of the spine, generally lumbar with the convexity as one looks anteriorly.

**lumbo-pelvic-hip complex**—Anatomical structure of the lumbar, thoracic, and cervical spine, pelvic girdle, and hip joint; core muscle groups.

**macrocycle**—Long-term periodized cycle ranging from several months up to one year.

**maternal endothelial dysfunction**—Abnormal function of cells lining the blood vessels and heart, believed to play a role in preeclampsia.

**menarche**—Onset of menses; the first menstrual period or flow.

**mesocycle**—Periodized cycle that ranges anywhere from 3 to 12 weeks.

**microcycle**—Periodized cycle consisting of a single workout session.

**multijoint**—Referring to movements in which more than one joint is involved in the action.

**neuromuscular efficiency**—Ability of the neuromuscular system to allow agonists, antagonists, stabilizers, and neutralizers to work synergistically to produce, reduce, and dynamically stabilize the entire kinetic chain in all three planes of motion.

**neuropathy**—Any disorder affecting the nervous system.

**autonomic**—Referring to nerve damage causing inability of the heart to keep up with the body's needs. May also cause inability of the intestines to digest food.

**peripheral**—Characterized by numbness (loss of feeling) or painful tingling in parts of the body.

**neutralizing muscles**—The muscles contracting to prevent unwanted movement of other muscles.

**nulliparous**—Having borne no children.

**overload**—Work at a greater intensity than the body is accustomed to; there must be a training stimulus that exceeds the current capabilities; specific adaptations to imposed demands (SAID) principle.

**passive stretch**—Form of static stretching in which the joint is moved to its maximal range without any voluntary muscle contraction.

**pattern overload**—Many repetitions performed in the same pattern of movement; can lead to soft tissue overload.

**peripheral vascular disease or peripheral arterial disease (PAD)**—A problem with blood flow in the arteries. Usually the arteries have become narrowed by atherosclerosis.

**planes of motion:**

**frontal plane**—Divides the body into front and back. Movements are abduction and adduction.

**multiplanar**—Referring to movements in more than one plane of motion.

**sagittal plane**—Divides the body into right and left halves. Movements are flexion and extension.

**transverse plane**—Divides the body into top and bottom halves. Movements are rotation and circumduction. Also known as the horizontal plane.

**plant sterol**—Soy extracts used as ingredients in a number of fat-based foods on the market including salad dressings and margarines. Potential dietary benefits of plant sterols include cholesterol reduction.

**plyometric training**—Power training programs commonly used for enhancing sport- or activity-specific performance by utilizing eccentric contractions immediately followed by explosive concentric contractions (jump training).

**posterior**—Referring to a position toward or on the back of the body.

**prolapse (uterine or bladder)**—The sinking or dropping of an organ.

**pronation**—Palms down in anatomical position.

**proprioception**—Neural input to the central nervous system that senses limb movement, location, and position; allows one to know where one is in space.

**proprioceptive neuromuscular facilitation (PNF)**—Stretching technique that focuses on the contract–relax and hold–relax mechanisms; a muscle group is passively stretched, then contracted against resistance while in the stretched position, then passively stretched again with increased range of motion; usually requires a partner; facilitates increased range of motion, increased strength, and movement pattern control.

**prospective study**—A type of scientific study in which subjects are followed forward in time, as opposed to a retrospective study, in which subjects recall prior history and events.

**randomized controlled clinical trial**—A very robust type of research study in which two similar groups of people are randomized to a study or control group in order to test a medication or intervention.

**scleroderma**—An autoimmune disorder with thickening of the skin caused by swelling and thickening of fibrous tissue.

**self-myofascial release**—Soft tissue release technique; pressure point release. SMR devices include foam roller, thumb pressure, the Stick, tennis ball, etc.

**specificity training**—Performing exercises or activities that mimic or are very similar to the required movement of a specific activity; transfer-of-training effect.

**stabilization**—Ability to control the body both statically and dynamically.

**stabilizing muscles**—The muscles that secure a joint or support the body while primary muscles produce a movement.

**static stretching**—A controlled, passive movement taken to the point of first resistance, which is held for a desired length of time (usually 15-30 seconds).

**supination**—Palms up in anatomical position.

**synergists**—Muscles that assist prime movers during functional movement patterns.

**types of muscle contraction:**

**concentric**—Isotonic phase in which the muscle is shortened while resisting a load (positive work).

**eccentric**—Isotonic phase in which the muscle is lengthened while resisting a load (negative work).

**isometric**—Contraction of a muscle with no joint movement.

**vastus lateralis**—Lateral muscle of the quadriceps.

**vastus medialis**—Medial muscle of the quadriceps.

**$\dot{V}O_2$max**—The maximal ability of a person to take in, transport, and use oxygen.

**$\dot{V}O_2$peak**—Peak oxygen uptake during an activity, not necessarily equal to $\dot{V}O_2$max.

**$\dot{V}O_2$R**—Equals maximal oxygen uptake minus resting oxygen uptake.

# References

Ahmed C, Hilton W, Pituch K. 2002. Relations of strength training to body image among a sample of female university students. *J Strength Cond Res* 16(4):645-648.

Akuthota V, Nadler SF. 2004. Core strengthening. *Arch Phys Med Rehabil* 85(3):S86-92.

American Academy of Orthopaedic Surgeons. 2000a, June. Knee ligament injuries. www.orthoinfo.aaos.org.

American Academy of Orthopaedic Surgeons. 2000b, June. Preventing ACL injuries in women.www.orthoinfo.aaos.org.

American Academy of Orthopaedic Surgeons. 2002a, April. Orthopaedists research female knee problems. www.orthoinfo.aaos.org.

American Academy of Orthopaedic Surgeons. 2002b, February. Women and ACL injuries. www.orthoinfo.aaos.org.

American College of Obstetrics and Gynecology (ACOG) Committee opinion. 2002. *Obstet Gynecol* 99:171.

American Diabetes Association. 2002. Gestational diabetes mellitus. *Diabet Care* 25:S94-S96.

American Diabetes Association. 2004. Position statement: diagnosis and classification of diabetes mellitus. *Diabet Care* 27:suppl 1.

American Psychiatric Association. 1994. *Diagnostic and statistical manual of mental disorders, fourth edition.* Washington, DC: American Psychiatric Association.

Anderson GL, Limacher M, et al. (The Women's Health Initiative Steering Committee). 2004. Effects of conjugated equine estrogen in postmenopausal women with hysterectomy. *JAMA* 291(14):1701-1712.

Anorexia Nervosa and Related Eating Disorders, Inc. 2004, November. Eating disorders statistics. www.anred.com.

Arruda-Olson AM, Juracan EM, Mahoney DW, et al. 2002. Prognostic value of exercise echocardiography in 5,798 patients: Is there a gender difference? *J Am Coll Cardiol* 39:625-631.

Audrain-McGovern J, Rodriquez D, Moss HB. 2003. Smoking progression and physical activity. *Cancer Epidemiol Biomarkers Prev* 12:1121-1129.

Babyak M, Blumenthal JA, Herman S, et al. 2000. Exercise treatment for major depression: Maintenance of therapeutic benefit at 10 months. *Psychosom Med* 62:633-638.

Baker KR, Nelson ME, Felson DT, et al. 2001. The efficacy of home based progressive strength training in older adults with knee osteoarthritis: A randomized controlled trial. *J Rheumatol* 28:1655-1665.

Barnes DE, Yaffe K, Satariano WA, et al. 2003. A longitudinal study of cardiorespiratory fitness and cognitive function in healthy older adults. *J Am Geriatr Soc* 51:459.

Batterham AM, Birch KM. 1996. Allometry of anaerobic performance: A gender comparison. *Can J Appl Physiol* 21:48-62.

Bergen JL, Smith HH, Caballero K, et al. 2003. Incremental exercise responses for females during three different phases of the menstrual cycle. *Med Sci Sports Exerc* 35(5):S332.

Bergmark A. 1989. Stability of the lumbar spine: A study in mechanical engineering. *Acta Orthop Scand* 230(suppl):20-24.

Bernstein L, Henderson BE, Hanisch R, et al. 1994. Physical exercise and reduced risk of breast cancer in young women. *J Natl Cancer Inst* 86:1403-1408.

Bertone ER, Newcomb PA, Willett WC, et al. 2002. Recreational physical activity and ovarian cancer in a population-based case-control study. *Int J Cancer* 99(3):431-436.

Bertone ER, Willett WC, Rosner BA, et al. 2001. Prospective study of recreational physical activity and ovarian cancer. *J Natl Cancer Inst* 93(12):942-948.

Binder EF, Schechtman KB, Ehsani AA, et al. 2002. Effects of exercise training on frailty in community-dwelling older adults: Results of a randomized controlled trial. *J Am Geriatr Soc* 50:1921-1928.

Blair SN, Goodyear NN, Gibbons LW, Cooper KH. 1984. Physical fitness and incidence of hypertension in healthy normotensive men and women. *JAMA* 252:487.

Blair SN, Kampert JB, Kohl HW 3rd, et al. 1996, July 17. Influences of cardiorespiratory fitness and other precursors on cardiovascular disease and all-cause mortality in men and women. *JAMA* 276(3):205-210.

Blair SN, Kohn HW, Paffenbarger RS, et al. 1989. Physical fitness and all-cause mortality: A prospective study of healthy men and women. *JAMA* 262:2395-2401.

Blum JW, Beaudoin CM, Caton-Lemons L. 2004. Physical activity patterns and maternal well-being in postpartum women. *Matern Child Health J* 8(3):163-169.

Blumenthal JA, Babyak MA, Moore KA, et al. 1999. Effects of exercise training on older patients with major depression. *Arch Intern Med* 159:2349-2356.

Boscaglia N, Skouteris H, Wertheim EH. 2003. Changes in body image satisfaction during pregnancy: A comparison of high exercising and low exercising women. *Aust NZ J Obstet Gynaecol* 43(1):41-45.

Boule NG, Haddad E, Kenny GP, et al. 2001. Effects of exercise on glycemic control and body mass in type 2 diabetcs mellitus: A meta-analysis of controlled clinical trials. *JAMA* 286:1218.

Brankston GN, Mitchell BF, Ryan EA, Okun NB. 2004. Resistance exercise decreases the need for insulin in overweight women with gestational diabetes. *Am J Obstet Gynecol* 190:188-93.

Brill PA. 2004. *Functional fitness for older adults*. Champaign, IL: Human Kinetics.

Bruyere O, Pavelka K, Rovati LC, et al. 2004. Glucosamine sulfate reduces osteoarthritis progression in postmenopausal women with knee osteoarthritis: Evidence from two 3-year studies. *Menopause* 11(2):138-143.

Bugianesi E. 2005. Review article: Steatosis, the metabolic syndrome and cancer. *Aliment Pharmacol Ther* 22(suppl 2):40-43.

Campbell AJ, Robertson MC, Gardner MM, et al. 1997. Randomised controlled trial of a general practice programme of home based exercise to prevent falls in elderly women. *BMJ* 315:1065-69.

Campbell L, Marwick TH, Pashkow FJ, et al. 1999. Usefulness of an exaggerated systolic blood pressure response to exercise in predicting myocardial perfusion defects in known or suspected coronary artery disease. *Am J Cardiol* 84:1304.

Centers for Disease Control/National Center for Health Statistics, National Household Education Surveys Program, and National Health and Nutrition Examination Survey. 2004. Prevalence of overweight among children and adolescents ages 6 to 19 years. www.cdc.gov/nchs/products/pubs/pubd/hestats/overwght99.htm.

Center for Science in the Public Interest. 1977, July 31. CSPI press release—caffeine content of foods and drugs chart. www.cspinet.org.

Chan SP, Hong Y, Robinson PD. 2001. Flexibility and passive resistance of the hamstrings of young adults using two different static stretching protocols. *Scand J Med Sci Sports* 11:81-86.

Chang JT, Morton SC, Rubenstein LZ, et al. 2004. Interventions for the prevention of falls in older adults: Systematic review and meta-analysis of randomized clinical trials. *BMJ* 328:680-686.

Chek P. 2001. *The golf biomechanics manual, second edition*. Encinitas, CA: C.H.E.K. Institute.

Chen Y, Fredericson M, Smuck M. 2002. Sacroiliac joint pain syndrome in active patients. *Physician Sportsmed* 30(11):30-38.

Chen Y, Henson S, Jackson AB, Richards JS. 2006. Obesity intervention in persons with spinal cord injury. *Spinal Cord* 44(2): 82-91.

Chiarelli P, Cockburn J. 2002. Promoting urinary continence in women after delivery: Randomized controlled trial. *BMJ* 324:1241.

Clapp JF 3rd, Capeless EL. 1990. Neonatal morphometrics after endurance exercise during pregnancy. *Am J Obstet Gynecol* 163(6 pt 1):1805-1811.

Clapp JF 3rd, Kim H, Burciu B, Lopez B. 2000. Beginning regular exercise in early pregnancy: Effect on fetoplacental growth. *Am J Obstet Gynecol* 183(6):1484-1488.

Clark MA. 2000. *Integrated flexibility training*. Thousand Oaks, CA: National Academy of Sports Medicine.

Clark MA. 2001. *Integrated training for the new millennium*. Thousand Oaks, CA: National Academy of Sports Medicine.

Clark MA. 2005. Advanced core stabilization training for rehabilitation, reconditioning, and injury prevention. American Physical Therapy Association, Strength and Conditioning Course. Unpublished.

Clark MA, Parracino L. 2003. *Advanced integrated flexibility: Course manual, first edition*. Thousand Oaks, CA: National Academy of Sports Medicine.

Clark N. 2003. *Nancy Clark's sports nutrition guidebook, third edition*. Champaign, IL: Human Kinetics.

Clark SR, Jones K, Burkhart CS, Bennett R. 2001. Exercise for patient with fibromyalgia: Risk versus benefits. *Curr Rheumatol Rep* 3(2):135-140.

Colbert LH, Lacey JV Jr., Schairer C, et al. 2003. Physical activity and risk of endometrial cancer in a prospective cohort study (United States). *Cancer Causes Contr* 14(6):559-567.

Colditz GA, Cannuscio CC, Frazier AL. 1997. Physical activity and reduced risk of colon cancer: Implications for prevention. *Cancer Causes Contr* 8:649-667.

Colditz GA, Feskanich D, Chen WY, et al. 2003, September 1. Physical activity and risk of breast cancer in premenopausal women. *Br J Cancer* 89(5):847-851.

Cooper KH. 1968. *Aerobics*. New York: Bantam Books.

Cooper M, Cooper KH. 1972. *Aerobics for women*. New York: Bantam Books.

Cooper Clinic Nutrition Department. 2005, revised; 1997, copyright. Sources of calcium-rich foods. Dallas: Author.

Cooper Institute. 2005. *Physical fitness specialist course and certification.* Dallas: Author.

Cowlin AF. 2002. *Women's fitness program development.* Champaign, IL: Human Kinetics.

Cox KL, Burker V, Morton AR, et al. 2001. Long-term effects of exercise on blood pressure and lipids in healthy women aged 40-65 years: The Sedentary Women Exercise Adherence Trial (SWEAT). *J Hypertens* 19:1733.

Cramer JT, Housh TJ, Johnson GO, Miller JM, Coburn JW, Beck TW. 2004. Acute effects of static stretching on peak torque in women. *J Strength Cond Res* 18(2):236-241.

Da Costa D, Rippen N, Dritsa M, Ring A. 2003. Self-reported leisure-time physical activity during pregnancy and relationship to psychological well-being. *J Psychosom Obstet Gynaecol* 24(2):111-119.

Daniels SR, Morrison JA, Sprecher DL, et al. 1999. Association of body fat distribution and cardiovascular risk factors in children and adolescents. *Circulation* 99:541-545.

DeBusk RF, Stenestrand U, Sheehan M, Haskell WL. 1990. Training effects of long versus short bouts of exercise in healthy subjects. *Am J Cardiol* 65:1010-1013.

Devlin JT. 1992. Effects of exercise on insulin sensitivity in humans. *Diabet Care* 15:1690.

Dempsey JC, Butler CL, Williams MA. 2005. No need for a pregnant pause: Physical activity may reduce the occurrence of gestational diabetes mellitus and preeclampsia. *Exerc Sport Sci Rev* 33:141-49.

Dewey KG, Lovelady CA, Nommsen-Rivers LA, et al. 1994. A randomized study of the effects of aerobic exercise by lactating women on breast-milk volume and composition. *N Engl J Med* 330(7):449-453.

Diabetes Prevention Program Research Group. 2002. Reduction in the incidence of type 2 diabetes with lifestyle intervention or metformin. *N Engl J Med* 346(6):393-403.

Dirks AJ, Leeuwenburgh C. 2006. Caloric restriction in humans: Potential pitfalls and health concerns. *Mech Ageing Dev* 127(1): 1-7.

Dunn AL, Trivedi MH, Kampert JB, et al. 2005. Exercise treatment for depression. *Am J Prev Med* 28:1-8.

Edgerton VR, Wolf SL, Levendowski DJ, Roy RR. 1996. Theoretical basis for patterning EMG amplitudes to assess muscle dysfunction. *Med Sci Sports Exerc* 28(6):744-751.

Epstein LH, Roemmich JN, Paluch RA, Raynor HA. 2005. Influence of changes in sedentary behavior on energy and macronutrient intake in youth. *Am J Clin Nutr* 81(2):361-366.

Exercise prescription for older adults with osteoarthritis pain: Consensus practice recommendations. A supplement to the AGS Clinical Practice Guidelines on the management of chronic pain in older adults. 2001. *J Am Geriatr Soc* 49:808-823.

Fagard RH. 1995. The role of exercise in blood pressure control: Supportive evidence. *J Hypertens* 13:1223.

Farrell SW, Cheng YJ, Blair SN. 2004. Prevalence of the metabolic syndrome across cardiorespiratory fitness levels in women. *Obes Res* 12:824-830.

Feskanich D, Willett W, Colditz G. 2002. Walking and leisure-time activity and risk of hip fracture in postmenopausal women. *JAMA* 288(18):2300-2306.

Fleg JL, Morrell CH, Bos AG, et al. 2005. Accelerated longitudinal decline of aerobic capacity in healthy older adults. *Circulation* 112:674-682.

Foti T, Davids JR, Bagley A. 2000. A biomechanical analysis of gait during pregnancy. *J Bone Joint Surg* 82-A(5):625-632.

Foye PM, Stitik TP. 2004, June 14. Plantar fasciitis. www.emedicine.com.

Franklin BA, Swain DP. 2003. New insights on the threshold intensity for improving cardiorespiratory fitness. *Prev Cardiol* 6:118-121.

Franklin BA, Whaley MH, Howley ET, eds. 2000. *ACSM's guidelines for exercise testing and prescription, sixth edition.* Baltimore: Lippincott Williams & Wilkins.

Frezza EE, Wachtel MS, Chiriva-Internati M. 2006. The influence of obesity on the risk of developing colon cancer. *Gut* 55(2): 285-291.

Frid A, Ostman J, Linde B. 1990. Hypoglycemia risk during exercise after intramuscular injection of insulin in thigh in IDDM. *Diabet Care* 13:473.

Fried LP, Tangen CM, Walston J, et al. 2001. Frailty in older adults: Evidence for a phenotype. *The Journals of Gerontology Series A: Biological Sciences and Medical Sciences* 56:M146-M157.

Gardner AW, Montgomery PS. 2004. Sex differences in physical function, physical activity, and falling history in older men and women. *Med Sci Sports Exerc* 36(5)suppl:S29.

Gardner MM, Robertson MC, Campbell AJ. 2000. Exercise in preventing falls and fall related injuries in older people: A review of randomized controlled trials. *Br J Sports Med* 34:7-17.

Garshasbi A, Faghih ZS. 2005. The effect of exercise on the intensity of low back pain in pregnant women. *Int J Gynaecol Obstet* 88(3):271-275.

Giacomoni M, Thierry B, Olivier G, et al. 2000. Influence of the menstrual cycle phase and menstrual symptoms on maximal anaerobic performance. *Med Sci Sports Exerc* 32:486-492.

Gottdiener JS, Brown J, Zoltick J, Fletcher RD. 1990. Left ventricular hypertrophy in men with normal blood pressure: Relation to exaggerated blood pressure response to exercise. *Ann Intern Med* 112:161.

Gregg EW, Cauley JA, Seeley DG, et al. 1998. Physical activity and osteoporotic fracture risk in older women. *Ann Intern Med* 129:81-88.

Gregg EW, Gerzoff RB, Caspersen CJ, Williamson DF. 2003. Relationship of walking to mortality among US adults with diabetes. *Arch Intern Med* 163:1440.

Grundy SM, Blackburn G, Higgins M, et al. 1999. Physical activity in the prevention and treatment of obesity and its comorbidities: Evidence report of independent panel to assess the role of physical activity in the treatment of obesity and its comorbidities. *Med Sci Sports Exerc* 31(11):1493.

Haapanen N, Miilunpalo S, Vuori I, et al. 1997. Association of leisure time physical activity with the risk of coronary heart disease, hypertension and diabetes in middle-aged men and women. *Int J Epidemiol* 26(4):739-747.

Hannan LM, Leitzmann MF, Lacey JV Jr., et al. 2004. Physical activity and risk of ovarian cancer: A prospective cohort study in the United States. *Cancer Epidemiol Biomarkers Prev* 13(5):765-770.

Harmer P, Li F, Fisher KJ. 2002. Reducing fear of falling in the elderly through tai chi. *Med Sci Sports Exerc* 34(5)suppl:S29.

Hawley JA. 1998. Fat burning during exercise: Can ergogenics change the balance? *Phys Sports Med* 9:56-61.

Heinonen A, Oja P, Kannus P, et al. 1993. Bone mineral density of female athletes in different sports. *Bone Miner* 23:1-14.

Hewett TE, Myer GD, Ford KR. 2004. Decrease in neuromuscular control about the knee with maturation in female athletes. *J Bone Joint Surg* 86:1601-1608.

Hills AP, Hennig EM, McDonald M, et al. 2001. Plantar pressure differences between obese and non-obese adults: A biomechanical analysis. *Int J Obes Relat Metab Disord* 25(11):1674-1679.

Holden C. 2004. An everlasting gender gap? *Science* 305:639-640.

Holschen JC. 2004. The female athlete. *South Med J* 97(9):852-858.

Horton MG, Hall TL. 1989. Quadriceps femoris muscle angle: Normal values and relationships with gender and selected skeletal measures. *Phys Ther* 69:897-901.

Hu FB, Li TY, Colditz GA, et al. 2003. Television watching and other sedentary behaviors in relation to risk of obesity and type 2 diabetes mellitus in women. *JAMA* 289(14):1785-1791.

Hu FB, Manson JE, Liu S, et al. 1999a. Prospective study of adult onset diabetes mellitus (type 2) and risk of colorectal cancer in women. *J Natl Cancer Inst* 91:542-547.

Hu FB, Sigal RJ, Rich-Edwards JW, et al. 1999b. Walking compared with vigorous physical activity and risk of type 2 diabetes in women: A prospective study. *JAMA* 282(15):1433-1439.

Hu FB, Stampfer MJ, Colditz GA, et al. 2000. Physical activity and risk of stroke in women. *JAMA* 283(22):2961-2967.

Hu FB, Stampfer MJ, Solomon C, et al. 2001. Physical activity and risk for cardiovascular events in diabetic women. *Ann Intern Med* 134:96.

Hutchinson PL, Cureton KJ, Outz H, Wilson G. 1991. Relationship of cardiac size to maximal oxygen uptake and body size in men and women. *Int J Sports Med* 12:369-373.

Ingraham SJ, Serfass RC, Walker AJ, Smiley J, Tews K, Chapman R. 2003. Menstrual cycle relaxin phase related to injury incidence and pain in female athletes. *Med Sci Sports Exerc* 35(5)suppl 1:S245.

Institute of Medicine, Food Nutrition Board. 2002. *Dietary reference intakes for energy, carbohydrates, fiber, fat, protein and amino acids (macronutrients)*. Washington, DC: National Academy Press.

Ireland ML, Nattiv A. 2002. *The female athlete*. Philadelphia: Saunders.

Ireland ML, Ott SM. 2001. Special concerns of the female athlete. In *Sports injuries: mechanism, prevention, treatment, second edition*, edited by FH Fu and DA Stone. Philadelphia: Lippincott Williams & Wilkins.

Ireland ML, Ott SM. 2004. Special concerns of the female athlete. *Clin Sports Med* 23:281-298.

Jenkins DJ, Kendall CW, Marchie A, et al. 2003. Effects of dietary portfolio of cholesterol lowering foods vs. lovastatin on serum lipids and C-reactive protein. *JAMA* 290:502.

Johnson LG, Kraemer RR, Kraemer GR, et al. 2002. Substrate utilization during exercise in postmenopausal women on hormone replacement therapy. *Eur J Appl Physiol* 88:282-287.

Karper WB, Hopewell R, Hodge M. 2001. Exercise program effects on women with fibromyalgia. *Clin Nurse Spec* 15(2):67-73.

Kavanagh T, Mertens DJ, Hamm LF, et al. 2003. Peak oxygen intake and cardiac mortality in women referred for cardiac rehabilitation. *J Am Coll Cardiol* 42:2139-2143.

Kelley GA, Kelley KS, Tran ZV. 2001. Resistance training and BMD in women: A meta-analysis of controlled trials. *Am J Phys Med Rehabil* 80:65-77.

Kimm SY, Glynn NW, Kriska AM, Barton BA, Kronsberg SS, Daniels SR, Crawford PB, Sabry ZI, Liu K. 2002. Decline in physical activity in black girls and white girls during adolescence. *N Engl J Med* 347(10):709-715.

Kimm SY, Glynn NW, Obarzanek E, et al. 2005. Relation between the changes in physical activity and body-mass index during adolescence: A multicenter longitudinal study. *Lancet* 366:301-307.

Kocina P. 1997. Body composition of spinal cord injured adults. *Sports Med* 23:48-60.

Kohrt WM, Bloomfield SA, Little KD, et al. 2004. American College of Sports Medicine position stand: Physical activity and bone health. *Med Sci Sports Exerc* 36(11):1985-1996.

Koivisto VA, Felig P. 1978. Effects of leg exercise on insulin absorption in diabetic patients. *N Engl J Med* 298:79.

Kowalchik C. 1999. *The complete book of running for women.* New York: Pocket Books.

Kraemer WJ, Hakkinen K, Triplett-McBride T, et al. 2003. Physiological changes with periodized resistance training in women tennis players. *Med Sci Sports Exerc* 35(1):157-168.

Kraemer WJ, Ratamess NA. 2004. Fundamentals of resistance training: Progression and exercise prescription. *Med Sci Sports Exerc* 36(4):674-688.

Kraus WE, Houmard JA, Duscha BD, et al. 2002. Effects of the amount and intensity of exercise on plasma lipoproteins. *N Engl J Med* 347(19):1483-1492.

Larsson L, Lindqvist PG. 2005. Low-impact exercise during pregnancy—a study of safety. *Acta Obstet Gynecol Scand* 84(1):34-38.

Lawlor DA, Hopker SW. 2001. The effectiveness of exercise as an intervention in the management of depression: Systematic review and meta-regression analysis of randomized controlled trials. *BMJ* 322:1-8.

Lee IM, Rexrode KM, Cook NR, et al. 2001, March 21. Physical activity and coronary heart disease in women: Is "no pain, no gain" passé? *JAMA* 285(11):1447-1454.

Lee I-M, Sesso HD, Oguma Y, et al. 2003. Physical activity, body weight, and pancreatic cancer mortality. *Br J Cancer* 88:679-683.

Leetun DT, Ireland ML, Willson JD, Ballantyne BT, Davis IM. 2004. Core stability measures as risk factors for lower extremity injury in athletes. *Med Sci Sports Exerc* 36(6):926-934.

Le Foll-de Moro D, Tordi N, Lonsdorfer E, Lonsdorfer J. 2005. Ventilation efficiency and pulmonary function after a wheelchair interval-training program in subjects with recent spinal cord injury. *Arch Phys Med Rehabil* 86:1582-1586.

Leiferman JA, Evenson KR. 2003. The effect of regular leisure physical activity on birth outcomes. *Matern Child Health J* 7(1):59-64.

Li S, Holm K, Gulanick M, Lanuza D, Penckofer S. 1999. The relationship between physical activity and perimenopause. *Health Care Women Int* 20(2):163-178.

Littman AJ, Voigt LF, Beresford SA, Weiss NS. 2001. Recreational physical activity and endometrial cancer risk. *Am J Epidemiol* 154(10):924-933.

Lloyd T, Petit MA, Lin HM, Beck TJ. 2004. Lifestyle factors and the development of bone mass and bone strength in young women. *J Pediatr* 144(6):776-782.

Lowry R, Galouska DA, Fulton JE, Wechsler H, Kann L. 2002. Weight management goals and practices among U.S. high school students: Associations with physical activity, diet, and smoking. *J Adolesc Health* 31(2):133-144.

Lutter J, Jaffee L. 1996. *The bodywise woman.* Champaign, IL: Human Kinetics.

Lytle ME, Vander Bilt J, Pandav RS, et al. 2004. Exercise level and cognitive decline: the MoVIES project. *Alzheimer Dis Assoc Disord* 18(2):57-64.

Mahoney ET, Bickel CS, Elder C, et al. 2005. Changes in skeletal muscle size and glucose tolerance with electrically stimulated resistance training in subjects with chronic spinal cord injury. *Arch Phys Med Rehabil* 86:1502-1504.

Manson JE, Greenland P, LaCroix AZ, et al. 2002. Walking compared with vigorous exercise for the prevention of cardiovascular events in women. *N Engl J Med* 347:716.

Manson JE, Hu FB, Rich-Edwards JW, et al. 1999. A prospective study of walking as compared with vigorous exercise in the prevention of coronary heart disease in women. *N Engl J Med* 341(9):650-658.

Manson JE, Rimm EB, Stampfer MJ, et al. 1991. Physical activity and incidence of non-insulin-dependent diabetes in women. *Lancet* 338:774-778.

Marks R, Allegrante JP, MacKenzie CR, Lane JM. 2003. Hip fractures among the elderly: Causes, consequences and control. *Ageing Res Rev* 2:57-93.

Martinez ME, Giovannucci E, Spiegelman D, et al. 1997. Leisure-time physical activity, body size, and colon cancer in women. *J Natl Cancer Inst* 89:948-955.

Mazzeo RS. 1994. The influence of exercise and aging on immune function. *Med Sci Sports Exerc* 26:586-592.

McAuley KA, Williams SM, Mann JI, et al. 2002. Intensive lifestyle changes are necessary to improve insulin sensitivity: A randomized controlled trial. *Diabet Care* 25:445.

McGavock JM, Mandic S, Vonder Muhll I, et al. 2004. Low cardiorespiratory fitness is associated with elevated C-reactive protein levels in women with type 2 diabetes. *Diabet Care* 27:320-325.

McHam SA, Marwick TH, Pashkow FJ, Lauer MS. 1999. Delayed systolic blood pressure recovery after graded exercise: An independent correlate of angiographic coronary disease. *J Am Coll Cardiol* 34(3):754-759.

McHugh MP, Connolly DA, Eston RG, Kremenic IJ, Nicholas SJ, Gleim GW. 1999. The role of passive muscle stiffness in symptoms of exercise-induced muscle damage. *Am Orthop Soc Sports Med* 27(5):594-599.

McTiernan A, Tworoger SS, Ulrich CM, et al. 2004. Effect of exercise on serum estrogens in postmenopausal women: 12 month randomized clinical trial. *Cancer Res* 64(8):2923-2928.

Melton LJ III, Chrischilles EA, Cooper C, et. al. 1992. Perspective. How many women have osteoporosis? *J Bone Miner Res* 7:1005-1010.

Michaud DS, Giovannucci E, Willett WC, et al. 2001. Physical activity, obesity, height, and the risk of pancreatic cancer. *JAMA* 286(8):921-929.

Milani RV, Lavie CJ, Mehra MR. 2004. Reduction in C-reactive protein through cardiac rehabilitation and exercise training. *J Am Coll Cardiol* 43:1056-1061.

Milne L. 2003, October 28. Plantar fasciitis. www.emedicine.com.

Mittleman MA, Maclure M, Tofler GH, et al. 1993. Triggering of acute myocardial infarction by heavy physical exertion—protection against triggering by regular exertion. *N Engl J Med* 329:1677-1683.

Mock V, Pickett M, Ropka ME, et al. 2001. Fatigue and quality of life outcomes of exercise during cancer treatment. *Cancer Pract* 9(3):119-127.

Moore MA, Park CB, Tsuda H. 1998a. Implications of the hyperinsulinemia-diabetes-cancer link for preventive efforts. *Eur J Cancer Prev* 7:89-107.

Moore MA, Park CB, Tsuda H. 1998b. Physical exercise: a pillar for cancer prevention? *Eur J Cancer Prev* 7:177-193.

Morkved S, Bo K, Schei B, Salvesen KA. 2003. Pelvic floor muscle training during pregnancy to prevent urinary incontinence: A single-blind randomized controlled trial. *Am Coll Obstet Gynecol* 101(2):313-319.

Mundal R, Kjeldsen SE, Sandvik L, et al. 1994. Exercise blood pressure predicts cardiovascular mortality in middle-aged men. *Hypertension* 24:56.

National Heart, Lung, and Blood Institute, National Institutes of Health. 2001, May. Third report of the National Cholesterol Education Program (NCEP) Expert Panel on Detection, Evaluation, and Treatment of High Blood Cholesterol in Adults (Adult Treatment Panel III). NIH publication no. 01-3670. Washington, DC: NIH.

National Heart, Lung, and Blood Institute. 2005, March. High blood pressure in pregnancy. www.nhlbi.nih.gov.

National High Blood Pressure Education Program. 2003. The seventh report of the Joint National Committee on Prevention, Detection, Evaluation, and Treatment of High Blood Pressure (JNC 7), 03-5233. Washington, DC: NIH.

Naughton GA, Carlson JS, Buttifant DC, et al. 1997. Accumulated oxygen deficit measurements during and after high-intensity exercise in trained male and female adolescents. *Eur J Appl Physiol Occup Physiol* 76:525-531.

Needham BL, Crosnoe R. 2005. Overweight status and depressive symptoms during adolescence. *J Adolesc Health* 36(1):48-55.

Nelson ME, Layne JE, Bernstein MJ, et al. 2004. The effects of multidimensional home-based exercise on functional performance in elderly people. *J Gerontol A Biol Sci Med Sci* 59:M154-160.

Noreau L, Shephard RJ. 1995. Spinal cord injury, exercise and quality of life. *Sports Med* 20:226-250.

Otis CL, Goldingay R. 2000. *The athletic woman's survival guide.* Champaign, IL: Human Kinetics.

O'Toole ML, Sawicki MA, Artal R. 2003. Structured diet and physical activity prevent postpartum weight retention. *J Womens Health* 12(10):991-998.

Parracino L. 2004, December. Pregnancy trimesters and exercise. Personal training on the net. www.PtontheNet.com. Accessed April 2005.

Pate RR, Pratt M, Blair SN, et al. 1995. Physical activity and public health: A recommendation from the Centers for Disease Control and Prevention and the American College of Sports Medicine. *JAMA* 273:402-407.

Patel AV, Press MF, Meeske K, et al. 2003. Lifetime recreational exercise activity and risk of breast carcinoma in situ. *Cancer* 98:2161-2169.

Persinger R, Foster C, Gibson M, et al. 2004. Consistency of the talk test for exercise prescription. *Med Sci Sports Exerc* 36(9):1632-1636.

Pescatello LS, Franklin BA, Fagard R, et al. 2004. Exercise and hypertension: Position stand of the ACSM. *Med Sci Sports Exerc* 36:533-553.

Pilates J, Miller W, Robbins J. 1998. *Pilates' return to life through contrology.* Incline Village, NV: Bodymind Books.

Poehlman ET, Denino WF, Beckett T, et al. 2002. Effects of endurance and resistance training on total daily energy expenditure in young women: A controlled randomized trial. *J Clin Endocrinol Metab* 87:1004-1009.

Poirier P, Tremblay A, Catellier C, et al. 2000. Impact of time interval from the last meal on glucose response to exercise in subjects with type 2 diabetes. *J Clin Endocrinol Metab* 85:2860.

Pollock ML, Gaesser GA, Butcher JD, et al. 1998. The recommended quantity and quality of exercise for developing and maintaining cardiorespiratory and muscular fitness, and flexibility in healthy adults: Position stand. *Med Sci Sports Exerc* 30:975-991.

Prabhakaran B, Dowling EA, Branch JD, et al. 1999. Effect of 14 weeks of resistance training on lipid profile and body fat percentage in premenopausal women. *Br J Sports Med* 33:190-195.

Prentice AM, Jebb SA. 1995. Obesity in Britain: Gluttony or sloth? *BMJ* 311:437.

Protzman RR, Griffis CC. 1997. Comparative stress fracture incidence in males and females in equal training environment. *J Athl Train* 12:126-130.

Purdie DM, Green AC. 2001. Epidemiology of endometrial cancer. *Best Pract Res Clin Obstet Gynaecol* 15(3):341-354.

Rapp K, Schroeder J, Klenk J, et al. 2005. Obesity and incidence of cancer: A large cohort study of over 145,000 adults in Austria. *Br J Cancer* 93:1062-1067.

Redman LM, Hamdorf P, Norman RJ, et al. 2004. The menstrual cycle or oral contraceptive pill: Can it benefit or hinder exercise in women. *Med Sci Sports Exerc* 36(5):S280.

Redman LM, Weatherby RP. 2004. Measuring performance during the menstrual cycle: A model using oral contraceptives. *Med Sci Sports Exerc* 36:130-136.

Reichel W, ed. 1989. *Clinical aspects of aging, third edition.* Baltimore: Williams & Wilkins.

Reubinoff BE, Grubstein A, Meirow D, et al. 1995. Effects of low-dose estrogen oral contraceptives on weight, body composition, and fat distribution in young women. *Fertil Steril* 63:516.

Richardson C, Jull G, Hodges P, Hides J. 1999. Therapeutic exercise for spinal segmental stabilization in low back pain: Scientific basis and clinical approach. London, England: Churchill Livingstone.

Rich-Edwards JW, Spiegelman D, Hertzmark GM, et al. 2002. Physical activity, body mass index, and ovulatory disorder infertility. *Epidemiology* 13(2):184-190.

Ridker PM. 2001. High-sensitivity C-reactive protein: Potential adjunct for global risk assessment in the primary prevention of cardiovascular disease. *Circulation* 103:1813-1818.

Riggs BL, Melton LJ III. 1986. Involutional osteoporosis. *N Engl J Med* 314:1675.

Rikli RE, Jones J. 2001. *Senior fitness test manual.* Champaign, IL: Human Kinetics.

Robertson MC, Devlin N, Gardner MM, Campbell AJ. 2001. Effectiveness and economic evaluation of a nurse delivered home exercise programme to prevent falls. *BMJ* 322:1-6.

Robinson K, Ferraro FR. 2004. The relationship between types of female athletic participation and female body type. *J Psychol* 138(2):115-128.

Rockhill B, Willett WC, Hunter DJ, et al. 1998. Physical activity and breast cancer risk in a cohort of young women. *J Natl Cancer Inst* 90(15):1155-1160.

Rockhill B, Willett WC, Hunter DJ, et al. 1999. A prospective study of recreational physical activity and breast cancer risk. *Arch Intern Med* 159(19):2290-2296.

Rockhill B, Willett WC, Manson JE, et al. 2001. Physical activity and mortality: A prospective study among women. *Am J Public Health* 91(4):578-583.

Rooney BL, Schauberger CW. 2002. Excess pregnancy weight gain and long-term obesity: One decade later. *Obstet Gynecol* 100(2):245-252.

Rossouw JE, Anderson GL, Prentice RL, et al. (Writing Group for the Women's Health Initiative Investigators). 2002. Risks and benefits of estrogen plus progestin in healthy postmenopausal women. *JAMA* 288(3):321-333.

Saftlas AF, Logsden-Sackett N, Wang W, Woolson R, Bracken MB. 2004. Work, leisure-time physical activity, and risk of preeclampsia and gestational hypertension. *Am J Epidemiol* 160(8):758-765.

Samad AKA, Taylor RS, Marshall T, Chapman MAS. 2005. A meta-analysis of the association of physical activity with reduced risk of colorectal cancer. *Colorectal Disease* 7:204-213.

Samaras K, Kelly PJ, Chiano MN, et al. 1999. Genetic and environmental influences on total-body and central abdominal fat: The effect of physical activity in female twins. *Ann Intern Med* 130(11):873-882.

Schmitz KH, Holtzman J, Courneya KS, et al. 2005. Controlled physical activity trials in cancer survivors: A systematic review and meta-analysis. *Cancer Epidemiol Biomarkers Prev* 14:1588-1595.

Schwartz AL. 2004. *Cancer fitness: Exercise programs for patients and survivors.* New York: Fireside.

Shephard RJ, Rhind S, Shek PN. 1995. The impact of exercise on the immune system: NK cells, interleukins 1 and 2, and related responses. *Exerc Sport Sci Rev* 23:215-241.

Shultz SJ, Kirk SE, Johnson ML, Sander TC, Perrin DH. 2004. Relationship between sex hormones and anterior knee laxity across the menstrual cycle. *Med Sci Sports Exerc* 36(7):1165-1174.

Sinaki M, Itoi E, Wahner HW, et al. 2002. Stronger back muscles reduce the incidence of vertebral fractures: A prospective 10 year follow-up of postmenopausal women. *Bone* 30:836-841.

Singh JP, Larson MG, Manolio TA, et al. 1999. Blood pressure response during treadmill testing as a risk factor for new-onset hypertension. The Framingham heart study. *Circulation* 99:1831.

Singh NA, Clements KM, Fiatarone MA. 1997a. A randomized controlled trial of progressive resistance training in depressed elders. *J Gerontol A Biol Sci Med Sci* 52:M27-35.

Singh NA, Clements KM, Fiatarone MA. 1997b. A randomized trial of the effect of exercise on sleep. *Sleep* 20:95-101.

Smith DE, Lewis CE, Caveny JL, et al. 1994. Longitudinal changes in adiposity associated with pregnancy. The CARDIA study. Coronary risk development in young adults study. *JAMA* 271:1747.

Sorenson TK, Williams MA, Lee IM, Dashow EE, Thompson ML, Luthy DA. 2003. Recreational physical activity during pregnancy and risk of preeclampsia. *Hypertension* 41(6):1273-1280.

Stage E, Ronneby H, Damm P. 2004. Lifestyle change after gestational diabetes. *Diabet Res Clin Pract* 1:67-72.

Stefanick ML, Mackey S, Sheehan M, et al. 1998. Effects of diet and exercise in men and postmenopausal women with low levels of HDL cholesterol and high levels of LDL cholesterol. *N Engl J Med* 339(1):12-20.

Sternfeld B, Wang H, Quesenberry CP Jr., et al. 2004. Physical activity and changes in weight and waist circumference in midlife women: Findings from the Study of Women's Health Across the Nation. *Am J Epidemiol* 160(9):912-922.

Styne DM. 2005. Obesity in childhood: What's activity got to do with it? *Am J Clin Nutr* 81:337-338.

Symons Downs D, Hausenblas HA. 2004. Women's exercise beliefs and behaviors during their pregnancy and postpartum. *J Midwifery Womens Health* 49(2):138-144.

Taggert HM, Arslanian CL, Bae S, Singh K. 2003. Effects of t'ai chi exercise on fibromyalgia symptoms and health-related quality of life. *Orthop Nursing* (22)5:353-360.

Tanaka H, Bassett DR Jr., Howley ET, et al. 1997. Swimming training lowers the resting blood pressure in individuals with hypertension. *J Hypertens* 15:651.

Tarnopolsky MA, Atkinson SA, Phillips SM, MacDougall JD. 1995. Carbohydrate loading and metabolism during exercise in men and women. *J Appl Physiol* 78:1360-1368.

Tarnopolsky MA, Bosman M, MacDonald JR, et al. 1997. Postexercise protein-carbohydrate and carbohydrate supplements increase muscle glycogen in men and women. *J Appl Physiol* 83:1877-1883.

Tarnopolsky LJ, MacDougall JD, Atkinson SA, Tarnopolsky MA, et al. 1990. Gender differences in substrate for endurance exercise. *J Appl Physiol* 68:302-308.

Tarnopolsky MA, Zawada C, Richmond LB, et al. 2001. Gender differences in carbohydrate loading are related to energy intake. *J Appl Physiol* 91:225-230.

Thacker SB, Gilchrist J, Stroup DF, Kimsey Jr. CD. 2004a. The impact of stretching on sports injury risk: A systematic review of the literature. *Med Sci Sports Exerc* 36(3):371-378.

Thacker SB, Gilchrist J, Stroup DF, Kimsey Jr. CD. 2004b. Response. *Med Sci Sports Exerc* 36(10):1833.

Thomas KS, Muir KR, Doherty M, et al. 2002. Home based exercise programme for knee pain and knee osteoarthritis: Randomized controlled trial. *BMJ* 325:752-756.

Thompson DL, Rakow J, Perdue SM. 2004. Relationship between accumulated walking and body composition in middle-aged women. *Med Sci Sports Exerc* 36:911-914.

Thompson PD. 1996. The cardiovascular complications of vigorous physical activity. *Arch Int Med* 156:2297-2302.

Todd JA, Robinson RJ. 2003. Osteoporosis and exercise. *Postgrad Med J* 79:320-323.

Touchette N. 2002. *American diabetes association complete guide to diabetes, third edition*. Baltimore: Port City Press.

U.S. Department of Health and Human Services. 1996. *Physical activity and health: A report of the Surgeon General*. Atlanta: U.S. Department of Health and Human Services, Centers for Disease Control and Prevention, National Center for Chronic Disease Prevention and Health Promotion.

U.S. Department of Health and Human Services, Centers for Disease Control and Prevention, National Center for Health Statistics. 2002. *Nat Vital Stat Rep* 50, no. 15.

U.S. Department of Health and Human Services, Centers for Disease Control and Prevention. 2003. National diabetes fact sheet, United States. www.cdc.gov/diabetes/pubs/factsheet.htm.

U.S. Department of Health and Human Services, Centers for Disease Control and Prevention, National Center for Chronic Disease Prevention and Health Promotion. 2005. Promoting active lifestyles among older adults. www.cdc.gov/nccdphp/dnpa/physical/pdf/lifestyles.pdf.

U.S. Department of Health and Human Services, U.S. Department of Agriculture. 2005. *Dietary guidelines for Americans* (GPO 001-000-04719-1). Washington, DC: GPO.

van Baar ME, Assendelft WJ, Dekker J, et al. 1999. Effectiveness of exercise therapy in patients with osteoarthritis of the hip or knee. *Arthritis Rheum* 42:1361-1369.

Venables MC, Achten J, Jeukendrup AE. 2005. Determinants of fat oxidation during exercise in healthy men and women: A cross-sectional study. *J Appl Physiol* 98:160-167.

Verghese J, Lipton RB, Katz MJ, et al. 2003. Leisure activities and the risk of dementia in the elderly. *N Engl J Med* 348:2508-2516.

Vihko RK, Apter DL. 1986. The epidemiology and endocrinology of the menarche in relation to breast cancer. *Cancer Surv* 5:561-571.

Vincent KR, Braith RW, Feldman RA, Magyari PM, Cutler RB, Persin SA, Lennon SL, Gabr AH, Lawenthal DT. 2002. Resistance exercise and physical performance in adults aged 60 to 83. *J Am Geriatr Soc* 50(6):1100-1107.

Weissgerber TL, Wolfe LA, Davies GA. 2004. The role of regular physical activity in preeclampsia prevention. *Med Sci Sports Exerc* 36(12):2024-2031.

Weuve J, Kang JH, Manson JE, et al. 2004. Physical activity, including walking, and cognitive function in older women. *JAMA* 292:1454-1461.

Whaley MH, Brubaker PH, Otto RM, eds. 2006. *ACSM's guidelines for exercise testing and prescription, seventh edition*. Baltimore: Lippincott Williams & Wilkins.

Whelton SP, Chin A, Xin X, He J. 2002. Effect of aerobic exercise on blood pressure: A meta-analysis of randomized, controlled trials. *Ann Intern Med* 136:493.

White KP, Harth M. 2001. Classification, epidemiology, and natural history of fibromyalgia. *Curr Pain Headache Rep* 5(4):320-329.

Wiebe CG, Gledhill N, Jamnik VK, Ferguson S. 1999. Exercise cardiac function in young through elderly endurance trained women. *Med Sci Sports Exerc* 31:684-691.

Wilkerson GB, Colston MA, Short NI, Neal KL, Hoewischer PE, Pixley JJ. 2004. Neuromuscular changes in female collegiate athletes resulting from a plyometric jump-training program. *J Athl Train* 39(1):17-23.

Williamson DF, Madans J, Anda RF, et al. 1993. Recreational physical activity and ten-year weight change in a U.S. national cohort. *Int J Obes Relat Metab Disord* 17:279.

Williamson DR, Madans J, Pamuk E, et al. 1994. A prospective study of childbearing and 10-year weight gain in U.S. white women 25 to 45 years of age. *Int J Obes Relat Metab Disord* 18:561.

Wilson JD, Davis I, Ireland ML. 2004. The influence of lumbopelvic strength on lower extremity performance. *Med Sci Sports Exerc* 36(5):S100-S101.

Witt BJ, Jacobsen SJ, Weston SA, et al. 2004. Cardiac rehabilitation after myocardial infarction in the community. *J Am Coll Cardiol* 44:988-996.

Witzke KA, Snow CM. 2000. Effects of plyometric jump training on bone mass in adolescent girls. *Med Sci Sports Exerc* 32(6);1051-1057.

Woo SL-Y, Knaub MA, Apreleva M. 2001. Biomechanics of ligaments in sports medicine. In *Sports Injuries: mechanisms, prevention, treatment, second edition,* edited by FH Fu and DA Stone. Philadelphia: Lippincott Williams & Wilkins.

www.uptodate.com. Preventive cardiology: Obesity and weight reduction. January 4, 2005 (last updated).

# Index

# About the Authors

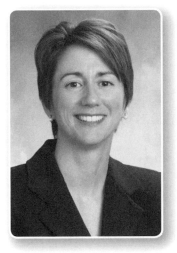

**Michele Anne Kettles, MD, MSPH,** is a physician at the world-renowned Cooper Clinic in Dallas, Texas. She is a graduate of the University of Pennsylvania School of Medicine (1990). She is a board-certified specialist in preventive medicine and practices clinical medicine full time with a focus on exercise counseling for better health and fitness. She has a particular interest in prevention and treatment of osteoporosis. Dr. Kettles is a member of the American College of Preventive Medicine and served in the U.S. Navy as a physician, where her mission was to maintain the health and fitness of the troops. She enjoys running, swimming, strength training, reading, travel and practicing yoga in her leisure time.

**Colette L. Cole, MS,** is an award-winning personal trainer and fitness coordinator with 18 years of experience in the health and fitness industry. She designs fitness programs and trains women with a variety of needs. Her clients include elite athletes, women recovering from serious injuries or surgeries, and those managing conditions such as breast cancer or osteoporosis, as well as women who see fitness as a means to improve daily function or appearance at any stage of life. Since 1994, she has worked at the Cooper Fitness Center in Dallas, Texas, where she is currently developing a women's lifestyle program called, "The Female Focus." She is a frequent lecturer on various health and fitness topics. Away from work, she enjoys exercise, the mountains, and her Harley-Davidson motorcycle.

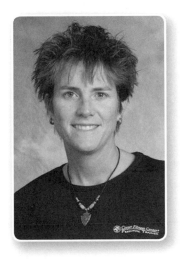

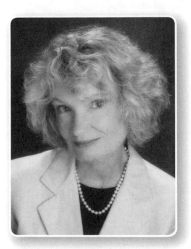

**Brenda Shepherd Wright, PhD,** is a health promotion consultant with more than 25 years of experience in the field, including her work as director of the Division of Behavioral Science and Health Promotion at the Cooper Institute. She has consulted with individuals and groups and has served as a developer and evaluator of school-based programs to increase physical activity among elementary and middle school students. She has also developed wellness programs for assisted living communities as well as numerous certification training programs and manuals for health professionals. She enjoys hiking in the mountains and jungles of Costa Rica, where she currently lives, and yachting.